# A History of Family Planning
# in Twentieth-Century Peru

# A History
# of Family Planning
# in Twentieth-Century
# Peru

RAÚL NECOCHEA LÓPEZ

THE UNIVERSITY OF NORTH CAROLINA PRESS    *Chapel Hill*

This book was published with the assistance of the
Lilian R. Furst Fund of the University of North Carolina Press.

The paper in this book meets the guidelines for permanence and durability
of the Committee on Production Guidelines for Book Longevity of the
Council on Library Resources. The University of North Carolina Press has
been a member of the Green Press Initiative since 2003.

Library of Congress Cataloging-in-Publication Data
Necochea López, Raúl.
A history of family planning in twentieth-century Peru / Raúl Necochea López.
pages cm
Includes bibliographical references and index.
ISBN 978-1-4696-1808-1 (pbk : alk. paper) — ISBN 978-1-4696-1809-8 (ebook)
1. Family planning—Peru—History—20th century. I. Title.
HQ766.5.P4N43 2014
363.9'609850904—dc23
2014017085

Portions of chapter 6 are drawn from "Priests and Pills: Catholic Family
Planning in Peru, 1967–1976." *Latin American Research Review* 43, 2
(2008): 34–56. Used with permission.

18 17 16 15 14   5 4 3 2 1

THIS BOOK WAS DIGITALLY PRINTED

*For my family, planned and unplanned*

# Contents

# Figures and Table

## Figures

## Table

# Acknowledgments

Associated Medical Services, Inc., the Social Sciences and Humanities Research Council of Canada, the UNC Institute for the Study of the Americas, and the Department of Social Medicine at the University of North Carolina at Chapel Hill funded the research for this project. I gratefully acknowledge the generosity of these organizations.

Numerous archives and individuals made their collections available to me during the time that it took to research and write this book. The complete list appears in the bibliography section. I would like to extend particular thanks to Dr. Carmen Delgado de Thays, Dr. Miguel Ramos Zambrano, Mrs. Graciela de Leidinger, Dr. Irene Santolalla Silva, Dr. Joseph Kerrins, and Mrs. Helen Kerrins for sharing materials with me that are not open to the general public. Likewise, every conversation I had with the people I interviewed made me realize just how much more there is still to be said about this topic. Some meetings were instrumental in finding needed clues for the story; others challenged me to keep my poise despite unsettling revelations; yet others made me realize I had received the wonderful gift of a friendship. Thanks to this project, I now count Consuelo Castillo, Fr. John Coss, Helen and the late Dr. Joe Kerrins, and Dr. Marie-Françoise Hall among my friends.

Spirited intellectual trade with many people went into the writing of this book. Steve Vallas and Marcos Cueto first inspired me to follow my nose with the idea of family planning in Peru. It was a great privilege to work and play at McGill University with Andrea Tone, Catherine LeGrand, George Weisz, and the lovely miscreants of the basement of the Department of Social Studies of Medicine, including Noémi Tousignant, Loes Knaapen, Hannah Gilbert, Pierre Minn, Dörte Bemme, Ari Gandsman, Jennifer Cuffe, Wilson Will, Hanna Kienzler, and Karine Peschard. Many others have helped me clarify my own ideas and contributed new ones along the way, particularly Stephanie Olsen, Lucho van Isschot, Lynn Morgan, Vinh-Kim Nguyen, Myron Echenberg, Jorge Lossio, Nuntxi Iguiñiz, Roger Guerra-García, Tasha Kimball, Anne-Emanuelle Birn, Barbara Brookes, Maren Klawiter, Nathan

Moon, Hannes Toivanen, Hyungsub Choi, Maggie Zegarra, Gisela Delgado, Michael McVaugh, and Gabriela Soto Laveaga. Cees Van Dijk translated from the Latin and Chelly Richards provided some research assistance at a crucial time. The sterling team at the UNC Press, especially Elaine Maisner, Alison Shay, Liz Gray, Dino Battista, Kim Bryant, and Paul Betz, guided me expertly as a novice author, and the press's two reviewers added helpful finishing touches.

I am lucky to be at the University of North Carolina at Chapel Hill for many reasons, foremost among them my gifted and lighthearted colleagues in the Department of Social Medicine. Conversations with Barry Saunders, Mara Buchbinder, Gail Henderson, Jon Oberlander, Sue Estroff, Eric Juengst, Annie Lyerly, Jeffrey Sonis, Deborah Porterfield, Stuart Rennie, Rebecca Walker, and the late Alan Cross have made me see the study of history as the beginning of something much greater and socially transformative. The seriousness with which the UNC School of Medicine treats its mission to care for the people of the state and to train physicians fills me with optimism, as does the warm welcome I have had from the Department of History and the exciting new partnerships that have sprouted with the Gillings School of Global Public Health and the Department of Anthropology. Heartfelt thanks to Lloyd Kramer, Fitz Brundage, Miguel La Serna, Jerma Jackson, Kathryn Burns, Cynthia Radding, Michelle King, Lou Pérez, Clare Barrington, Krista Perreira, Trude Bennet, Michelle Rivkin-Fish, Jocelyn Chua, and Peter Redfield.

My family is the best, and no words can express my gratitude and love for Lucy, Edgar, Alejandro, Lauren, Elsy, Flora, Raúl, Antuco, Ginucha, my cousins, aunts, uncles, nieces, and nephews, imprescindibles e impresentables. Last but not least, I thank Erica, Tomás, and Ansel. I am smitten by you and honored to be in your lives.

# A History of Family Planning
# in Twentieth-Century Peru

# Introduction

I cheered in 1995 when Peruvian president Alberto Fujimori gave a speech as the only male head of state at the Fourth World Conference on Women in Beijing.[1] There, Fujimori praised the skilled ways in which women were able to organize themselves to overcome economic hardship. To a standing ovation, he also announced the recent legalization of surgical sterilization as a contraceptive in Peru.[2] Just a few years later, the press began to publish a series of heartbreaking and indignant accusations about forced surgical sterilizations of hundreds of women in several rural areas of my home country. The reports involved officers from the Ministry of Health, directors of rural health centers, and even the U.S. Agency for International Development, and led to investigations by the Peruvian Ombudsman's Office and the U.S. House of Representatives.[3]

Yet, once more swung the pendulum when it became apparent that there was more to the story than powerful agencies and physicians victimizing poor, illiterate, indigenous, rural women. The same newspapers that brought the abuses to light reported details that made guilt seem less than straightforward. The Catholic Church, today an opponent of all contraceptive methods, had been behind many of the accusations of forced sterilization. Were the accusations less credible because of that association? Moreover, some local politicians lamented that sterilizations occurred in a country that they considered underpopulated. How did they determine such want of population? Physicians themselves were perplexed by accusations of abuse, as they believed they acted according to the standards of their profession in securing informed consent from women and in performing the surgeries. Finally, at least some of the women who had undergone the surgeries were satisfied with the outcomes. Not only had those women agreed to the operations voluntarily, but they had even traveled in search of the free-of-charge surgeries when these were not performed near their places of residence.[4]

Family planning has long been a contentious issue in Peru, and the book you are reading is about why this is so. Even today, the prevalence of modern contraceptive use in Peru hovers around 50 percent, a rate among the lowest in the Americas, next to that of Guyana (40 percent), Guatemala (34 percent),

Bolivia (34 percent), Belize (31 percent), and Haiti (24 percent).[5] The implementation of the first family planning programs in developing countries in the mid-twentieth century led to a rapid and understandable colonization of the field by policymakers, health and education activists, and demographers. Family planning, after all, involved changes in health care systems, the adoption of novel technologies, retraining of human resources, conflicts with existing religious institutions, and winning the trust of populations wary of the concept of contraception. Throughout the developing world, family planning held the promise of giving lay people a greater degree of control over their sexual and reproductive lives, and countries a host of opportunities to boost their economic fortunes through the management of population growth. It is no wonder the first and most poignant writings on family planning, as you will see later in this book, were aimed at defending and attacking specific technologies, ideas, and people. The stakes—the future of gender relations, individual autonomy, and national economies—were huge.

Fifty years after the implementation of these early family planning initiatives, the end of the Cold War and the availability of new archival sources allow greater historical perspective on the foundations and global implications of family planning. Recent works by historians of South Africa and India and of international relations, for example, acknowledge the role of the Cold War in exacerbating population debates but do not treat family planning as a simple by-product of Cold War antagonisms, instead tracing its origins further back, to the sociocultural ferment that shaped gender roles, racial stratification, scientific debates, and political activism in specific locales.[6] Scholars of Latin America too have been active in this field, addressing the links between family planning and imperialism, women's rights, the development of new contraceptives, and the governmental aspiration to population growth.[7] The regulation of fertility became an engrossing aspect of Latin America's public life during the twentieth century, a social and medical topic that is poised to become even more relevant with the increasing realization that the loftiest promises of family planning, greater economic development, more autonomy for women, and better maternal and infant health, have been fulfilled unevenly worldwide.

Unlike earlier stories of global family planning, mine does not just have policymaking at the core.[8] Instead, this book deals with the wide cast of actors and organizations that, at least since the late nineteenth century, have publicly dealt with the necessity and consequences of regulating fertility in Latin America: physicians, the eugenics movement, feminists, transnational birth control organizations, women and men who sought contraceptives and abortions, pharmaceutical companies, military leaders, and the Catholic Church. Family planning has been a constant and pivotal interest for all of the above actors. The twentieth century witnessed sharp and sharply contested changes in popular and professional thinking, from viewing large families and population growth as beneficial to national progress to viewing such phenomena as politically destabilizing, culturally backward, morally irresponsible, and unhealthy for women in various nation-states.

Among the latter, Peru stands out nowadays as the most unjust in the Americas when it comes to the provision of health care. Since 2001, its GDP growth has been the most robust in Latin America, remaining positive even during the global recession of 2008–9.[9] At the same time, Peru's maternal mortality rate, a key health indicator and long-term determinant of Peru's now-enviable macroeconomic performance, stood at 93 per 100,000 live births in 2011, lagging behind most countries in the region, save for much poorer Paraguay, the Dominican Republic, and Guatemala.[10] The index was, in fairness, an improvement over 2005, when the rate stood at 185 deaths per 100,000 live births.[11] That year, only Bolivia's and Haiti's maternal mortality rates were higher than Peru's, and yet Peru's 2005 per capita income was more than twice that of Bolivia and more than three times that of Haiti. With such dubious distinction, Peru illustrates well the limits of the optimistic view that greater economic wealth in developing nations will predictably lead to more equitable social relations.[12]

At the same time, many of the forces and ideas that have shaped Latin American health systems, beliefs, and resources have also shaped Peru's: the region's linguistic and religious similarities, its centuries-old medical institutions, its fusion of large native and immigrant populations of Europeans, Africans, and Asians, its longstanding history of violently clashing political interests, and its lopsided economic growth, wealth distribution, and educational opportunities. Much of what this book analyzes as Peruvian phenomena has correlates in other countries, which begs for both comparison and contrast. In that sense, this book is an invitation for Latin Americanists to think of the regional dimensions of health care, and for medical historians to consider new facets of the link between health and population, namely through the family planning lens.

## Enriching Demographic Transition Theory

For nearly a century now, the demographic transition theory has shaped our understanding of why population sizes change over time within a given territory and, more important for this book, how family planning played a role in fertility rate reductions in developing countries in the second half of the twentieth century.[13] Demographic transition theorists credited processes such as urbanization and industrialization with the weakening of pronatalist social conventions and used various names to refer to the process of completing the transition between "traditional" and "industrial" societies, particularly "modernization." In "modern" societies, having many children, whose labor might have been an advantage in preindustrial settings, could become a liability. This was so presumably because "modern" societies required greater expenditures in the education and health maintenance of children, and because people in "modern" societies had more ambitious individualistic aspirations to better health, wealth, and education for themselves, and they increasingly saw having many children as obstacles to those goals.[14]

Since the 1960s demographers have attempted to clarify the conditions under which the demographic transition theory is applicable to the developing world, particularly Latin America.[15] Three things are remarkable about this literature: first, it dates the onset of the Latin American demographic transition to the first half of the 1960s, a period during which Latin Americans presumably began to value smaller family sizes; second, it maintains that the reduction of birth rates in Latin America occurred not through the means Western Europeans most commonly used during their demographic transition in the nineteenth century (coitus interruptus, abortion, and the delaying of marriage), but through biomedical technologies used primarily by women; and third, it assumes that it was the United States that hegemonically extended the small nuclear family ideal and the technical-knowledge networks necessary to achieve this ideal.[16]

Interestingly, proponents of modernization theory in the 1960s argued that industrialization, the greater use of technology, urbanization, wealth generation, and the extension of educational opportunities were prerequisites for the sustainability of democratic institutions.[17] Writing in this vein, 1970s and 1980s public health experts criticized opposition to the use of contraceptives as a misinformed or, worse, irrational attitude, and an obstacle to development that must be overcome. In this context, the limitation of family size was no longer just a phenomenon to track and measure, but one to actively foment for the sake of democratic stability. The same experts credited biomedical contraceptive technologies with reducing population growth, easing economic development, and changing Latin American pronatalist mentalities. In other words, they associated the medical control of fertility with important population, economic, and cultural changes in the region.[18]

Far from disputing that biomedical technologies, knowledge networks, and transnational political actors have been important engines of social change in the developing world, I mean to refine and enrich demographic insights with new historical evidence. The mass distribution of contraceptives such as the pill and the intrauterine device, for example, certainly depended on the existence of U.S.-funded birth control organizations. However, as I will show, these birth control organizations did not justify their existence in Latin America solely in terms of the promotion of economic development, but also by making appeals to the integrity of the family and the domesticity of women, values that appealed to powerful patriarchal local actors, including the Catholic Church. In other words, foreign birth control organizations had to negotiate their interests with those of preexisting local actors in order to take root in the region, in the process helping consolidate the link between industrialization and small Catholic families (see figure 1).

A second challenge to demographic transition theory has to do with the sources of biomedical knowledge deployed to control fertility. Not all of this knowledge began to be applied in the early 1960s, nor did all of it originate in the United States or was oriented toward the limitation of birth rates. For example, a rich and mostly oral tradition about the fertility-enhancing or -limiting properties of certain plants exists in Latin America at least since the Colonial period, a topic I discuss in chapter 3. Likewise, French puericulture, a medical approach for the protection of pregnant women and infants that emphasized the enhancement of the quantity and quality of population, was popular among Latin American physicians and other health workers beginning in the late nineteenth century. Moreover, knowledge about fertility control produced by Latin American physicians circulated in regional conferences since the early twentieth century and influenced local policymakers' views about the importance of both increasing and limiting fertility.[19] The latter two topics are crucial themes in chapter 1. In addition, homegrown, not foreign, Catholic social reformers in the early twentieth century focused a tremendous amount of attention on the quality of the work that parents (mothers especially) put into raising and providing for their children, singling out this endeavor as the most important human duty, one well worth an alliance with the detestably Protestant family planning establishment. This is the subject of chapter 2.

A third critique to demographic transition theory concerns its assumption that financial calculations by people of reproductive age were the primary reason for the prevention or spacing of births. While children certainly required time, energy, and financial investments, Peruvian women who had

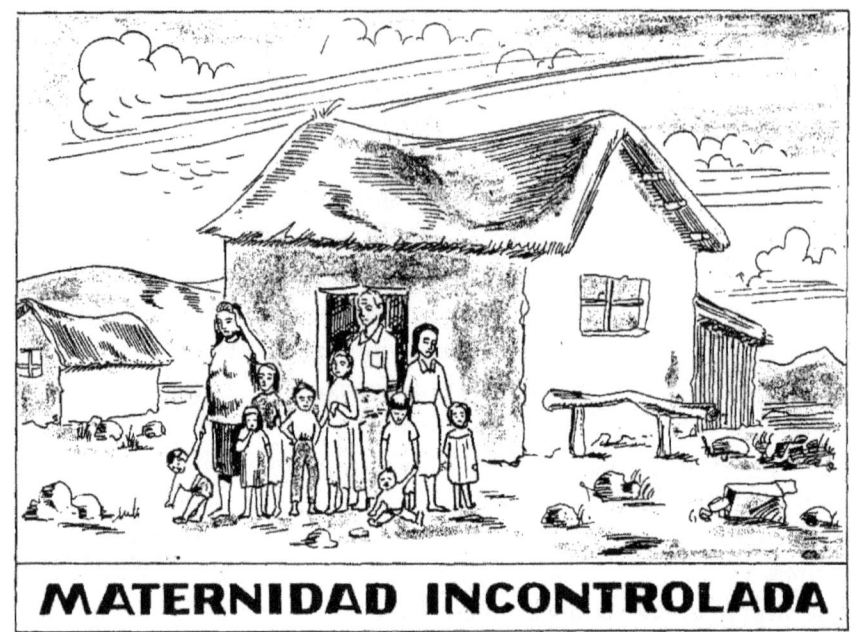

**MATERNIDAD INCONTROLADA**

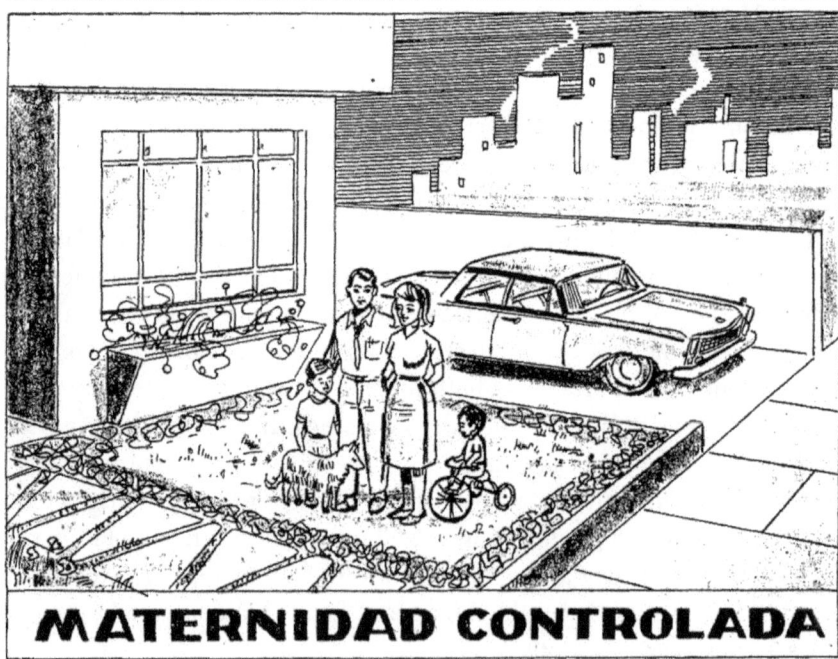

**MATERNIDAD CONTROLADA**

Figure 1. "Out of Control Maternity" vs. "Controlled Maternity." From Salvador Robles Ramírez, *Páginas de la Vida Real: Guía Matrimonial, Control de la Natalidad, Para Que?* (Lima: Ediciones Luz, 1967), 4–5.

abortions teach us that fertility limitation often had more to do with other reasons, such as the troubled interpersonal relations between sexual partners. Likewise, the financial-calculations-by-users argument leaves out the history of the health workers who first advocated for the prevention and spacing of births. This heterogeneous group worked hard to sell a very novel idea, and little by way of changing anyone's mind (let alone behavior) would have been accomplished without their exertions. These workers entered the field for different motives: to arrest the growth of poor, nonwhite immigrants in urban areas, in some cases; to advance clinical careers by testing out new contraceptives, in others; and, of course, in response to popular demand. The stories of women who had abortions and those of health workers who first supported birth control are central to chapters 3 and 4, respectively.

This all amounts to a need to address family planning as something that reaches deep into the past, certainly before the 1960s, when different social actors began to reflect publicly on the implications of their fertility. The number of offspring a woman has is not the only important dimension of fertility. Male and female infertility, and the physical changes in a woman's body as a result of a pregnancy, for example, remind us that fertility is also a biological phenomenon and not simply a statistical one. Different events can disrupt fertility from what societies deem organically normal; hence the longstanding link between fertility, health, and healing that gave rise to the knowledge of birth attendants and faith healers in multiple contexts. These specialists developed ways to care for bodily ailments such as impotence, hemorrhages during birth, and the transmission of genetic defects.[20] Nevertheless, the disruption of an organic function need not be automatically deemed a disease. Some changes linked to fertility, such as menopause, point less to a quantitative loss of or increase in health, than to what Georges Canguilhem dubbed "new dimensions of life," that permit or precede new behaviors and experiences while precluding others.[21] To make matters still more complex, fertility involves not only statistical and biological dimensions, but also social and cultural ones. The socioeconomic status of parents, the timing and geographic location of births, the assistance of certain individuals before, during, and after birth, as well as the reasons for the spacing of births, among other considerations, make fertility socially meaningful and tie it to the waxing and waning of wealth and prestige.[22]

Since the 1990s, a growing body of literature connects fertility to elite projects to "civilize" Latin Americans along Western lines.[23] This process coincided, not by chance, with the acceleration of Latin American nation-states' insertion into transnational capitalist networks in the nineteenth century. Latin American countries participated in these networks mostly as producers of raw materials, which generated new prosperity (for a minority), attracted new immigrants, encouraged population growth, and promoted urbanization.[24] In this context, Latin American elites embraced science, Positivism, and European tastes as markers of high culture, and as prerequisites for national progress.[25] My story begins in this period.

The topic of gender is especially salient within this historiography. As several scholars have pointed out, Latin American women played various roles in the nineteenth and twentieth centuries: as heads of households, political activists, salespeople, domestic and agricultural workers, soldiers, and writers, among others.[26] We also know that Latin American women commonly partook in the dispensation of potions to enhance sexual potency and in the procurement of abortions, and that many women regularly used contraceptive potions and juggled multiple sexual partners before and after marriage.[27] None of this is consistent with the exhortations of some nineteenth-century professionals and intellectuals that civilized and decent women had best keep to the Catholic domestic sphere, lest they ruin their valuable reproductive potential and thus hurt the nation.[28] Confining female participation to the private realm of the family, or enforcing strict gendered honor codes would have been the equivalent of restraining a genie that had never met the bottle. Conflicts emerged in the early twentieth century over new attempts (by the state, professionals, and lay activists) to manage this reproductive potential when material, legal, and cultural factors of older vintages pointed in different directions.

This rich and growing literature on gender history connects the process of state formation to fertility. Yet there are gaps that have only begun to be addressed. Among these is the period after World War II. Population size became a strategic factor during the Cold War, and the growth of a U.S.-backed network of advocates of population limitation disproportionately affected women through the widespread promotion of female contraceptives. This network relied on the ingenuity of health workers for the large-scale production and distribution of birth control, as well as on the prestige and political power of different experts to implement government policies to limit population growth. Transnational medical networks were not new in Latin America by the onset of the Cold War. In fact, the epistemic and financial resources embedded in these networks had helped urban physicians of the late nineteenth century coalesce into politically strong collectives in different countries. Latin American physicians benefited from foreign innovations such as vaccines, anesthesia, x-rays, and the germ theory, as well as from the support of philanthropic organizations such as the Rockefeller Foundation, which provided support to battle several diseases, including yellow fever and hookworm.[29] These contributions from without enhanced the prestige and, to some extent, effectiveness of medical science at home and cemented its links to increasingly better-organized government agencies.[30]

Latin American physicians became interested in fertility thanks in part to advances in European medical technologies, namely the introduction of anesthesia to midwifery in 1863, Lister's invention of antisepsis in 1867, and the development of the dilation and curettage operation to induce abortions and treat incomplete ones in 1874.[31] The medical inclination to intervene in pregnancy and birthing did not necessarily mean safer deliveries or surgeries, however. In fact, before the widespread use of sulfa drugs in the mid-1930s and penicillin in the mid-1940s, physicians worldwide were troubled by high maternal mortality rates due to sepsis, hemorrhage, and eclampsia. This situation strengthened propositions to increase medical surveillance over women, such as the prohibition of dangerous activities (including physical work and strenuous exercise), and greater postbirth state support (through neonatal clinics and laws providing maternity leaves from work). Such initiatives also became popular in Latin America.[32]

During the Cold War, various U.S.-based social scientists and government agents, as well as institutions such as the Milbank Memorial Fund, the Population Council, and the International Planned Parenthood Federation, contributed knowledge and funding to treat what they deemed an unhealthy and dangerous trend, rapid population growth, in Latin America. Their preferred solution to this threat was technical, in the form of the mass promotion of contraceptives such as the pill and the intrauterine device to cut down birth rates. We must pay more attention than we have so far to the U.S. experts who created the representations of 1960s Latin America as a demographic danger zone, as well as to their Latin American allies. Their predilection for simple technical solutions to complex social problems suggests continuities between population-limitation campaigns and the worldwide campaigns to eradicate infectious insect-borne diseases through the use of DDT while paying relatively less attention to the social and environmental contexts in which diseases emerged and spread.[33] Likewise, Cold War population experts' inability and unwillingness to see the neocolonial attitudes and consumption habits of U.S. citizens or wealthy Latin Americans as part of the problems they sought to address are eerily reminiscent of the contemporary region-wide antinarcotics strategy that disproportionately penalizes the poor. Thus, my analytical incorporation of the Cold War era, up to the late 1970s transition from military to civilian rule, is as much about extending our historiographical reach as it is about understanding a style of intervention that has characterized U.S.–Latin American relations from the late 1940s on.

On the other hand, Western biomedicine has not been the only way in which to intervene in fertility matters in Latin America. Practitioners such as faith healers, herbalists, and traditional birth attendants have successfully taken part in this enterprise and continue to exert considerable power among health consumers.[34] This medical pluralism, in addition to the chronic financial and organizational limitations of public health care institutions, helps explain why biomedical knowledge is not the only epistemic resource for people to make sense of fertility. Lay understanding of one's own body is also a crucial resource, one that underscores the longstanding significance of self-care when experiencing pain or discomfort. As Arthur Kleinman notes, human beings view their own bodies as subject to manipulation (by oneself or by others) and as knowledge-producing organizers of experiences.[35] We regularly tap into this knowledge of our own bodies to care for ourselves and to explain our bodily shortcomings in ways that are shared with people in circumstances similar to our own. These forms of personal and local lay knowledge production can be and have been at odds with allopathic knowledge.[36]

Abortion, the subject of chapter 3, allows for lay knowledge to enter the realm of fertility control in a dramatic, visceral way. Seeking or performing an abortion was not only illegal but also taboo in most of Latin America throughout the nineteenth and twentieth centuries. Yet, undoubtedly, abortions have been and continue to be sought and carried out nowadays, often using more subtle and ambiguous language to capture the attention of interested consumers only.

By learning more about why and how women sought to help themselves by getting rid of unwanted pregnancies we learn much about people's social-support networks, as well as their sometimes-embattled relations with lovers, neighbors, physicians, and the police. This means seeing women seeking abortions not only as criminals or victims of injustice, but also as people making the best of the bad hands that fortune sometimes dealt them, including their shame and anger at failing to manage parenthood in ways they deemed morally appropriate. It also means recognizing that the meaning of "abortion" is a heavily contested one.[37] This leads us to consider scarcely addressed issues, including the way in which women seeking to end their pregnancies made sense of what they did, the public's reaction to these actions, and the connections between the world of abortion seekers and providers, and that of family planning policymakers.

Anyone writing a history of family planning in Latin America has to be mindful of the lessons the demographic transition theory has taught, particularly concerning the role biomedical technologies and transnational political actors have played as catalysts of social change. On the other hand, some of the received wisdom needs to be revised, particularly the assumption that the logic for the prevention or spacing of births is primarily financial, and the discounting of local actors' interests and dispositions as subordinate to those of foreign actors. Still other elements of the demographic transition theory have become obsolete, as applied to Latin America at least. Changes in mentality that led people to reflect on the value of a large number of offspring, the "independent variable" in the demographic transition model, long predate the 1960s. In the context of the late nineteenth century's accelerated insertion of Latin American nation-states into transnational capitalist networks, the control of one's own individual fertility and the state's ability to manage its population gave fertility-oriented biomedical interventions, alternative healing traditions, and self-care greater public visibility. The same issues are evident during the Cold War. Thus, throughout the twentieth century the management of fertility has been at the center of debates about the nature of modern nationhood, and about the proper and improper ways to be a parent. In this way, Latin American notions of citizenship have been strongly informed by one's qualities as a parent.

It is also high time to shed the demographic transition theory–inspired association between "pronatalist" mentalities and "traditional" societies, opposed to the equally spurious association between "antinatalist" mentalities and "modern" societies. Such language rightfully sought to underscore that real transformations occurred, and that they were conflictive, given the way in which the control of fertility redrew existing boundaries between experts and lay people, between men and women, and between nation-states. However, it is also a language that all too simplistically introduces both artificial distinctions and linkages that are more richly understood through empirical studies, and that fails to explain why "pronatalist" mentalities persist in "modern" societies, and how "antinatalist" mentalities emerge in "traditional" societies.[38] This language also glosses over the specific motivations of social actors for using and promoting family planning. Jennifer Johnson-Hanks's and Caroline Bledsoe's work on Africa shows, for example, that "fertility control" cannot be reduced to the strategies used to have fewer children and that, in fact, women may use family planning to maximize how many children they beget.[39] As I will show in chapter 6, when the Catholic Church in Peru embraced the pill in the 1960s, it did so on its own terms, that is, to nourish the growth of Catholic families, not to reduce birth rates and not to give women more contraceptive choices.

## Plan of the Book

Each subsequent chapter delves into the conundrums family planning posed from the point of view of, respectively, medical experts in the early twentieth century, Peru's first feminists, the women and men who sought abortions, the health workers and contraceptive users who supported birth control initiatives, governmental agencies (civilian and military alike) and their foreign allies, and the Catholic Church. Each topic weaves together Peruvian, Latin American, and U.S. histories and actors.

Chapter 1, "The Reproductive Potential of the Nation," focuses on the legacy of eugenically inspired advice and laws to regulate female and male sexuality so as to maximize the fertility of the "right" kind of population in order to unleash the vast economic potential of the country. Chapter 2, "Irene Silva de Santolalla and the Well-Constituted Family," discusses how experts' advice and interventions described in chapter 1 were an integral aspect of the first women's movement in the country to explicitly raise the issue of reproduction as politically problematic. Chapter 3, "Abortion and Accusation: Experts and Lay People between Crime and Custom," contrasts starkly with chapter 2, as the main characters are not women defending motherhood but women resorting to criminal acts to avoid having children, in medical, legal, and social environments that enabled a series of strategies for these women (and men) to protect themselves from prosecution. Chapter 4, "Contraception Crucible: Health Workers Encounter Family Planning," explains how a combination of the noxious devaluation of recent immigrants from rural areas into urban ones and the benign concern with maternal health, negatively affected by the widespread use of abortion as a contraceptive, prompted a change between the 1930s and the 1960s among health workers who began to embrace the value of smaller families for all, and the use of family planning to accomplish this goal. Chapter 5, "The Government Steps In (and Out): Family Planning and Population Policymaking," analyzes how family planning became an aspect of civilian and military government policies aiming for greater socioeconomic development and improved health for women and children amid the Cold War fear of rapid population growth in developing countries. Chapter 6, "Priests and

Pills: Catholic Birth Control in Peru," takes up the issue of how Catholic authorities in the 1960s, neither believing that religious doctrine was in conflict with the control of one's fertility nor willing to treat fertility control as a prerogative of individuals, set up a program to provide birth control pills while emphasizing the communal and national implications of the use of family planning.

## CHAPTER ONE

# The Reproductive Potential of the Nation

In the summer of 1933, the Callao Rotary Club readied for "Child's Week," an event the club sponsored in Peru's most important port city, west of Lima. Under the enthusiastic leadership of Dr. Alberto Sabogal, Child's Week consisted of a series of activities to kindle interest in all things toddler. Luisa Arróspide Bueno won the contest for the child with the best "vital traits." At two years, eleven months, and seventeen days, Luisa had uncommonly good physical proportions, according to the judges: she stood just over a meter tall, weighed twenty-one kilos, and had a sixty-two centimeter thoracic perimeter. She had also been exclusively breastfed during her first two months of life. An article in *La Reforma Médica* emphasized Luisa's mother's clever and careful food choices for her daughter, as well as Luisa's father's complete devotion to his family. In an accompanying photo, a naked Luisa stared at the camera with a vacant look, making obvious what the article left unsaid: she was a white child, all brown locks and chubbiness. The article's message, explicit in its final lines, was that children such as Luisa, with her white skin, doting parents, and scientifically monitored development, were urgently needed for the progress of the nation.[1]

This chapter deals with experts such as Dr. Sabogal and their passion for eugenic progress. How did their ideas and initiatives shape the earliest national approaches to family planning? Early twentieth-century physicians believed that the country's population was under siege from multiple enemies: high rates of infant mortality, the backwardness of indigenous peoples, venereal diseases, alcoholism, the ignorance of women who neglected their maternal duties, and the carelessness of two-timing men who fathered children out of wedlock. Few among these experts saw population growth as a threat before the 1950s. In fact, one of their key concerns since the eighteenth century had been how to increase such growth.[2] From strategic positions within university and government circles, physicians helped popularize the idea that sexual and reproductive behaviors of both men and women were a matter of the utmost social importance, given that these behaviors could determine the long-term well-being of the nation even more decisively than national elections. Just as notable, however, was these physicians' will to circumscribe their attention to urban areas, a bias that exerted a powerful influence over the framing of later family planning debates.

## Academic Medicine Rises Again

The medical experts who rose to prominence advocating the link between eugenic pronatalism and national progress in the early twentieth century were all linked to the Faculty of Medicine in Lima, invigorated since the 1890s after a period of stagnation and decay. Until 1961, medical training was available in Peru only at San Marcos University. The university had been founded in 1551, while Peru was still a Spanish colony, and its first medical courses began in 1571, with the earliest dissections conducted in 1711 at San Andrés Hospital.[3] Dr. Hipólito Unanue, the chair of anatomy in 1792, however, deemed contemporary training at the university woefully out of date. Unanue was one of the foremost promoters of the adaptation of European science to Peru's needs, through organizations such as the Sociedad de Amantes del País, of which he was a founding member, and the newspaper *El Mercurio Peruano*, which he published.[4] His lobbying to the Viceroyalty finally brought about the construction of a new anatomical amphitheater and curricular modifications emulating the highly regarded Paris Medical Faculty.

The newly structured Faculty of Medicine, renamed the Real Colegio de Medicina y Cirugía de San Fernando, was inaugurated in 1811. The 1810s, however, were politically turbulent. Agitation in favor of independence had begun in Spanish America, resulting in a smaller budget for the Faculty of Medicine, diminished enrollments, and fewer instructors. General José de San Martín, commander of one of the independentist armies of South America and self-titled Protector of Peru, renamed the Faculty of Medicine the Colegio de la Independencia in 1821. However, with much of the country in financial difficulties, the Faculty of Medicine went through frequent periods of inactivity after independence in 1824.[5]

Medicine as an institution began to recover in the mid-nineteenth century, as the Peruvian government became, albeit briefly, wealthier through the revenues generated by the export of guano. President Ramón Castilla signed off on the budgetary allocation for the Faculty of Medicine in 1856, renaming it the Facultad de Medicina de San Fernando, and appointed anatomy professor Dr. Cayetano Heredia as dean. Like Unanue before him,

Heredia looked to Europe when he reorganized physician education to include more training in areas such as biochemistry and pathology.[6] The diffusion of this type of knowledge was the goal of the *Gaceta Médica de Lima*, the first periodical published by Peruvian academic physicians, edited by Heredia himself.[7]

Thanks to the 1856 reforms, medicine became the first profession in Peru to establish a unified standard curriculum for its trainees, doing away with the distinction between physicians and surgeons and creating instead a new type of hybrid specialist, the *médico-cirujano* (physician-surgeon). Inspired by the work of scientists such as Claude Bernard and Louis Pasteur, Heredia funded study-abroad trips for some of his most promising students, with other Peruvian physicians following suit and using their own funds to travel to Europe to further their education.[8] These trips were important not only because of the advanced training acquired, but also because the young physicians made it a point to send back books and pedagogical materials for the university library. Perhaps more crucially, these physicians returned to take up teaching jobs at the Faculty of Medicine.[9]

The War of the Pacific against Chile (1879–83) truncated these efforts and left the country, and the Faculty of Medicine, in financial ruin. Nevertheless, as the nineteenth century came to a close, Peru experienced yet another bonanza, this time underwritten by the export of copper, sugar, cotton, oil, wool, rubber, coffee, and silver: "four unprecedented decades" of economic growth and production diversification, according to economic historian Carlos Contreras.[10] The period between the mid-1890s and 1919, known as the "Aristocratic Republic," was characterized by the growing power of a small, tight-knit oligarchy that defended economic liberalism, scientific Positivism, and bureaucratic improvements.[11] The Civilista Party was the leading political arm of the Peruvian elite, and included coastal hacienda owners, noted university professors, and wealthy urban merchants from the Lima area as its most prominent members. Under Civilista leadership, the central government acted vigorously to improve tax collection, the army, primary education, and public health, and to place these activities under its control. To the Civilistas, the upgrading of the central administrative apparatus was essential to make a cohesive whole out of Peru's natural and human diversity. Yet, only coastal cities and their inhabitants, not the majority of Peruvians at that time, were the biggest beneficiaries of Civilista initiatives.

This new cycle of prosperity and governmental centralization was the backdrop for the increase in medical courses, often taught by Peruvian specialists returning from Europe, including bacteriology and microscopy, gynecology and obstetrics, pediatrics, and ophthalmology, all begun in the 1890s. Paris-trained Constantino T. Carvallo, chair of obstetrics and gynecology, introduced techniques such as asepsis and the use of rubber gloves in surgical practice, as well as radium therapy for cancer in 1896. He even took an x-ray, the first one in the country, of Peruvian president Nicolás de Piérola's hand just a year after Wilhelm Roentgen's development of this technology. Courses in treatment of the ear, nose, and throat and in urology began in the 1900s; dermatosyphilis, psychiatry, tropical medicine, and hygiene in the 1910s.[12]

In addition to creating new specialties, Peruvian physicians at the turn of the twentieth century began attending regional professional conferences such as the Pan-American Medical Congresses and the Latin American Medical Congresses.[13] A related development was the foundation of new periodicals, including *La Crónica Médica* (1884), *El Monitor Médico* (1885), *Anales de la Facultad de Medicina* (1915), *La Reforma Médica* (1915), and *La Acción Médica* (1927).[14] International meetings and periodicals not only helped colleagues exchange scientific information but also aided local professional organization efforts, which led to the establishment of new interest groups, such as the Academia Nacional de Medicina (1888), which launched the *Anales de la Academia Nacional de Medicina* in 1897.[15]

Even more indicative of the rising power of academic medicine in early twentieth-century Peru was the establishment of the Dirección de Salubridad Pública (Office of Public Sanitation, DSP), forerunner to Peru's Ministry of Health.[16] Physicians had been elected to Congress since the formation of the Peruvian legislative branch in 1822.[17] This demonstrated, however, a degree of individual and not corporate influence. Then, in 1903, the Ministry of Economic Development wrested control of all sanitary initiatives away from municipalities and brought them under the jurisdiction of the newly created DSP. Led by Julián Arce, professor of tropical medicine at the Faculty of Medicine, the DSP's upper management and board of advisers were dominated by academic physicians.[18] The agency's main function was to coordinate national efforts against tuberculosis, plague, yellow fever, and malaria as a means to promote population growth. Indeed, the DSP's 1905 programmatic statement envisioned population as a national economic resource that must be cared for and harnessed to produce more wealth. In their efforts to protect this "human capital," the DSP promoted the control of epidemics, the teaching of hygiene courses in schools, the creation of health clinics and milk distribution centers for newborns, and the building of hygienic housing for workers.[19]

Thus, by the 1900s, Peruvian academic physicians had capitalized on yet another cycle of national prosperity and transformed themselves into an elite that exerted a significant influence based out of the expanding and specializing Faculty of Medicine, with students and instructors who received part of their training abroad and networked with colleagues throughout the Americas. Physicians also founded new medical associations and journals, and their expertise was not only in demand in Congress but had been institutionalized in the executive branch of government. To this elite, sexual and reproductive behaviors were emerging as a crucial area of intervention, alongside their established concerns with epidemic diseases and sanitation. This was so not only because of the link between reproduction and the long-standing political yearning for population growth, but because of the prevalence of factors that could negatively affect sexuality and lead to the growth of the "wrong" kind of population, the degenerate kind.

## Degeneration and Puericulture in Translation

Racial degeneration had been a concern of European and American intellectuals at least since the eighteenth century, and its prevention would underwrite the discursive and practical participation of Peruvian physicians in sexual and reproductive matters well into the twentieth century. Ill defined, and all the more versatile for it, the concept of racial degeneration pointed both to individual and collective traits transmitted over generations and leading to and/or causing immorality, idiocy, criminality, and, ultimately, premature death. A vast range of physical deformities, alcoholism, sterility, and madness were the pathological symptoms accompanying racial degeneration, which, if unchecked, could engulf entire societies. Although degenerate individuals were beyond help, degeneration as a population-level phenomenon advanced slowly, which could presumably give national leaders opportunities to intervene in a timely manner and arrest its progression.[20]

In the late nineteenth century, racial degeneration animated national debates in Latin America. Fear of it was implicated in diverse reform proposals of governments in the region: European immigration, urban renewal, sanitary campaigns, the regulation of prostitution, and the promotion of sports, for example.[21] Peruvian intellectuals felt ambivalent about the source of a creeping degeneration that, they agreed, was at the core of Peru's want of population and its defeat in the War of the Pacific. Essayist Manuel González Prada, for example, blamed Peruvian leaders' resolute refusal to embrace the influence of northern European immigrants for the loss. In contrast, José Gálvez lamented the corruption of beloved Iberian-inspired traditions through the rising influence of northern Europe and the United States. Some, including Joaquín Capelo, Carlos Lissón, Alejandro Garland, and Francisco Graña saw little of value in Iberian culture, claiming it instilled laziness and conservatism, while they castigated Spain for the catastrophic depopulation of the Inca Empire during the conquest and colonial periods. In Clemente Palma's opinion, however, it was the Inca Empire and Andean cultures that were at the root of Peru's degenerative tendencies.[22]

Peruvians also placed responsibility on some of the new immigrants, Chinese ones in particular. Chinese settlers began arriving in large numbers in the mid-nineteenth century as farm hands, guano collectors, and railroad workers and created a vibrant society within urban Peruvian society.[23] Yet several Peruvian physicians claimed that miscegenation with the Chinese weakened the national hereditary stock, and they did not hesitate to blame Chinese immigrants' "filthy habits" for the 1903 plague epidemic in Lima.[24] Dr. Julián Arce, soon to become head of the DSP, was one of the few medical experts to support Chinese immigration, though exclusively on the grounds that their inexpensive labor could consolidate the economic growth of coastal haciendas.[25] Congress took notice of the ill will toward the Chinese and twice, in 1909 and in 1916, tried unsuccessfully to pass laws to limit Chinese immigration to the country.[26] By the 1930s, *Anti-Asia* and *Fuera Chinos*, the two newspapers that agitated against Chinese immigration, stopped circulating.

In contrast, the promotion of European immigration as a way to strengthen national racial qualities had broader support. *Diputado* for Lima Matías Manzanilla, for example, promoted Italian immigration through a bill introduced at the behest of the Sociedad de Inmigración y Colonización Italiana en el Perú.[27] But European immigration, although much desired and touted, failed to effect significant demographic growth for the country.[28] Instead, the position that gained purchase among academic physicians was the one seeking to increase endogenous population growth, without heavy reliance on immigrants. As Julio Egoaguirre, physician and former minister of economic development, put it, "Peru is underpopulated, and we had better defend the lives we produce naturally. . . . Our inhabitants must be healthy, robust, capable of procreating healthy children, because the nation's territory demands workers for fields, mines, industry, and civic life. It is not appropriate to seek this growth through other races, which often do not blend well with our ethnic traits, and prevent us from fulfilling the maxim 'to govern is to populate.'"[29]

The 1905 DSP directorship summarized what would become one of its main new areas of involvement for the next four decades: "in recent years there have been attempts to restrict the freedom to marry, by giving the physician the power to control the health of those called to propagate the human race. This is certainly one of the most logical remedies against degeneration."[30] With a view to raising a healthy, robust, and fertile population, the medical elite deemed that its mandate to protect endogenous population growth ought to go beyond improving the local sanitary environment, and this led them to adopt rhetoric and implement actions to regulate the more intimate realms of mate selection and reproduction. Thus, the desire for population growth and the fear of degeneration became the lenses through which physicians first envisioned the question of the reproductive potential of the nation. However, even though managing the fertility of Peruvians was their goal, gender informed their approaches. While physicians treated women primarily as potential mothers in need of protection, they saw men as lusty and irresponsible, less in need of protection than containment and even intimidation. Different strategies flowed from this gendered characterization. Some of these came to fruition, while others failed, but they all hinged on the adoption of puericultural assumptions.

Parisian physician Alfred Caron coined the term "puericulture" in 1865 to refer to the improvement of the health of newborns. However, the notion did not catch on until Adolphe Pinard, head of the Baudeloque Maternity Clinic and chair of clinical obstetrics at the Paris Medical Faculty, revived it in the 1890s. Inspired by the weight gains among infants born to mothers who spent time in a maternity clinic before giving birth, Pinard began to advocate for special care and rest for pregnant women before delivery. Based on these findings, French pediatricians and obstetricians supported Pinard, as they worried that physical exertion and psychological stress could provoke the premature expulsion of the fetus. Premature infants, if they survived, would presumably grow to become weak individuals prone to disease and degeneration.[31]

From the outset, puericulture was deeply concerned with the theme of national decline and degeneration in France, something that resonated strongly with the priorities of Latin American intellectuals in the 1920s. In his address to the Sixth Latin American Medical Congress that met in Lima in 1922, Dr. Leonidas Avendaño, chair of legal medicine at San Marcos University, echoed the tenets of puericulture as he zeroed in on the high infant mortality that did not permit an optimal endogenous demographic growth in Peru. Excessive work for women in urban factories and the inheritability of tuberculosis, alcoholism, and syphilis were the main culprits for this infant mortality, according to Avendaño. Nevertheless, he also blamed lecherous men who did not care for the children they fathered, the "despicable" providers of abortions, and the voluntary practice of "*el birthcontrol.*"[32]

To physicians such as Avendaño, threats to the nation's reproductive potential were everywhere. The mother of all dangers, Avendaño argued, was a comfort-induced relaxation of morals that seeped into dress styles, manners, the dailies, and even informal conversations, awakening disorderly appetites, especially among women. "There are no mothers," Avendaño declared, because women instead had their minds filled "with worry and ignorance. . . . How can we make her abandon obsolete routines and the advice of the so-called wise old women?" To him, this was best accomplished through scientifically managed state assistance to pregnant women.[33]

Physicians had been interested in these services since the late nineteenth century, particularly the control of the quality of milk served in hospices and orphanages. Was the milk collected from donkeys? From black wet nurses, "known for their bad habits, excesses and unsanitariness"? From sick or overworked women?[34] Only oversight by the medical profession, in the self-serving opinion of physicians, could guarantee the nutritiousness, hygiene, and volume of the supply of milk given to infants by charitable organizations. Dr. Alejandro Lawezzari lavished praise on the "healthy tripod" sustaining the health of young children: milk, physician, and mother (in that order).[35] Wealthy Lima philanthropist Mrs. Juana Alarco de Dammert had advice like this in mind when she founded the Sociedad Auxiliadora de la Infancia (Society for the Protection of Children) in 1894, a charitable organization that hired physicians to monitor the health of children under seven, and that oversaw the operation of the country's first daycare center (founded in 1901) and pasteurized milk distribution center (founded in 1908).[36] Dr. Francisco Graña, chair of hygiene at the Faculty of Medicine, used his influence at the Beneficence Society of Lima to create another milk distribution center in the city in 1912.[37] The same year, Mrs. María de Piaggio, a Callao philanthropist, founded a daycare center overseen by physicians on the second floor of the town's central market.[38]

Puericulturists scored another victory with the 1918 legalization of paid leaves from work for pregnant women, which stipulated that women would receive up to 60 percent of their wages from twenty days before to forty days after they gave birth. In addition, the law mandated that workplaces with more than twenty-five female workers over the age of seventeen must provide daycare for infants. This law was the brainchild of *diputado* for Lima

Matías Manzanilla, a member of the Civilista Party and a strong advocate of workplace safety, the curtailment of female and child labor, and the eight-hour day for female workers. Unfortunately, the law, which employers did not always obey, only applied to women working in the industrial sector in urban areas and not to women in rural areas or to domestic workers.[39] In other words, it excluded the majority of working women in Peru.

It was the administration of President Augusto B. Leguía (1919–30) that turned the modest and piecemeal puericultural initiatives to protect infants and pregnant women into nationwide projects. In 1920, Leguía sponsored Dr. Enrique León García, recently appointed chair of pediatrics at the Faculty of Medicine, when the latter proposed to conduct the nation's first survey of hospital infant mortality. The sobering conclusion was that, between 1919 and 1924, 37.4 percent of all babies born at the Santa Ana Hospital, the busiest maternity hospital in Peru, died within a year.[40] That hospital was closed in 1924. Most of its operations were taken over by the newly created Arzobispo Loayza Hospital, but its obstetrics and gynecology ward moved to a new specialized hospital, the Hospital de Maternidad, later known as the Maternidad de Lima.

Leguía also created the Junta de Defensa de la Infancia (Board for the Defense of Children) in 1922, the first state agency dedicated to the protection of low-income mothers and children. Professor of hygiene Carlos Enrique Paz Soldán lobbied for the establishment of the board after his election to Congress for Lima. The board organized its first conference in July 1922, with Paz Soldán as secretary general, and President Leguía as honorary speaker.[41] One of the main conclusions of this conference was the need to create an Instituto Nacional del Niño (National Child Institute), with more power and responsibilities than the Board for the Defense of Children wielded. Once again, President Leguía offered his support, and the institute was created in 1925, with Paz Soldán as director. By 1930, the institute had replaced charitable organizations in the management of infant health clinics, daycare centers, and milk distribution centers. The institute's personnel also began to lobby for the creation of a specialized hospital. President Leguía backed this initiative as well and founded the Hospital del Niño (Children's Hospital) in 1929.

The National Child Institute's mandate to represent the state in all matters relating to the protection of children extended to what was termed "extra-uterine puericulture." It was not enough to protect pregnant women to ensure healthy and abundant offspring. The institute sought to have a hand in the design of education curricula, the promotion of sports, sexual education, and home economics for women. This outreach mission was to be carried out by its corps of *visitadoras sociales*, female social workers who knocked on doors and delivered information to women about proper feeding and hygiene habits and exhorted them to marry the men with whom they lived. Charged with propagating ideas about hygiene to the farthest and most neglected areas of Peru, the *visitadoras* also staffed the National Child Institute's six pregnancy-consultation clinics, thirteen milk distribution centers, six daycare centers, and two children's hospices, dispersed throughout Peruvian cities.[42]

The first *visitadora social* program began at the National Child Institute in September 1925. Their training emphasized their role as the foot soldiers of the nation's "demogénesis," or "the cluster of biosocial phenomena that determine how a race is to endure within a geographical area."[43] Graduates valiantly took an oath "for maternity, home, and fatherland," and swore to "ensure the life and health of the new seedlings."[44] The most common form of intervention by *visitadoras* consisted of simple advice to women about the importance of appropriate clothing, nutritious food, physical exercise, and marriage. This advice was geared toward making women aware that their main function in life was to bear many children within formalized unions, and that just about every aspect of their behavior and physical state could affect such a delicate mission.[45]

The training was designed as a specialization course for midwives.[46] However, the program's budget was small, and personnel education suffered as a result. Between 1927 and 1933 only seventeen new *visitadoras* graduated.[47] Meanwhile, population continued to increase. Between 1876 and 1940 the population of Lima alone grew more than fourfold, from 129,000 to 595,000 inhabitants, and that of the country as a whole more than doubled, from 2.65 million to more than 7 million.[48] Like *visitadoras*, midwives worked under strict performance standards enforced by supervising physicians. The DSP demanded that midwives working for the government report on their activities every six months, established how much midwives could charge for their services, and, in 1909, stipulated that they must provide assistance free of charge "to poor women who need their help, at any time of the day or night."[49]

This strict management and the low pay dissuaded midwives from working for the state, either as midwives or as *visitadoras sociales*, and, some physicians believed, pushed midwives to provide abortions as a way to make ends meet.[50] The situation was especially dire in the country's smallest cities. The town of Huanuco, for example, could not attract a university-trained midwife in 1917, even though the DSP ordered it to do so.[51] By 1940, although the Faculty of Medicine's School of Midwives had 273 graduates, 210 of them worked in Lima. Meanwhile not a single university-trained midwife could be found in Tumbes, Amazonas, San Martin, Ancash, Huancavelica, Apurimac, Madre de Dios, or Moquegua. Not surprisingly, most births in Peru between the 1910s and the 1930s occurred without the assistance of a university-trained expert.[52]

Greater moneymaking possibilities drove the Lima-centric midwifery labor market. However, we must also consider the effects of an insidious health worker bias against serving rural and indigenous populations, which were more abundant outside the capital. Since colonial times, administrators had posited the distinctiveness of Spanish and indigenous cultures. Although miscegenation among indigenous peoples, Europeans, and Africans complicated this simple dichotomy, leading to a caste system with many fluid categories of race mixtures, the original binary definition endured.[53] The actions and inaction of different indigenous groups during the War of the Pacific further intensified the insecurities the Peruvian white elite harbored about indigenous culture as an untrustworthy yet numerically dominant element of the nation.[54] Even after the war, as the external threat lessened, indigenous civil uprisings and regional rebellions worried this elite.[55] Not surprisingly, by the 1890s many among them were convinced of indigenous Peruvians' lack of patriotism and civic virtues.

Elites' beliefs in their political difference from, and superiority to, the indigenous population received legal support in the Peruvian Penal Code of 1924, valid until 1991, which divided Peruvians into categories of "civilized," "semi-civilized," and "savages" and meted out punishments that varied depending on the guilty party's degree of "civilization," treating "savages" more leniently.[56] This attitude had a medical counterpart that described indigenous peoples as reluctant to embrace the advance of science, indigenous health knowledge as invalid, indigenous languages as barriers to intellectual and moral development, and indigenous women as capable of experiencing pain and fear in exclusively bestial ways.[57] At their most benign, these discriminatory attitudes were couched in a paternalistic rhetoric that recognized Peru's indigenous peoples as heirs of the mighty Inca Empire and blamed the brutality of the Spanish conquest and colonial periods for their contemporary prostration and poverty. Physicians did value the growth of the indigenous population of Peru as well as acknowledge the country's reliance on indigenous labor for key economic and geopolitical activities such as agriculture, mining, and the military. Nevertheless, indigenous demographic growth, physicians held, required institutions such as medicine, the military, and contract agricultural work to act as civilizing and disciplining forces to "redeem" and "rebuild" the Indian into a "utilizable building block of the nation."[58]

Given the lack of economic incentives to work in rural areas and the endurance of prejudices among university-trained health care workers against serving and understanding indigenous populations, it is not surprising that, in the 1920s and 1930s, plans to protect pregnant women to ensure healthy and abundant offspring remained largely an urban phenomenon. A similar process unfolded throughout Latin America. As Ana María Carrillo, Kim Clark, and Soledad Zárate have shown in the Mexican, Ecuadorean, and Chilean cases, respectively, it was mainly cities that benefitted from the presence of university-trained midwives.[59] Moreover, the eugenic will to rank people based on phenotypes was notable in academic medicine elsewhere in Latin America. Yet, Peru stands out as a place where the medical elite's animosity against nonwhites was especially fierce. Such a deeply ingrained attitude could still be discerned in the professional lack of outrage over the forced sterilization accusations of the mid-1990s. The few physicians who engaged with the systemic discrimination that shortchanged women in rural areas in the early twentieth century were, not surprisingly, rural physicians, but their pleadings went unanswered for the most part.[60] Puericultural initiatives, as mentioned above, unfolded with great publicity in Lima, promoted by academic physicians such as Paz Soldán and Avendaño in the 1920s. Notably, urban puericultural projects converged with eugenic ideas and did not exclude men.

## Restraining Male Sexuality

The first Peruvian eugenics organization was the Liga Nacional de Higiene y Profilaxis Social (National League of Hygiene and Social Prophylaxis, hereafter referred to as the Liga). Several individuals and institutions convened to form it in 1923, including the Peruvian chapter of the Red Cross, Faculty of Medicine professors such as Miguel Aljovín, Leonidas Avendaño, and Rómulo Eyzaguirre, and female activists such as San Marcos University educator Esther Festini de Ramos Ocampo.[61] Peruvian eugenicists supported the National Child Institute as it strove to educate women about the importance of hygiene and of their choice of a marriage mate. Yet, they also pioneered interventions in men's lives. Emblematic of this was their early antialcoholism campaign, undertaken long before the Liga's establishment. In 1896 the

Ministry of Justice, Religion, and Education sponsored the formation of a commission to tackle the issue of public drunkenness. The commission included a group of distinguished physicians from the Faculty of Medicine and produced a far-reaching bill that called for talks on the effects of alcohol to be given in schools, universities, parishes, police and military units, warships, hospitals, and prisons, as well as for all people registering births, deaths, and marriages.

The bill forbade employers from paying wages in alcoholic beverages. It also banned alcoholic beverages in theaters, circuses, churches, bullfighting arenas, and other public places. The initiative reduced taxes for restaurants that did not serve alcohol and called for police surveillance of all businesses that did, forbidding them to cover their windows with paint or curtains. It also ordered businesses that sold alcohol to close from Saturday at 6 p.m. until Monday at 9 a.m. The remaining days of the week such businesses were to stay open only until 11 p.m., always barring entrance to minors, members of the police and armed forces, women, clergy, and government workers. The bill even ordered the increase of taxes on alcohol imported to produce pharmaceutical compounds.

Supporters of this draconian legislation claimed that alcohol made up a "deadly trinity" alongside syphilis and tuberculosis, causing the hereditary degeneration of the race and "damaging up to the fourth generation of alcoholics." They explicitly targeted males, noting the sad spectacle of men spending their wages on Saturday nights instead of spending that time with their families. Proponents argued that alcohol "turns the popular masses into brutes, weakening their family values, already underdeveloped among our people, and thus leading to the nation's depopulation."[62] The bill was defeated in Congress in 1901. However, two decades later, during the heyday of Peruvian puericulture, President Augusto B. Leguía resuscitated two weakened portions of the same bill. One forbade the drinking of alcohol in brothels, as intoxicated customers might be less likely to demand a prostitute's health certificate. The other mandated the institution of a course in high schools about hygiene, contagious diseases, alcoholism, and puericulture.[63]

The National League of Hygiene and Social Prophylaxis also dared to bring men into a discussion of prostitution for the first time in Peru. Prostitution grew during the boom-bust cycle of guano production of the mid-nineteenth century.[64] Authorities deemed it a necessary evil, as they saw male sexuality as too ardent to withstand inactivity.[65] However, the government attempted to regulate the trade in 1910 through the Servicio Sanitario de la Prostitución (Office for Prostitution Hygiene, SSP). The SSP organized the medical corps of the police in May 1914, which began to register and subject prostitutes to weekly genital exams to detect venereal diseases.[66] Many academic physicians ridiculed the policing campaign. These strong-arm tactics, they accused, made prostitutes fear medical men and encouraged a flourishing business of fake registration identifications. More important, the campaign only dealt with prostitutes working in known brothels and did not affect freelance prostitutes at all. In addition to supporting the creation of free treatment clinics, physicians were strong proponents of the use of condoms by all clients of prostitutes, especially members of the armed forces.[67]

Still, the campaign continued, and prostitutes were subjected to increasingly brutal police harassment in the name of public health. Peru's harsh treatment of prostitutes was hardly unique in this period. Beginning in the second half of the nineteenth century, antivice campaigns in Europe, the United States, and Latin America also targeted prostitution as a threat to public health, good morals, and the safety of women and attempted to regulate it.[68] As elsewhere, antiprostitution campaigns in Peru did not single out the male clients of prostitutes for monitoring. Focusing attention on the sexual lives of men was the most significant contribution to the prostitution regulation debate that the National League of Hygiene and Social Prophylaxis made in the 1920s. As Dr. Pando put it, men's behaviors could not be exempted from responsibility: "the problem is very complex: coquettishness, love of luxury, poverty, insufficient education, etc, are crucial factors in prostitution. But, it is men's selfish bachelorhood that is the ultimate cause of it."[69]

In addition to supporting the establishment of venereal disease clinics, the first of which opened in Lima in 1923, the Liga supported academic research on the occupations, racial backgrounds, and marriage status of prostitutes' clients and launched an educational campaign using fliers and public speakers to educate men about their role in the production of healthy offspring.[70] Liga supporters deemed married men the vanguard of healthy citizenship, men such as little Luisa Arróspide Bueno's father, whose virtuous behavior had been rewarded with a precious child. The Liga promoted the view that married men's greatest interest was the preservation of the health of their family members. In contrast, they assumed that unmarried men lived with no one to care for, and thus willingly severed the ties between themselves and society. In their view, single men were tormented by their freedom, lived shorter and more disorderly lives than married men, and had unusual sleep and eating patterns, in addition to sexual habits that only prostitutes tolerated.[71]

On September 10, 1926, President Leguía issued a special decree creating the Liga Nacional Antivenérea (National Antivenereal League, LNA), just months after the country's first national conference on venereal diseases, to coordinate all initiatives for the regulation of prostitution and the control of sexually transmitted infections. Thus, Leguía threw the weight of his office behind yet another eugenics project, as he had previously with the National Child Institute. Medical experts, eugenics promoters, political appointees, and Leguía himself worked together on the LNA's board of directors, board of advisers, and executive council.[72] In 1929, Leguía made the LNA's activities an official part of the DSP, creating within the latter a Hygiene and Social Prophylaxis Section. Even after Leguía's fall from power, this DSP section continued its work, establishing the National Museum of Antivenereal Prophylaxis in September 1932 in Lima's red-light district, Huatica. The museum, located inside the venereal disease clinic of La Victoria, explicitly catered to boys of high school age, urging them to become acquainted with "the horrors caused by venereal contagion."[73]

Managing male sexuality through fear and disgust persisted as a strategy of the local public health establishment into the 1930s and 1940s. General Oscar Benavides (president from 1933 to 1939) elevated the DSP to the level of a ministry in 1935, dubbed the Ministry of Public Health, Work, and Social Welfare.[74] Its Dirección General de Salubridad (General Office of Sanitation, DGS) was in charge of hospitals and health posts, including venereal disease clinics.[75] Within just six months in 1935, the DGS staged thirty lectures on the contagion of sexually transmitted infections. It also distributed fliers, screened the film *El Azote de la Humanidad* (*The Scourge of Humanity*), and made an itinerant exhibit out of the wax statues of the National Museum of Antivenereal Prophylaxis. The DGS praised the Ministry of Education for "all the forms of help" it provided transporting 2,460 male students over sixteen years of age to attend its functions. The DGS also reported reaching 1,820 male workers, 900 male patients of venereal disease clinics, and 555 "young men" through its antivenereal education campaign.[76]

As was the case for women, however, the vigorous campaign was based out of Lima, for Lima's benefit. Exemplary of this provincialism was the celebration of the "National Antivenereal Day," preparations for which started in August 1936. The minister of public health, work, and social welfare, Dr. Fortunato Quesada, came to support the event after intense pressure from the National League of Hygiene and Social Prophylaxis.[77] The mobilization of resources was significant, as organizing this special day on September 4, 1938, required the participation of the navy's cadets and students from the Faculty of Medicine.

In addition, Dr. Carlos Bambarén, president of the Liga, Dr. Victor Eguiguren, chief medical officer of the antivenereal disease campaign, and Dr. Guillermo Almenara, minister of public health, spoke about the importance of prenuptial health certificates, the role of the state in fighting venereal diseases, and the promotion of moral and physical education as a means to curb male lasciviousness. These lectures were broadcast by radio. Moreover, the film *The Scourge of Humanity* was screened at least six times, and the film *Let Us Open Our Eyes* (*Abramos los Ojos*) at least four times in different venues in Lima. In the evening, the theatrical company of actor Angel Sebratti performed *The Deadly Kiss* (*El Beso Mortal*), a morality play written by the French playwright Gouredice, at the Municipal Theater of Lima. Tickets for the play had been distributed free at the three male venereal disease clinics in Lima.[78]

The wide deployment of personnel required to celebrate National Antivenereal Day is a good indicator of the political clout wielded in Lima by the Liga and its allies in the Faculty of Medicine by the late 1930s. To them, the reproductive potential of men was not to be squandered. In fact, because this reproductive potential had a tendency to waste away in single life, and to contaminate women and offspring, men's behavior had to be restrained through exhortation, repetition, and even intimidation. Of course, the Liga's antialcoholism campaigns, lobbying for prenuptial certificates, and antivenereal disease initiatives implicated women too. Women were, after all, the domestic partners who suffered if men's wages were spent at the bar, the unwitting recipients of crippling diseases, and the potential mothers of degenerate children. To women, puericulturists offered concrete solutions in daycare centers and milk distribution centers, as well as advice on the importance of appropriate clothing, nutritious food, physical exercise, and marriage.

The achievements and limitations of this gendered way of safeguarding the reproductive potential of the nation say more about the proponents of these puericulture and eugenics interventions than about their target audiences. Above all, they reveal that defining and defending a proper male role was as cherished a goal of eugenicists as was shaping a proper female role. Men and the management of their emotions such as fear and disgust have been important and neglected aspects of the history of Latin American fertility control.[79] In addition, considering how culturally entrenched male behaviors such as heavy drinking and having multiple sex partners and children out of wedlock (and failing to support either) were since colonial times, one marvels at the quixotic Liga and the people within it.[80] Their goal, to get men to measure up to a single manhood model, was as audacious as their contempt for and ignorance of indigenous Peruvians in rural areas was deep.

## An Enduring Urban Bias

Like most elite Peruvians, academic physicians believed the nation needed more inhabitants to take full advantage of the new opportunities provided by its participation as an exporter of raw materials in a transnational capitalist economic system. This was a particularly persuasive view during the years of economic growth between 1890 and 1930. Within this framework, the Peruvian elite to which academic physicians belonged saw indigenous peoples as a determined fixture of rural areas: working for the greater good of the nation as agricultural and mining workers, as soldiers, and as colonizers of the farthest reaches of the country, civilized by whites, and politically subordinate to them.[81] The steps taken to protect the reproductive potential of Peruvians were, before the 1940s, almost exclusively urban institutions, out of the reach of rural populations. Peru's pre-1940s medical writings and health policies reveal the institutionalization of a deeply racist national demographic culture that reproduced reductionist stereotypes about women as potential mothers in need of protection and men as potential fathers in need of tough guidance.

Yet, the 1940s ushered in important transformations. Constantino J. Carvallo increased the government's attention to rural health during his long and stable tenure as minister of public health. Carvallo established twenty-five of the forty-two venereal disease clinics that existed in Peru by 1944, most of them, at last, outside of Lima. Carvallo also relaunched the national corps of *visitadoras sociales* and increased the number of physicians working for the state from 260 in 1939 to 600 in 1945.[82] In addition, the Ministry of Public Health continued requiring prenuptial medical certificates, particularly to screen out syphilis, although it acknowledged how difficult it was to enforce this throughout the country.[83] Furthermore, between 1940 and 1960, Peru added 213 health centers and 177 rural health posts. The number of medical students also increased, from approximately 680 in 1940 to 2,045 in 1956. That year there were 479 physicians practicing in the country.[84]

These changes and the greater availability of medical human resources proved timely. Between 1876 and 1940, Peru's population grew from 2.6 million to over 7 million inhabitants.[85] Cities such as Lima grew the most, particularly as a result of internal migrations from rural areas.[86] Some, such as demographer Alberto Arca Parró, organizer of the 1940 census, celebrated this growth and the migrations because they believed that Peru's cities, with some careful planning, could harness the vigor of the new workforce and enter a stage of rapid industrialization.[87] Still, rural migrations spurred the growth of medical research on the risks the new migrants posed to Lima. Between 1953 and 1956, San Marcos University physicians published over one hundred works on this topic, mainly as theses.[88] With titles such as "An Urban Concentration Dangerous to the Health of Lima," the genre reveals the animosity and repugnance that the migrant indigenous provoked among the elite.[89] The San Cosme hill settlement, for example, struck "a dissonant note in the capital's harmonic flourishing, challenging the fatherland's civilization."[90] It is important to note that it was the settlers themselves, and not only the glaring lack of health or sanitation services in the area, that elicited these diatribes.

Facing what they believed was an invasion from people abandoning their legitimate places of residence in rural areas, academic physicians started advocating the use of eugenic birth control measures among the new arrivals as a tool to somewhat soften the polluting blow to their environs. If physicians could not stem the tide of immigrants, perhaps they could prevent further damage caused by the effluents of "substandard sources," made up of "families of masons, bakers, and the unemployed, [who] are more prolific than those of lawyers and physicians."[91] Whereas previously they had been content to promote the adoption of prenuptial health certificates for brides and grooms, physicians of the 1950s demanded the inquiry be extended to include the parents of the brides and grooms.[92]

The professional mentality of the medical elite underwent an important transformation around the mid-twentieth century. Before the acceleration of internal migration, eugenics discourse among physicians was limited to paternalistic calls for the improvement of the social and hygienic environment, with a view to enhancing the reproductive potential of men and women. This was, according to Nancy Stepan, the distinguishing feature of Latin American eugenics.[93] But eugenics was a dynamic creature, and Peruvian eugenicists after the 1940s had finally come face to face with other Peruvians, younger, poorer, and recently emigrated, demanding a place in a city that they too claimed as theirs, starting with the peripheral areas north of the Rimac River and south of the fancy Miraflores district. To the ongoing, if slow and inefficient, sanitary initiatives to improve the physical surroundings of this new population, the new eugenicists joined a pedagogical project to demonstrate how a "proper family" navigated city life, one that was energetically and self-righteously taken up by a new breed of female activist, the subject of the next chapter. Looming in the background of this pedagogical project was the wider utilization of birth control.

## CHAPTER TWO

# Irene Silva de Santolalla
# and the Well-Constituted Family

The Schering Pharmaceutical Corporation of Germany conducted the first clinical trials of injectable hormonal contraceptives for Peruvian women in the mid-1960s. The locale was the Hacienda Huando, an agricultural estate located in the province of Huaral, north of Lima. The opportunity had materialized when Peruvian physician Alfredo Larrañaga introduced Schering Peru's clinical director, the Hungarian-Argentine Istvan ("Esteban") Kesserü, to Larrañaga's friends, the brothers Fernando and Antonio Graña, owners of Huando, in 1962. Between 1966 and 1969, while the trials lasted, it was family educator Elsa Lescano's responsibility to determine the fitness of individual women to participate in the trial. Encouraged by the Grañas' confidence in her skills, Lescano decided that only married women, or those living in stable unions with men, were eligible, as long as they already had at least one child. "I imposed moral guidelines," she asserted proudly, "they had to be well-constituted families [*familias bien constituídas*]."[1]

The notion that some families are better than others runs deep in the history of Latin America. Colonial elites, for example, celebrated the purity of the blood of their ancestors from non-Spanish and non-Christian elements and offered it as a sign of moral superiority and a justification for their high socio-economic status.[2] Yet, nonelites and mixed-race individuals also claimed being morally upstanding, stressing traits such as honesty and hard work rather than their family backgrounds.[3] These plebeian bids for greater social regard are interesting because they raised the possibility that worthy traits could be passed on to later generations through the examples set and education provided by parents, rather than through the less laborious process of bequeathing a last name to one's offspring. Thus, one of the most important social legacies of the late Colonial period has been the emergence of the "well-constituted family" as both a moral imperative and the result of parental work.

Moreover, the adscription of a specific kind of socially valuable labor to parents, namely the raising of a manageable and productive population, was bound to a form of gendered specialization that permeated racial and class boundaries, with men responsible for their families in the public sphere and women doing the same in the private one. Such specialization, for women at least, can be traced to what little education convents and teaching orders made available for women in sixteenth-century Iberia, an education that focused on turning wealthy pupils into good Christians and wives for men. Not surprisingly, the first Peruvian women to publicly question the domestic female ideal in the mid-nineteenth and early twentieth centuries, including Flora Tristán, María Jesús Alvarado Rivera, Zoila Aurora Cáceres, Clorinda Matto, Mercedes Cabello, and Elvira García y García, did not reject childrearing as a primary female responsibility and source of respectability.[4] This devotion to domesticity constitutes, as Francesca Miller put it, "the heart of feminist movements in Latin America."[5] Following this view, hindrances to the traditional duty to care for home and children justified forceful public female condemnation. In fact, Peru's first female demonstrations took place in 1919 to protest price increases of basic foodstuffs. Such taking over of the public sphere by women in order to protect their home lives adds a politico-economic layer to the complexities of the Latin American "well-constituted family."

At the same time, as seen in the introduction, Latin American women have worn hats other than that of housewife for centuries. This makes it all the more fascinating to see how, in the 1930s, women began to explicitly address fertility as an issue that complicated their duties to home and children. One of the most prominent figures in this process in Latin America was Mrs. Irene Silva de Santolalla, the first woman elected to the Peruvian Senate in 1956. Mrs. Santolalla achieved notoriety starting in the 1930s for her advocacy of "family education," which moved from the pedagogical periphery toward generalized diffusion in high schools and postsecondary institutions in the 1950s. By the 1960s, family educators were university-trained specialists that regularly joined the staff of birth control clinics throughout Peru; and family education became a vehicle to portray family planning as an important duty of "well-constituted families."

Mrs. Santolalla's career and the trajectory of the field of family education between the 1930s and the 1970s illustrate how reproduction concerned social actors besides physicians. Mrs. Santolalla's entrepreneurial approach, blending Catholicism and heterosexual procreative marriage as guiding values, readily reinforced the notion that the "well-constituted family" was a rewarding product of hard work, a national necessity, and a primarily female responsibility. Consistently, family educators within the birth control establishment did not portray contraception only as a right, nor as something to be offered to individual women, but rather as a means to better accomplish the job of raising children properly, an approach that still echoes in the contemporary national policy of support for "responsible parenthood." The very term *familia bien constituída* is still liberally used as praise for married couples with well-cared-for children, including the family of Peru's president, Ollanta Humala.[6]

## The Rise of a Public Intellectual

Irene Silva Linares was born in Cajamarca in 1902, the first of thirteen siblings. Her Catholic, middle-class upbringing, complete with piano lessons, culminated with her marriage to Fausto Santolalla Bernal, an engineer twelve years her senior, when she was twenty years old.[7] From the moment of marriage, young Irene was expected to competently manage her new family's home, first in Chiclayo, on Peru's northern coast, and finally in the capital city of Lima. Her own frustrations with her new role likely contributed to her later interests. "My mom," eldest daughter, Irene, commented, "married without even knowing how to boil water. She had a bad time of it at first. She suffered from not knowing how to be a wife and a housewife. The whole idea about preparing people for marriage came out of that."[8]

Though mainly devoted to her homemaker duties and her four children, Mrs. Irene Silva de Santolalla enjoyed publishing her writing locally, using the pseudonym "Renova." Her earliest works, unfortunately, have not survived, which makes her rise to prominence seem rather abrupt. In 1938, the popular Argentinian child psychology magazine *¡Hijo Mío . . . !* requested contributions by parents on their experiences disciplining their children. As Mrs. Santolalla later claimed, "the idea of helping youth regarding marriage and family life already fluttered within me," and she submitted an article entitled "Correcting Adult Behaviors to Educate Children."[9] The editors of *¡Hijo Mío . . . !* published the article and, impressed with the quality of the writing, asked her to become a regular contributor and encouraged her to sign her articles with her own name rather than with a pseudonym.[10] Santolalla not only took this advice but also began to pitch her articles to similar magazines, including *Margarita*, in Chile, and *Personalidad y Cultura Mental*, in Cuba.

In the 1930s, Peruvian women were at the center of a national debate regarding the right to vote. Following the collapse of the regime of Augusto B. Leguía in 1930, a congressional assembly gathered to draft a new constitution and call for general elections. A committee of nine recommended not granting women the right to vote in national elections. It had been a narrow defeat, with four congressmen submitting a minority report stating that "women today partake of diverse occupations. This large presence makes it urgent for them to assume political responsibilities." The dissenters' opinion was that the right to vote ought to be granted to female professionals, university students, factory workers, writers, and industrial, commercial, and public administration employees, as long as they were at least twenty-one years old and literate.[11] Though liberal for the 1930s, this initiative excluded the rural female electorate in a country that was still predominantly rural. Approximately 66 percent of Peru's 5.65 million inhabitants lived in rural areas in 1930.[12]

Congressional dissenters had an ally in Magda Portal, the most influential woman within APRA, the political party with the greatest popular following at the time. Like the congressmen, Portal was wary of "society girls" whose reliance on the status quo and Catholic clerics might make them unwilling to support reformist causes.[13] She believed in the value of studying and working outside the home as means to make women aware of the grave injustices committed against the poor and indigenous in the country. Ultimately, in 1933 the congressional assembly granted the right to vote in municipal, but not national, elections to literate women age twenty-one and older and to literate women over eighteen who were already married or lived in stable heterosexual unions.[14]

Neither worker nor scholar, deeply Catholic, and dependent on her husband's income, the comfortably middle-class Irene Silva de Santolalla may have benefited from the change, but she did not participate in the debate leading up to it. In fact, the publication of her articles arose in her a tremendous fervor to defend the role of women not as voters, or as workers, but as pillars of home life. In 1940 she published her first book of advice on childrearing, *For Our Children's Happiness*, a compilation of her columns in *¡Hijo Mío . . . !*[15] That year, the Bulletin of the Chilean Ministry of Health, Prevention, and Social Welfare reprinted one of Santolalla's articles. In addition, Ernesto Goldschmidt, president of the Uruguayan Association for the Education of Mothers, invited Mrs. Santolalla to join their efforts to internationalize the "Crusade to Educate Future Mothers," an annual week-long series of educational events Goldschmidt had sponsored since 1934.[16] Santolalla's star was on the rise.

Santolalla's Peruvian branch of this pan–Latin American crusade consisted mainly of her purchasing airtime in radio stations to deliver speeches.

Male professionals abroad (physicians, lawyers, teachers, and journalists) who, like her, were distraught at women's presumed flight from domesticity orchestrated by political radicals and female suffragists, began to correspond with Santolalla, impressed with her resourcefulness and energy. In 1943, she published her second book of advice to parents, *Towards a Better World*, based on her radio addresses. In it, Santolalla questioned the "senseless fashion" of working outside the home and claimed that training women to become better mothers and valuing such labor was the best way to honor them and raise new generations.[17]

This opinion had been common in upper-crust circles (and those who emulated them) since private secondary education became available to women in the second half of the nineteenth century, with a warning of impending decadence for the nations whose women refused to fulfill their "natural" domestic duties.[18] Teresa Gonzalez de Fanning, who opened an elite school for girls following Peru's defeat in the War of the Pacific (1879–83) against Chile, for example, argued that "as long as there are mothers who do not understand the magnitude of their mission, we will not have citizens capable of lifting the fatherland from its debased present state."[19] As Fanning had done decades before, Santolalla too reflected on the mission of properly trained mothers given the context of war, World War II this time: "Europe has spent its money and ingenuity preparing armies to kill, destroy, and inflict pain," Santolalla wrote, "we must prepare armies of Christian mothers capable of changing this through education."[20]

The trope of the decadence of the world and the need for its redemption was certainly inspired by Catholicism, but not all of Santolalla's ideas were. She opposed, for example, the demands for governmental support for child and maternal welfare institutions advanced by the Pan American Child Congresses and supported by charitable Catholic orders: "A self-respecting nation teaches people to help themselves, to assume their responsibilities, and fulfill their duties. . . . Protecting children consists not of healing sick proletarian kids, feeding the hungry, and clothing the naked, but of preparing mothers to look after the development of their children."[21]

Complementing Santolalla's repudiation of charity and her liberal emphasis on personal responsibility was her appreciation for eugenics, particularly the puericultural tradition that idealized the reproductive potential of men and women as the means to build a strong nation. During the 1940s Santolalla was active in the eugenics movement, as vice president of the Liga Nacional de Higiene y Profilaxis Social (National League for Hygiene and Social Prophylaxis), which encouraged, among other things, the raising of children within "well-constituted families," defined as a heterosexual marriage with a male breadwinner and a female homemaker, disease free both.[22] Indeed, in Santolalla's eugenic vision, a crucial aspect of the preparation of potential mothers was an understanding of how undesirable traits and diseases could be passed on to future generations. Hence, Santolalla argued, a young woman's first important duty was to choose a marriage partner well: someone with whom she could get along and who was free of diseases such as tuberculosis and syphilis as well as of deleterious habits such as excessive alcohol consumption. Not surprisingly, Santolalla favored the enforcement of prenuptial medical certificates, since the choice of a marriage partner was "the key to responsible parenthood" and a prerequisite for the establishment of "an environment in which [children] can be perfected in all respects."[23]

In the 1940s, the Bolivian Eugenics Society and the Argentinian Eugenics Society named Santolalla an honorary member, and she began a mutually flattering correspondence with Paul Popenoe, founder of the American Institute of Family Relations and human sterilization advocate turned marriage counselor.[24] Yet, Santolalla's adamant position that women needed only better instruction, and not necessarily an improvement in the material conditions of their lives, to raise their children properly jarred even fellow eugenicists such as Elvira García y García, who urged Santolalla to pay greater attention to initiatives to build affordable and sanitary housing for workers' families, for example, lest "all good advice becomes meaningless."[25] Even more surprising than Santolalla's unrealistic prescriptions was her seeming lack of awareness of fundamental facts about Peruvian families at the time. Female income earners had been cornerstones of domestic economies at least since the seventeenth century.[26] Moreover, as the 1940 census indicated, 41 percent of all children in Peru had been born to parents who were not married. In *departamentos* such as Loreto and Madre de Dios, the proportion rose to 68 and 75 percent, respectively.[27] Santolalla's worldview did not match the lived realities of most Peruvian families.

Between 1946 and 1948 Santolalla taught at the Instituto Femenino de Estudios Superiores, a non-degree-granting unit directed by fellow Catholic Action member and future colleague in Congress Mrs. Matilde Pérez Palacio, located within the rapidly expanding Pontifical Catholic University of Peru.[28] It was as a teacher that Santolalla began to develop the idea of formalizing the field of family education. She publicized her proposal at the First International Congress of Mothers, which met in Buenos Aires in 1948, on the heels of the Eighth Pan American Child Congress, held in Caracas, which Santolalla pointedly snubbed.[29] "Women," she told a Chilean interviewer on her way back from Argentina, "must receive stronger educational foundations than men. [However], such foundations must always be geared toward motherhood." Her words "provoked gestures of astonishment and perplexity" among members of the Chilean Federation of Women's Institutions, who had chosen that week to mobilize in favor of granting women the vote.[30]

Santolalla's next book came out in 1948, shortly after her return from the Congress of Mothers. *The Great Problem!* presented Santolalla's vision for women's postsecondary education, based on a series of courses on nutrition and first aid, puericulture, home decor and administration, toy manufacturing, and the establishment of close links between home and school. Importantly, this curriculum did not preclude working outside the home, or the right to vote. However, Santolalla deemed these activities peripheral to a woman's life, and legitimate only when a woman's male relatives could not provide for her materially. Social institutions such as divorce laws, child welfare societies, prisons, insane asylums, and daycare centers were, to Santolalla, mere palliatives that could not address the deep harm caused to children by a woman's poor choice of a husband who suffered from defective hereditary traits, or one with whom a harmonious home life was impossible.[31]

By the late 1940s, however, the eugenics discourse was becoming increasingly unpopular throughout the Western world, and the once-prestigious Peruvian Liga de Higiene y Profilaxia Social was in decline.[32] On the defensive following the widespread condemnation of Nazi atrocities, Santolalla railed against "the negative eugenics" that wished to "make one race prevail above all others through sterilizations, abortions, artificial insemination, and the promotion of birth control," and upheld a "positive [eugenics]" that sought "the improvement of all races without distinction" and was "the best ally" of Catholic morals as it struggled to strengthen mankind. "Christ was the first eugenicist," she wrote, as his teachings "had no purpose other than to purify man's body and soul." The coupling of Catholicism and this form of eugenics was not only a rhetorical coup. It was a succinct manifesto that Santolalla tried to implement when she became a public officer, one that emphasized a couple's responsibility to raise healthy and dutiful children in the Catholic faith, and the leading role that women had in the enterprise to renew humanity's body and soul.[33]

## The First Female Senator

Energized by the attention she received at home and abroad, Santolalla finally presented her idea for a school course in family education training to the Ministry of Education in 1950, but her effort did not prosper despite the support of Cardinal Juan Gualberto Guevara.[34] This failure is significant. General Manuel Odría had deposed democratically elected president José Bustamante y Rivero in 1948, ostensibly because of the latter's willingness to strengthen social reforms and his increasing closeness to the APRA party. The Catholic Church was an important backer of Odría's, yet Odría declined to support the family education initiative advanced by his ally until after he relinquished power and reinvented himself as a candidate in the 1956 presidential elections, as head of the aptly named Unión Nacional Odriísta (National Odría Party, UNO). Women figured prominently in Odría's political calculations. Shortly after announcing the 1956 elections, Odría submitted a bill to the Congress he controlled, a bill that had received public endorsements from female lawyers, women in the slaughterhouse trade union of Lima, and the Legión Feminista Pro-Cultura, a women's rights organization.[35] The bill became Law 12391, promulgated in September 1955, and it extended the reforms initiated in 1933, granting the right to vote in national elections to literate women age twenty-one and older and to women over eighteen who were already married. This development put Odría on Santolalla's path, to their mutual benefit.

Between her failed attempt to sway the Ministry of Education and the passing of Law 12391, Santolalla looked for alternative ways to bring her family education curriculum to life, and finally committed to establishing her own postsecondary school to train family educators, the Instituto de Orientación Matrimonial y Familiar (Institute for Marriage and Family Education), founded in 1952 in the up-and-coming Lima district of Miraflores. As with most new ventures, the beginning was difficult. The institute had at first only seven students, and its first twelve employees were, like Santolalla herself, "Lima society ladies" without formal training. It was "an emergency measure, while specialized teachers were being trained."[36] Things changed dramatically, however, once Odría set in motion his plans to grant women the vote. "Odría did not know my mother," acknowledged Santolalla's daughter, "but he sent for her and asked her to popularize voting among women."[37]

Santolalla's closeness to Odría gave her new influence. Between 1954 and 1955 she received invitations to address female high school students at elite private high schools in Lima such as Villa María, San José de Cluny, Santa Ursula, and Rosa de América, as well as the nurse trainees at the Archbishop Loayza Hospital. In 1955 she acquired her own show, *La Hora de la Familia* (*The Family Hour*) on Radio Nacional.[38] By the end of the year, the number of students at her school had grown to seventy.[39] Topping it all off, Odría offered Santolalla the chance to become a candidate to the Senate for her native Cajamarca. Just a few months later, in 1956, the Union of American Women (UAW) awarded Santolalla the Woman of the Americas prize because of her pioneering work in the field of family education. The UAW prize had honored a motley group of women since the mid-1940s, including Chilean poet Gabriela Mistral (1946), U.S. suffragist Carrie Chapman Catt (1947), Dominican diplomat Minerva Bernardino (1948), and former U.S. First Lady Eleanor Roosevelt (1949).[40]

Congratulations were arriving still from different quarters when Santolalla learned that she had been elected to Congress, the sole female senator, along with eight other women, the first to be elected to the Chamber of Deputies (see figure 2).[41] In her new role, Santolalla successfully supported legislation to censor children's books, establish a training center for industrial workers, legalize shantytowns in Lima's periphery, and regulate polluting industries. She did not succeed in creating a training center for domestic workers, installing gardening courses in public schools, or establishing the Universidad Femenina del Norte in Cajamarca.[42] A member of the conservative UNO bloc, Santolalla spoke out against "Communist atheism" at the Third Congress against Soviet Intervention in Latin America, held in Lima in 1957, and applauded President Manuel Prado's breaking off diplomatic relations with Cuba in December 1960, following Fidel Castro's overthrow of Fulgencio Batista.[43] Santolalla's most cherished project, however, remained the institutionalization of family education. To that end, she successfully pushed legislation in 1957 to create a new course for all public elementary and high schools to train girls "to understand and fulfill their roles as wives, mothers, housewives, and citizens."[44] The course was made possible by eliminating portions of the existing curriculum, especially in the fields of mathematics and science. After all, in Santolalla's opinion, it was a mistake to "encourage women to dedicate themselves to occupations besides mothering."[45]

Congress approved of the initiative, though it was to be only the first part of a more ambitious agenda. When Santolalla informed historian Jorge Basadre, then minister of education, of her intention to extend the course to male public schools, Basadre told her that the resources for such an expansion were not available.[46] Although the ministry was unresponsive, Santolalla managed to enroll fourteen young men from the National Engineering University at her school. Their training, however, never started. For this she blamed satirical journalist Luis Felipe Angell, better known as Sofocleto, and his persistent mockery of the idea that men too needed to prepare for

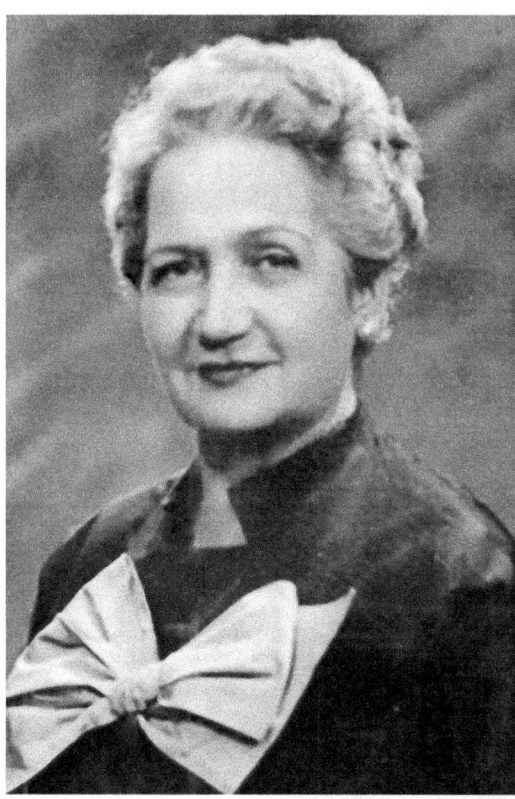

Figure 2. Senator Irene Silva de Santolalla in 1956. Photograph from the website of the Congress of the Republic of Peru (http://www.congreso .gob.pe/_ingles/historia.htm), accessed July 16, 2010.

marriage.[47] Although it failed to involve young men, family education became an established school subject for Peruvian girls. Legislators in Argentina, Brazil, Colombia, Uruguay, Venezuela, Mexico, and Costa Rica modeled similar bills after Santolalla's, cementing her reputation as "the pioneer in family education in Latin America."[48]

Aware that state support alone would not fulfill her vision, Santolalla sought to further cultivate her private institute. In 1959, thanks to Santolalla's diligence, the Ministry of Education officially authorized it to train family educators, belatedly, it turns out, as Santolalla had been doing this informally since 1952. The postsecondary course of study comprised four years of preparation in topics including psychology, sex education, relations between the family and the nation, and interior decoration. Between 1964 and 1968, Santolalla opened new schools in Trujillo, Chiclayo, Piura, and Cajamarca, due to increased demand that spilled beyond Peru's borders and into Bolivia and Brazil.[49] By 1971, there were 500 family educators in Peru. They later organized as the Peruvian Association of Family Education

Professionals; one of them, Susana Villarán, became mayor of Lima in 2010, running as the candidate of a leftist coalition.[50] That Santolalla's crusade to keep women in the home resulted in the creation of a women's professional advocacy group and helped train a left-of-center mayor are ironies fitting the career of a woman who became a senator to prevent other women from embracing public life.

## Challenge and Response

If Santolalla's defense of women's domesticity was strong, it was precisely because the forces against that position were robust. Laws awarding women paid pregnancy leaves date from 1918. Of course, those provisions protected the traditional role of motherhood, not women in general. Moreover, the law excluded female agricultural workers and was poorly enforced to boot. However, it acknowledged that women already constituted an important sector of the industrial workforce.[51] Worker mobilization experienced a high point in the late 1910s, with massive strikes that helped pass laws granting the eight-hour workday. These laws, however, did not address the high cost and scarcity of foodstuffs and housing. In response, the anarchist Comité Pro-Abaratamiento de las Subsistencias formed in April 1919; its women's committee organized the first public protest by women in Lima.[52]

Female intellectuals had carved important parallel spaces for political expression since the 1910s, with Maria Jesús Alvarado's Evolución Femenina, Lucie Rynning's Sociedad Bien del Hogar, Elisa Rodríguez Parra's Legión Feminista Pro Cultura, and Zoila Aurora Cáceres's Feminismo Peruano.[53] Moreover, the Peruvian Communist Party established its Commission on Women in 1930 at the behest of party leader José Carlos Mariátegui. In 1936, Communists Alicia del Prado and Adela Montesinos founded Acción Femenina, an organization that Odría's government declared illegal and persecuted. The Odría years were difficult for feminist and, especially, Communist organizing. Odría's authoritarian presidency was popular among low-income Peruvians in Lima and counted on a disciplined congressional bloc. The APRA party, for its part, had become an antagonist of Communism, despite its popular appeals to social justice.[54]

APRA women, however, also sought political outlets by the mid-1950s, through institutions such as the Escuela Sindical Autónoma, nested within the Confederación de Trabajadores del Perú (Free Union School of the Workers' Federation of Peru). Delia Delgado, one of its organizers, celebrated the fact that "old prejudices that made the home a woman's sole sphere have diluted. . . . New opportunities urgently require women to acquire practical higher education, and leadership and management skills to become more confident and autonomous." Significantly, this movement grew just as Santolalla became a senator, and it echoed her view that women were "managers of their home," in addition to deserving workers, in need of training in child nutrition, first aid, and puericulture.[55] Male critics failed to engage with this dual vindication of women as workers and mothers and instead locked onto women's aspirations to financial and educational autonomy as a dangerous slippery slope: "Women who work, whether or not they have children, no longer fear their husbands might leave them. They know perfectly well they can make a living on their own. This confidence in their own skills and hard work, while beneficial, can slowly undermine their femininity."[56]

Santolalla's brand of family education, which enshrined domestic Catholic femininity, countered these trends in the mid-twentieth century. Yet, family education as a field of study also began to change in the 1960s, challenging Santolalla's organization as the leading provider of this kind of instruction. The Inter-American Institute of Agricultural Sciences of the Organization of American States, for example, organized a seminar for family educators in Lima in 1967. Taking a swipe at Santolalla, the workshop leaders raised the issue of whether existing family education programs took into account social changes sweeping through Latin America, including new parenting roles, rapid urbanization, and agrarian reforms. Santolalla, in attendance along with current students and graduates of her school, registered her displeasure with the way in which "traditional values were being swept aside without justification" by new university-based family education courses, which were offered as part of social science and education programs at the National Agrarian University and the Pontifical Catholic University of Peru.[57]

Changes in the field of family education during the 1960s coincided with national debates about population growth and the use of new contraceptives. Between 1964 and 1968, while Santolalla's Institutes for Marriage and Family Education expanded nationwide, the government of Fernando Belaúnde created the Centro de Estudios de Población y Desarrollo (Center for the Study of Population and Development, CEPD), and the International Planned Parenthood Federation (IPPF) established its first affiliate in Peru, to be discussed in greater detail in chapters 4 and 5. The former aimed to conduct and disseminate demographic research linking phenomena such as population growth and migrations to national development, while the latter was involved in the direct provision of family planning services through an expanding network of clinics and agreements with physicians, universities, and hospitals.

When controversies about contraception intensified in the 1960s, Santolalla responded by extending invitations to foreign experts such as Avabai Wadia, president of the Family Planning Association of India, to address her students. Though better funded than Peru's family planning establishment and more overtly concerned with limiting population growth, experts such as Wadia demonstrated their eagerness to build bridges by insisting that the interest "in the field of marriage and the family [was] not alien to the work being done by the IPPF."[58] Family size, after all, critically affected the quality of care mothers could devote to their children. Santolalla never spoke either for or against voluntary family planning. Yet, at least according to observers such as Wadia, Santolalla's outlook changed with the times and the openness of her own daughter, Irene, to birth control. A decisive shift was underway for upper- and middle-class Peruvian women. "Belonging as they did to a Spanish, aristocratic, Catholic culture, these women nevertheless felt the need to move with the times, and they welcomed hearing of distant lands and new ideas," Wadia reflected.[59]

Santolalla's cautiously liberalizing position only partly matched that of the military regime that took control of Peru's political life in 1968. The so-called Revolutionary Government of the Armed Forces, led by General Juan Velasco Alvarado, paid foremost attention to ending discrimination against women in the workplace, in marriage, and as citizens.[60] In this regard, one of Velasco's first actions was to appoint a National Commission on Peruvian Women to study the main obstacles to women's greater civic involvement. It was during Velasco's rule that the legal distinction between children born within or outside a marriage ended. More ambitious gender-equality proposals, such as the implementation of a national program on sex and health education in schools, failed to draw Velasco's attention.[61] Moreover, in late 1973 Velasco led an offensive against the IPPF in Peru, leading to the organization's ending direct provision of contraceptive services through clinics.

Velasco's reticence and lack of imagination concerning sex education and family planning disappointed the energized nucleus of feminist intellectuals that came of age in the late 1960s, a group of university-educated urban middle-class women who identified with a pan–Latin American Left and who played an important role in the new family education and social science curricula taught at universities.[62] Their reception of Velasco's National Commission on Peruvian Women was cool, as the commission attempted to bring under its umbrella all women's organizations, including those associated with

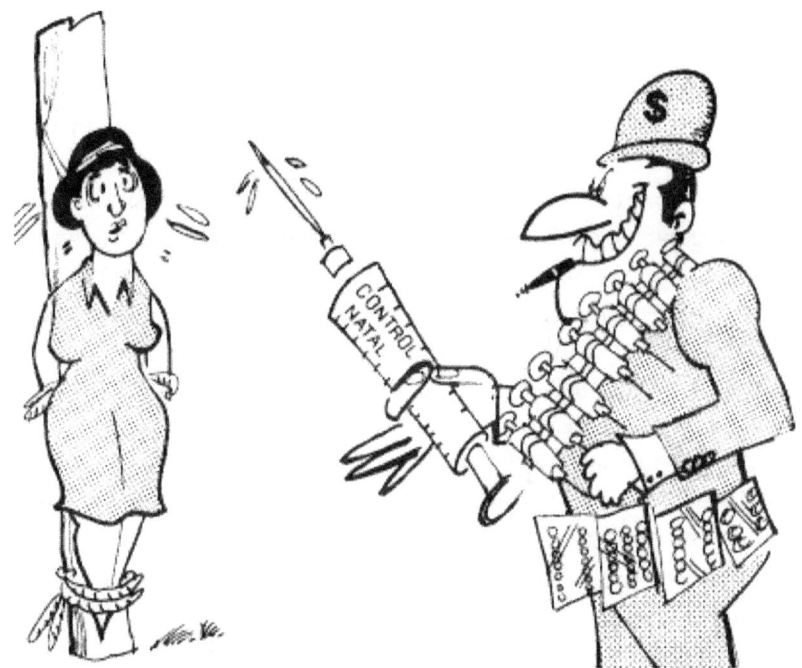

Figure 3. Unequal match between woman and contraceptive-toting capitalist, through a 1970s Latin American feminist lens. From Centro de Documentación de la Historia de la Mujer, Lima, "La Educación Popular con Mujeres en América Latina" (1981): 10.

conservative women such as Irene Silva de Santolalla.[63] By the early 1970s, this group of feminist intellectuals had grown and created associations such as Acción para la Liberación de la Mujer Peruana (ALIMUPER), Movimiento de Promoción de la Mujer, and the Taller de Trabajo Flora Tristán, organizing their first street protests.[64]

Early on, these organizations defended positions Velasco did not embrace, including the legalization of abortion, women's need for greater education in sexual matters, and their autonomy to make reproductive decisions. Yet none of these issues could be addressed, as sociologist Violeta Sara-Lafosse indicated, until women began to understand and demand their rights as citizens, something women were less likely to do if motherhood remained their only aspiration.[65] Some activists took a rather confrontational approach, accusing husbands, the government, the Catholic Church, physicians, and pharmaceutical companies of preventing women from exercising their rights and controlling their own fertility (see figure 3).[66] This new group of female leaders also acquired a more self-conscious identity as feminists, particularly after abandoning left-wing parties when these parties demonstrated the same low level of solidarity with women's causes that General Velasco had shown.

This trenchant critique did not spare the Santolallan defense of women's "natural" domesticity, calling it a "hypocritical idealization" and "one of the most skillfully constructed weapons to make women conform to the maternal role."[67] Admittedly, according to some of these feminists, women's demands for greater equality in the home and beyond would "lead to the failure of many marriages." For women, it was a sacrifice worth making, however, as facing and overcoming these conflicts could open up "new opportunities for personal and societal fulfillment."[68]

Santolalla's prominence made her an easy target for feminist critics who longed for women's greater autonomy from patriarchal power. Yet, her definition of women's labor as encompassing motherhood, caring for children, and the strengthening of communal bonds was shared by women on the Peruvian Left, workers and peasants who did not self-identify as feminists. Despite setbacks, organizing by Communist women persisted beyond the 1950s. The Peruvian Communist Party, for example, created the Unión de Mujeres Peruanas in 1958, which changed its name to the Unión Popular de Mujeres Peruanas (UPMP) in 1970. Unlike the disillusioned feminists, the UPMP tried to carve a space for itself within Velasco's military government's priorities, namely, the agrarian and educational reforms. The 1972 educational reform, for example, stressed the importance of raising a "new man, free within a just society."[69] In response, Grimaldina Vera, one of the UPMP's officers, played up the important role of peasant women not only as leaders in rural areas but also as "forgers of new men through their children."[70] Attuned to Velasco's personal views, the UPMP also decried the expansion of birth control services as an imperialist ploy to consolidate the economic interests of the United States in Peru, and aligned the importance of childrearing to the internationalist goal of achieving world peace. As the UPMP's Zoila Gutierrez wrote in her poem commemorating International Women's Day in 1971,

> yes to procreation, but not to sow
> destruction,
> we must avert wars.[71]

Interestingly, even as these activists emphasized the value of motherhood, they, like the self-described feminists, demanded greater equality with men and even downplayed their duty to act as the self-effacing, pious, and faithful bedrocks of harmonious married couples, contrary to what Santolalla prescribed. Concepción Quispe, leader of the Confederación Campesina del Perú (Peasant Federation of Peru), thus explained her relation with her male "compañero" (partner): "We didn't marry saying 'I love you, you love me, our love will last 'til death.' I married to acquire the responsibility for a house, a home, and children."[72]

It is clear, however, that Santolalla's rhetoric about the importance of women as children's caregivers was shared more widely than 1970s feminists cared to acknowledge. Santolalla was also a more pragmatic educator than her feminist antagonists made her out to be, helping train a cadre of specialists who eagerly joined the ranks of providers of birth control services not only in Peru but also in Brazil.[73] These specialists made their most distinctive mark as family educators who persuaded women that the use of birth control was a key responsibility for women in well-constituted families.

## Family Education in the Clinic

The first birth control clinics established in Latin America in the 1960s portrayed themselves in public as fundamentally concerned with protecting families from poverty and illness, hence names such as the Puerto Rican Association for Family Welfare (Asociación Puertorriqueña Pro-Bienestar de la Familia), the Mexican Association for Family Welfare (Asociación Mexicana Pro-Bienestar de la Familia), Colombia's Profamilia, the Chilean Association for Family Protection (Asociación Chilena para la Protección Familiar), and the Civil Association for Family Welfare of Brazil (Sociedade Civil de Bem-Estar Familiar no Brasil, BEMFAM). The IPPF in Peru, established in 1967, adopted the name of Asociación Peruana de Protección Familiar (Peruvian Association of Family Protection, APPF). Similarly, Peru's Instituto Marcelino was named to honor the memory of a boy who passed away allegedly because his parents lacked the knowledge and resources to care for him.[74] The concern with the quality of the fabric of family life did not stop with organizational nomenclatures but extended to the turning of family educators into members of the team of experts who delivered family planning services.

In the Peruvian context, it was the APPF that developed the most sophisticated approach to harnessing the talents of family educators for the birth control enterprise. Much of the credit for this belongs to Dr. Carmen Delgado de Thays, the APPF's director of education. An anthropologist by training, Delgado was charged with the design of strategies to deliver information about sexuality and contraception to women and men and with establishing rapport with community, political, and business leaders to further the popularity of family planning. Her first interventions took place with groups of women, whom Delgado prompted to open up about their experiences having children, raising them, and living with their male partners. Although Delgado focused on women, she pointedly avoided portraying family planning as a strictly individual issue. As she put it, "it was always a family issue. The mother was not the only one who mattered. After all, where would she be without a husband who fulfills his obligations?"[75]

These early experiences shaped the role of the family educator within the clinic as an expert who reinforced the message that contraception was necessary to carry out the important work of caring for a woman's children. Elsa Lescano, for example, a family educator at Instituto Marcelino, routinely chastised single women who approached the clinic to obtain contraceptives to avoid getting pregnant. "I would tell them 'this is a *family* planning office. It is not a place where you will find *that* kind of freedom.'"[76] The respect for the maternal role and the labor it demanded extended from the interview protocol, to the arrangement of the environment of the clinic, down to the furniture and plants, to make the clinic appear homey, welcoming, and clean, pleasing to both clients and visiting journalists.[77]

Family educators greeted new clients, noted their social and sexual histories, and estimated their income level. They also led group educational sessions on the implications of population growth and the kinds of birth control methods available, followed by individual interviews with women, "trying, obviously, to win them over," as one put it.[78] Group meetings to discuss sex and contraception proved very popular. In 1969, family educators reached 88 people in this manner at the various APPF clinics, 6,170 in 1970, 15,653 in 1971, and 18,335 people in 1972. During the same period, family educators' visits to potential clients' homes grew from 125 in 1969 to 1,285 in 1972.[79] In addition, family educators repeated physicians' instructions to clients and conducted outreach activities to obtain the support of critical actors in the communities they served, men in particular.[80]

Family educators stressed that women's understanding of their sexuality and the promotion of contraception would ultimately help women provide better care for their existing children to a greater extent than did the midwives and physicians also employed by birth control clinics. The latter two kinds of professionals were certainly aware of the challenges involved in the popularization of birth control, and they often participated in group presentations and film showings. The main role of physicians and midwives in the birth control establishment, however, was the direct provision of medical services, and they tended to have more liberal attitudes toward the distribution of contraceptives than family educators did.[81] Some physicians, male ones in particular, even sought to influence family educators by introducing them to ailing patients who induced their own miscarriages under dangerous circumstances, and even by bullying them into admitting clients who sought birth control simply to have occasional sex without the fear of pregnancy.[82] Physicians' attempts to use their professional status and gender identity as means to make female family educators comply with their desires occasionally backfired. Elsa Lescano, for example, quit after being harassed by the clinic director over her unwillingness to admit single women as clients. More broadly, though, these attempts illustrate the subordinate position that family educators, even very senior ones, occupied within family planning clinics. Given their equally entrenched views, some family educators opted for flight before compromise.

If medical personnel often found family educators to be recalcitrant underlings not sufficiently attuned to the health consequences of excessive childbearing, 1970s Peruvian feminists avoided engaging with their maternalist rhetoric altogether. There are no empirical studies about the work of family educators, nor accounts of Irene Silva de Santolalla's life in the volumes produced by established feminist organizations such as the Movimiento Manuela Ramos, Centro de la Mujer Peruana Flora Tristán, or Promsex. This coolness is understandable, for, despite her accomplishments and popularity, Senator Santolalla used her position to insist on the primacy of women's domesticity and to set back young girls by curtailing their mathematics and science instruction. Peruvian feminists abhorred those messages. Even today, Santolalla's career evokes neither pride nor admiration among feminists, but silence; a silence made all the more awkward because, throughout her career, Santolalla always defined herself as a staunch defender of women. It is important to conduct a critical reappraisal of this well-behaved woman's work and ideas, given her large imprint on Latin American history. Doing so enriches our understanding of feminism as a dynamic intellectual tradition, capable of encompassing seemingly incommensurable ideologies that heighten our awareness of gender differences and the social consequences of those differences.[83]

From the standpoint of medical history, it is vital to acknowledge the importance of the maternalist discourse that existed alongside the medicalizing one in family planning clinics from their inception. Family educators partook of a tradition reaching back to the Colonial period that described "well-constituted families" as the result of parental work, with distinct and complementary male and female contributions, with women specializing in child care, nurturance, and (more recently) the regulation of fertility and men financially supporting their families and representing them publicly.[84] The birth control organizations that emerged in mid-twentieth-century Latin America made strategic use of the status quo by equating birth control with the protection of families and, in Peru at least, by hiring family educators and designing their community outreach activities as family oriented and not individual interventions. In so doing, the family planning establishment acquired committed and energetic members for their staff, as well as a greater degree of social legitimacy.

At the same time, the pairing of an assertive medical arm that favored a wide distribution of contraceptives to individuals with the more conservative and family-oriented educators within the clinics underscores the extent to which heterogeneous ideologies and professional standards made up the Peruvian family planning establishment during the 1960s and 1970s, a topic to which I will return in chapter 4. When Velasco's government soured on the large-scale provision of family planning services, to be discussed in chapter 5, it did not renege on its commitment to sex education.[85] However, the educators who partook of the debates leading up to the Education Reform Law of 1972 knew that discussing sex in schools would be controversial. Such topics, they argued, should be addressed by parents and, when addressed in schools, must be couched within broader discussions of family life education, maternal and child care, hygiene, nutrition, interpersonal relations, and national development.[86] This position is indicative of the continuous vitality of the arguments Santolalla defended. A similar phenomenon, the pedagogization of sexuality to broach the subject of birth control, may have occurred in other countries. As Ford Foundation consultants Cecilia Cardinal and Bruce Carlson coyly wrote in 1974, "sex education is to Latin America what population education is to the United States."[87] Unfortunately, at least in Peru, sex education curriculum development in the 1970s wound up not in the hands of personnel specialized in facilitating conversations about human reproduction, as family educators were, but in those of policymakers who sidestepped themes such as coitus, pleasure, and physiology in favor of others, such as the link between population and development, which, while necessary, still did not offer young Peruvians all they needed to understand their sexuality.[88]

Yet we know that there was more to women's and men's lives than acting as potential and actual caregivers to children. Throughout this period,

Peruvian women and men met for fun, economic convenience, and paid sex in bars and on the street, and they formed domestic alliances with each other without the mediation of health certificates and without interest in procreating, much less in the work of parenting.[89] New problems arose for these men and women when an unwanted pregnancy occurred, as we shall see in the next chapter.

## CHAPTER THREE

# Abortion and Accusation

*Experts and Lay People between Crime and Custom*

An abortion? Not just one, but several. This is one of the greatest problems for women, because it turns out abortions are used as contraceptives. And in my days? Of course, and the majority were done in secret.
—Magda Portal (1901–89), Peruvian poet and leader of the APRA party

The Peruvian medical establishment considered pregnancy losses from abortion an important cause of demographic stagnation already in the eighteenth century. By the mid-twentieth century, this establishment also construed unsafe illegal abortions as a cause of maternal mortality that suggested the need to improve the medical care of women and to popularize family planning.[1] Indeed, by the 1960s physicians throughout Latin America and elsewhere warned of the grave risks women ran when attempting to end a pregnancy through an unsafe illegal abortion. Whether women were coerced into getting an abortion or whether they sought one out, the 1960s and 1970s medical literature tended to portray women as victims, either of their own misguided actions or of unskilled or dishonest abortion providers.[2]

Present-day public health practitioners and the popular press have not deviated from the above portrayal.[3] Yet, this "women as victims" message buries much of the social complexity of abortion. My intention in this chapter is to connect abortion to different layers of everyday social life, the very same ones Magda Portal alluded to: the practice's secretiveness, the problems it caused, and the role women played seeking it out.[4] It also pushes us to acknowledge that the meaning of "abortion" is historically contingent on the way in which women seeking to end their pregnancies made sense of what they did, the public's reaction to these actions, and the connections between the world of abortion seekers and providers and that of family planning workers, advocates, and policymakers.

Laws, medical and lay knowledge, cultural norms about proper behavior for men and women, and sexual violence shaped the understanding of abortion throughout the twentieth century as a ghastly, professionally problematic, and widespread crime. Despite the fact that physicians witnessed many instances of pregnancy loss, they rarely instigated criminal accusations of abortion. Even when physicians and state authorities advanced such charges, several obstacles stood in the way of a conviction. Among these obstacles were socially sanctioned violence against women, as well as the precept that "honorable women" who had abortions deserved forgiveness and reformation rather than punishment. Meanwhile, lay Peruvians, unable or unwilling to openly resort to abortions to end unwanted pregnancies, dealt with uninvited scrutiny into their sexual and reproductive lives through a variety of strategies to derail medical and police investigations and protect themselves from embarrassment and criminal charges, including withholding the truth from physicians and accusing others of causing their miscarriages.

## Medico-Legal Knowledge and Debates about Abortion

Throughout the nineteenth and early twentieth centuries, Peru's medical profession deemed pregnancy loss a social, medical, and legal problem with difficult solutions and grave consequences for population growth, the prestige of the profession, and the stability of the family. Abortion first entered the Peruvian legal lexicon through the 1836 penal code, Republican Peru's first, which classified it as a homicide. This was consistent with the Catholic idea that male fetuses over forty days and females over eighty days had souls and were, therefore, persons.[5] According to the 1836 penal code, knowingly assaulting or giving food or drink to a pregnant woman to make her miscarry was considered an abortion. Successful attempts were more severely punished than unsuccessful ones (four to eight years in jail, as opposed to two to four years, respectively). Importantly, a woman's consent lessened the punishment, cutting the jail time in half. The law was relatively lenient to all women. They were deemed criminals only if they succeeded in ending their pregnancies. Even then, the penalty for women was not jail time but rather internment in a moral reform institution for a period between one and two years. Moreover, a woman might not be interned at all if a judge determined that she was "single, or a non-corrupt widow, and honorable," whose only motive had been to cover up her having sex outside of marriage.[6] Physicians, surgeons, pharmacists, and midwives who provided abortions were treated more harshly. The law barred these specialists from practice if found guilty of providing abortions. Still, they were spared any jail time. In other words, the only people the 1836 law punished with incarceration were unlicensed abortion providers and those who physically assaulted women known to be pregnant.

Peru's next penal code, promulgated in 1862, treated abortion in greater detail than the previous one and introduced two important changes.[7] First, women who obtained abortions could end up in jail for up to two years. Still, like the 1836 law, the 1862 law was lenient toward "women of good repute" who sought only to cover up extramarital sex. The second important change was the harsh punishment doled out to physicians, surgeons, midwives, and pharmacists "who abuse[d] their art" by performing abortions. The jail terms for these practitioners could be as long as five years, longer than the punishment for potions manufacturers and assailants who caused miscarriages. The severity of the penalties in 1862 extended to infanticide, which had not been previously regulated.[8] Women found guilty of this crime could receive jail sentences of up to five years. The sentences for people who assisted them varied between four and twelve years' imprisonment.[9]

Medical treatises in the late nineteenth century described miscarriage as a complex, unintended, and, unfortunately, common pathology determined by genetics, the environment, a woman's temperament, and the frequency of her sexual activity. According to this view, physical trauma and disease further debilitated the body's ability to hold on to the fetus and led to its premature expulsion.[10] Tuberculosis and syphilis were among the most dreaded diseases, because of their links to stillbirths, premature births, and the birth of weak and low-weight infants, which in turn affected the quality and quantity of the country's population.[11] Dr. Eduardo Basadre, for example, criticized the use of corsets, which prevented proper oxygenation of the body and could cause miscarriages. He urged women to remember that "lack of air leads to the weakness of important organs" needed to nurture a fetus and give birth, and that children born under these circumstances would be "incapable of fulfilling their duties to the fatherland."[12]

There was little for physicians to do for women hospitalized after miscarrying, beyond curettage and bed rest. Parisian gynecologist Joseph Récamier had introduced the curette to scrape off infected tissues in the uterus around 1850.[13] Peruvian gynecologists embraced Récamier's device and publicized the dilation and curettage procedure enthusiastically in the late nineteenth century, celebrating it as a radical step forward in surgical therapy, thanks to its ease and low cost. Dr. Wenceslao Molina, for example, touted its potential to revitalize the uterus by arguing that the dilation and curettage procedure "fertilized barren fields; thanks to the scraping technique many marriages that had lost all hope for offspring have fulfilled their ambitions."[14] Physicians such as A. A. Beraún went further, indicating that anesthesia was not always necessary for the dilation and curettage to succeed, as the uterus, in his view, was not a very sensitive organ.[15]

These early medical works on pregnancy loss reveal the importance of French puericulture on Peruvian medicine in two ways. First, pregnancy loss was defined as a kind of pathology characterized by a female body's inability to hold on to and nourish a growing fetus. Instead of treating instances of pregnancy loss as deliberate, physicians tended to consider these losses as unintended and adopted leading French puericulturist Adolphe Pinard's penchant for metaphorically linking pregnancy loss to failed agricultural production: stillbirths and the prematurely born became unripened fruits, curettes became fertilizers, and childless women's uteruses became barren fields. Second, physicians believed that physical weakness was a crucial reason for the female body's inability to protect the fetus. Diseases such as syphilis, tuberculosis, and malaria, mental strain, and bodily exertion through excessive toil and sexual activity purportedly caused this weakness. Thus, Peruvian physicians, like their French colleagues, began to promote the avoidance of weakness-inducing factors in women's lives as a matter of national interest, since population growth was at stake. I will return to the notion of physical strain later, since some women invoked it as the reason why they miscarried.

By the 1910s there was a decisive shift in the methodology and tone of medical investigations of abortion, determined by the emergence of the gynecology and obstetrics specialization in the 1890s and the awareness of physicians of the importance of population growth to national politics.[16] Gynecologists began to leverage the topic of pregnancy loss to gain political notoriety. Their new works emphasized the collection of hospital statistics, and no longer just the presentation of clinical cases. Likewise, medical texts from this period strongly condemned abortion providers and infanticides and made policy recommendations to prevent further population losses that included, not surprisingly, more medical oversight of pregnancies.

The new generation of specialists focused also on the city of Lima. In 1917, for example, Dr. Leoncio Chiri became the first to attempt a statistic of pregnancy losses in the country. He based his calculations on the medical histories collected at the Maternidad de Lima, the Santa Ana Hospital, the Bellavista Maternity Hospital in Callao, and the San Juan de Dios Hospital, also in Callao. Chiri found that an average of thirty-four miscarriages occurred every year between 1908 and 1916 in these hospitals. In every single case, the reason that led to the miscarriage was listed as unknown.[17] It is possible that poor record keeping was responsible for researchers' failure to identify the specific causes of the miscarriages they counted. Dr. Humberto Portillo, for example, did not indicate how he determined the difference between stillbirth and infanticide, yet some of his colleagues worried that the two could be confused.[18] The feature that defined a newborn was whether the child had ever breathed air. It was a standard adopted from Napoleonic France, one that likely predated 1811.[19] The standard was based on the notion that, although fetuses grew and developed in the womb, they were still dependent on a woman's body for nourishment, and thus not separate from that body. This changed the moment infants were born and were able to breathe on their own. Although infants were still unable to fend for themselves, the air in their lungs and their ability to expel it through crying was a turning point in their achieving personhood status, medically speaking. The distinction had legal implications as well, according to the 1862 penal code: killing a breathing infant was considered infanticide, a severely punishable crime, whereas the death of a newborn that had not breathed was considered a stillbirth, a tragic accident.[20]

The suspicion that abortion and infanticide often occurred led well-known physicians to suggest legal changes. Dr. Leonidas Avendaño, professor of legal medicine at the Faculty of Medicine of Lima, supported mandatory public registration of all pregnancies and the liberalization of paternity lawsuits.[21] Earlier, Avendaño had made a proposal to the Fifth Latin American Medical Congress of 1913 to mitigate the guilt of "women of good repute" who killed their newborns "at birth or immediately after" so they would not be humiliated when it became publicly known that they had conceived outside the bounds of marriage.[22] Avendaño was not the only one to support leniency for women who committed infanticide. In 1915, led by Lima's *diputado*, Víctor Maúrtua, the Peruvian Congress began work to upgrade the 1862 penal code. Maúrtua himself introduced an infanticide bill that exempted women from responsibility if they acted within the period that immediately followed a birth. Maúrtua suggested that the strain of labor left women temporarily physically and mentally unable to care for an infant and made it more likely for some to commit "unnatural" acts.[23] Maúrtua's proposal was different from Avendaño's in that it did not make a woman's "good repute" a prerequisite to benefit from the law.

Congress's work on a new penal code began in 1915. It continued after the election of Augusto B. Leguía as president in 1919 and concluded in 1924. The new penal code stipulated jail penalties for women who caused their own miscarriages (up to four years), for abortion providers who had the woman's consent (up to four years, and up to six if the woman died as a result of the intervention), for providers who acted without a woman's consent (up to ten years), and for those who caused a woman to miscarry unintentionally through a physical assault (up to two years).[24] In addition, the code adopted a modified version of Víctor Maúrtua's infanticide bill. Women who killed their newborns during birth or "under the influence of the puerperal state" could be jailed for up to three years.[25] Unfortunately, the code did not specify the duration of the "puerperal state," a loophole that could in theory open the door to gross abuses.

An important change introduced in the 1924 penal code was the legalization of therapeutic abortion, which was defined as an abortion carried out by a physician with a woman's consent, "if there is no other way to save the mother's life or avoid a permanent and grave injury."[26] Unfortunately, the Archivo del Congreso did not record the debates of the congressional commission that crafted the 1924 penal code and that led to the legalization of therapeutic abortion. However, this legal change was in keeping with changes in penal law in other Latin American countries. Between 1916 and 1931, for example, Argentina, Uruguay, and Chile legalized therapeutic abortions when a pregnancy endangered a woman's life. Moreover, as previously shown, medical research on the frequency of miscarriages, stillbirths, and infant deaths in the 1910s suffered because of the incompleteness of records showing the cause of death. Physicians were aware of their colleagues' practice of omitting this data when they suspected or, worse, had themselves induced an abortion, as I will show in the next section. It is possible that these researchers thought the legalization of therapeutic abortion would encourage a more complete and honest recording of clinical histories. In addition, as shown above, physicians considered dilation and curettage a safe, inexpensive, and fast procedure. Allowing this to be an alternative for women might bolster physicians' prestige and incomes and would also dissuade women from attempting other, presumably more dangerous, ways to end a pregnancy.

These possibilities notwithstanding, there was little debate in Peruvian medical circles about the need for physician-controlled therapeutic abortion before 1924 or advocacy by physicians to secure the privilege. This makes it difficult to determine how desirable the monopoly of therapeutic abortion was for Peruvian physicians. In fact, some medical doctors did not celebrate the legalization of therapeutic abortion because they feared it could lead to greater popular demand for abortion services. As professor of legal medicine Guillermo Fernández Dávila put it in 1926, "long past are the times when an abortion was the result of the desperation of honest women following a moment of weakness. . . . Today, women of all social classes ask us directly and almost daily for abortions, giving banal and untrue justifications, with the same equanimity and assertiveness with which they demand remedies for common discomforts. Our refusal irritates them; it makes them hold us in contempt and mistrust us. . . . The carefree procreators will always find someone to get rid of the seedling we respected, because these days criminal abortions are a lucrative industry and its practitioners are legion."[27]

It is clear, then, that some physicians worried about two potential consequences of the legalization of therapeutic abortion. One was an increase in the demand for abortions that would overwhelm the capacity of medical professionals to provide these services, and thus encourage the growth of a profitable black market in which the participation of nonphysicians would be inevitable. The other was the strengthening of a carefree attitude regarding procreation, as safe abortions could separate sex from pregnancy and encourage men and women to see each other erotically and not as long-term partners in a Catholic marriage.

Faced with a presumed potential explosion in the demand for abortions, a few professionals thought it important to document and denounce cases of illegal abortion. Daniel Fosalba y Muro analyzed 2,831 clinical histories of women hospitalized after miscarrying at the Arzobispo Loayza Hospital and the Bellavista Maternity Hospital between 1923 and 1928. He found that 3.3 percent of these women had complied with the criteria specified for the performance of a therapeutic abortion by a physician (to save the mother's life or avoid a permanent and grave injury). An additional 13.84 percent miscarried due to complications arising from malaria; 9.56 percent miscarried due to some form of physical trauma; 8.06 percent miscarried due to syphilis; and only 1.16 percent miscarried due to abortions performed illegally. Significantly, Fosalba y Muro classified the causes of most miscarriages as unknown, due to the incompleteness of medical records.[28]

The same incompleteness of medical records beleaguered Fosalba y Muro's colleague Dr. Juan Escudero. His analysis of clinical histories at the Arzobispo Loayza Hospital between 1925 and 1929 identified 1,174 cases of miscarriage. Yet, he was able to find complete records for only 83 patients. Of these, 27 women had spontaneous miscarriages; 9 were cases of therapeutic abortion; 17 women miscarried due to accidents, 24 due to various pathologies, and 6 due to physical trauma. Like Fosalba y Muro, Escudero suspected that the missing records hid a significant number of criminally induced abortions, but he went no further with his suspicions. However, Escudero was sympathetic to the reasons that drove women to seek abortions, including the fear of not being able to work or of being dishonored by an out-of-wedlock pregnancy.[29] In such cases, Escudero noted, women's partners played a role in helping them get abortions. Conversely, pregnancies resulting from the violent acts of partners who cheated on them and consumed drugs and alcohol were "repugnant" to women and also led them to seek abortion services, albeit on their own.[30]

Physicians between the 1930s and the 1950s quietly empathized with the economic and moral arguments that led women to seek abortions. By the early 1960s, some had become bold enough to own up to their collusion with these women. Dr. Carlos Olascoaga, for example, admitted that physicians seldom documented their suspicions regarding induced abortions, much less bothered to alert the police, when women were not forthcoming about the reasons for their hospitalization.[31] This helps explain, to some extent, the dearth of complete clinical histories that troubled researchers such as Fosalba y Muro and Escudero. Further, Escudero's compassion toward women who sought abortion reveals reasons why physicians would not bother making accusations even when they could. Without minimizing the demographic and ethical hazards posed by abortion, some physicians favored greater knowledge and not repression as a long-term solution. As professor of obstetrics Alejandro Busalleu put it in his inaugural 1938 lecture, "there are socially caused problems the future physician will face every day. One above all must be decidedly remedied: criminal abortions. Their frequency threatens our population and undermines our society's concepts of morality. This is a medical, social, moral, and even philosophical problem of such complexity that its solution will elude the mere enforcement of the [Penal] Code. Only understanding the factors that play a role in it will we be able to solve this problem."[32]

The call for greater understanding of the social determinants of abortion led some physicians to chastise Peruvians for their low rates of marriage. Marriage, these physicians believed, encouraged couples to stay together and raise children properly. Failure to marry encouraged men to abandon their homes, making it more likely for women to obtain abortions or become prostitutes and for their children to become criminals.[33] Others believed that a lack of sexual education made it difficult for young women to use their sexuality in a proper manner. For this, the Catholic Church's "deep-rooted inquisitorial prejudices" and its "false and archaic ideas about modesty" deserved part of the blame.[34] Also to blame were women's desires to be the equals of men, which led the former to abandon their homes in search of work and put them at the mercy of sexual predators.[35] Manuel Salcedo, director of the Ministry of Health's Department of Maternal and Child Protection in 1944, blamed both children's work and working women for "deforming the character" of new generations, rendering them more likely to commit crimes.[36] Salcedo's corollary was an exhortation to jump-start the civic education of men and women to understand their "natural" roles within a patriarchal family structure, a proposal that converged with the interests of prominent Peruvian female and Catholic intellectuals, as we saw in the previous chapter.

Of course, not all physicians were as keen to learn why people sought abortions, or to delve into the intricate links between familial anomie and delinquency. Professionals who only sought punishment for seekers and providers of abortion aimed their vitriol at midwives, traditional birth attendants, pharmacists, and some of their own colleagues, accusing them of practicing abortions liberally as a way to make a living.[37] Dr. Leonidas Avendaño, for example, reserved special contempt for the "ignorant women responsible for the horrible scenes seen in dark alleys and tenements, dirty and nauseating dives both, starring a rustic patient, resisting all hygienic practices, and a stupid woman who does not hesitate to sacrifice a life or two for a few cents snatched from the naïve family."[38] Dr. Luis Vargas Prada, director of the General Office of Sanitation, sent a cautionary memorandum to all hospital directors in April 1933, in which he stated that "abortions induced by unqualified personnel and without therapeutic goals are criminal practices that become more common every day, posing grave risks to pregnant women and society as a whole."[39]

Professor of social medicine Carlos Enrique Paz Soldán applauded Vargas Prada's official position. He accused "physicians and midwives without scruples, as well as ignorant curanderas [folk healers] who live and profit immorally, exploiting people's naïveté and disgrace," of being the culprits behind a supposed rising tide of abortion. With quixotic enthusiasm, Paz Soldán began a campaign to drag illegal abortion practitioners out in the open. Since he could not count on his colleagues to provide all the help he needed, he called on health workers in general to feed him tips "every time hospitals admit cases in which you suspect abortive maneuvers without therapeutic aim. We will investigate confidentially and make the appropriate accusation at the Public Defender's Office."[40] There is no evidence that Paz Soldán ever made a single accusation, much less one leading to an arrest or trial, at least in Lima, where he began his campaign in 1933.[41] Paz Soldán, however, was not the last to attempt to flush out illegal abortion providers. President José Luis Bustamante y Rivero established medical oversight committees in Peru's major hospitals in 1946.[42] One of the functions of these committees was to denounce the illegal practice of abortion by physicians. However, there is no evidence that any of these committees ever initiated a criminal abortion accusation either.

Physicians began to weigh in more explicitly on the nation's rates of maternal mortality in the 1940s, a shift in Peruvian medical practice that had two important consequences.[43] First, new research called attention to the fact that puerperal infections acquired in hospitals and health centers caused as many, if not more, maternal deaths than complications related to induced illegal abortions. Dr. Juan Landaburú, for example, found that ten out of the ninety-four parturient women who died at the Maternidad de Lima in 1945 died as a result of puerperal infections and thirteen as a result of abortion-related complications.[44] By 1950, postpartum infections at the same hospital were responsible for twice as many maternal mortalities as were abortion-related complications (twenty-two and eleven, respectively, out of a total of fifty-nine fatalities).[45] Second, the new research showed that abortion-related complications required surgery more often than any other obstetric complication. Landaburú found that 55 percent of all 5,887 surgical interventions on women between 1925 and 1945 at the Maternidad de Lima were dilation and curettage procedures required after a botched abortion.[46] Similarly, according to César Frías, the majority (44 percent) of all 1,470 surgeries at the Maternidad de Lima in 1950 were dilation and curettages following induced illegal abortions.[47]

The demand for dilation and curettage created pressures on hospital surgical services, not only for blood, anesthetics, and antibiotics.[48] The supply of antibiotics became more efficient throughout several Peruvian hospitals and health posts in the early 1950s, thanks to two related developments.[49] First, World War II increased the prices of commodities Peru produced and exported, and President Manuel Prado y Ugarteche's administration allocated some of the income generated to improve the country's medical services.[50] Second, U.S. president Franklin Roosevelt embraced a "Good Neighbor Policy" toward Latin America. As part of this new foreign policy, the United States funded what became known as the Inter-American Cooperative Service for Public Health (Servicio Cooperativo Interamericano de Salud Pública, or SCISP). The SCISP worked on a variety of health projects in Peru, including malaria control, water sanitation, obstetric care, the training of health personnel, and the management of health centers. The SCISP was also involved in setting up supply chains of medications, including antibiotics and sulfa drugs, to some of the poorest regions of rural Peru.[51]

In sum, in the first five decades of the twentieth century, the medical profession participated in national debates about pregnancy loss in a variety of ways. Some physicians continued to treat instances of miscarriage and abortion as causes of demographic stagnation. For others, deliberate pregnancy losses became opportunities to make moral judgments about Peruvians. Sometimes these judgments were somewhat benign, for example when they revealed physicians' sympathy for the plight of sexually scorned women or that of women and men concerned with the employment opportunities a new child would foreclose. Other times, the judgments were harsh, especially when physicians sought to distinguish themselves from the nonphysicians who also provided abortions without the legal protection that the 1924 penal code afforded to those who performed therapeutic abortions. It is important to place these harsh judgments in the context of the professionalization of Latin American medicine in the early twentieth century. Medical professionals attempted to assert their power by attacking potential competitors such as midwives and folk healers, who also provided abortions.

Abortion was a widespread means to avoid having children in Peru in this period, one used by women of different income and ethnic groups. Yet, by the late 1940s, the trend toward preventive medicine, exemplified by Peru's SCISP, helped raise the awareness of health professionals regarding maternal mortality. Abortion remained an important medical, social, and moral topic of discussion, but increasingly it also became part of a new public health discourse that emphasized its contribution to maternal mortality and morbidity rates. An important question concerns the translation of these medicolegal debates into practices of reporting the abundant suspected criminal abortion activities to public health and judicial authorities.

## Why Were Abortions So Rarely Investigated as Crimes?

Despite physicians' rhetoric about the threat abortion posed to the family, the profession, and the nation, their contribution to bringing abortion seekers and providers to justice was minimal between the 1890s and the 1970s. I came to this conclusion after reviewing the criminal records available at the five most populous *departamentos* in Peru, according to the 1940 census: Lima, Puno, Piura, Ayacucho, and La Libertad.[52]

Only 233 cases out of 26,402 dealt with suspicious miscarriages or abortions, and most occurred within the city of Lima between the early 1960s and

Table 1. Abortion Cases among Criminal Cases in Peru's Most Populous
*Departamentos*

| Archive | Years | Abortion cases | Total criminal cases consulted |
|---|---|---|---|
| Lima | 1895–1921, 1961–79 | 181 | 2,926 |
| La Libertad | 1895–1976 | 13 | 8,932 |
| Puno | 1919–75 | 20 | 12,960 |
| Ayacucho | 1920–65 | 17 | 828 |
| Piura | 1919–60 | 2 | 756 |
| | | 233 | 26,402 |

Source: Data compiled by the author.

the late 1970s (179 cases). Of the 233, only 20 began because of a physician's report to the authorities. Sympathy for hospitalized women and concerns for physicians' own careers were important reasons why physicians left out their suspicions about abortion from medical histories and did not report them to the police. In addition, hospitalized women's refusal to confirm physicians' suspicions of induced abortions through a confession made it difficult for physicians to prove these accusations. In fact, some women's accounts of their miscarriages fit medical explanatory schemes well, which also provided some protection from prosecution. A crucial change took place in the early 1970s, with the organization of the Department of Abortions (DA) within the Investigative Police of Peru's Division of Crimes against Life. The DA, with representatives in Lima's major hospitals, radically increased the number of reported cases of abortion in the capital, from an average of two cases every year between 1961 and 1969 to an annual average of sixteen between 1970 and 1979. In fact, of the twenty abortion cases physicians reported to the police between the 1890s and the 1970s, eighteen took place in Lima between 1970 and 1979.

As argued above, sympathy toward women who wished to keep their out-of-wedlock pregnancies secret and those who could not afford another child financially might have prevailed upon physicians' state-sanctioned duty to report a crime. Of course, making criminal accusations also required additional work, which physicians might have been glad to avoid. In addition, self-interest also made physicians reluctant to make accusations when they suspected an abortion had occurred. This was particularly clear when physicians dealt with an upper-class clientele keen on not making their private affairs public.

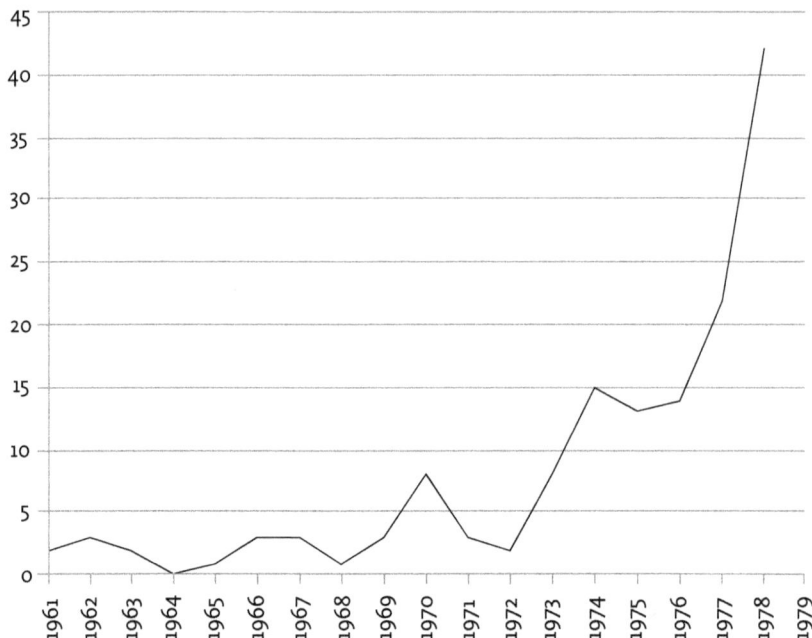

Figure 4. Abortion cases investigated by the police in Lima, 1961–1979.
Data compiled by the author.

Dr. José Montoya, for example, described in 1941 the case of Mrs. "N. N.," a well-off thirty-seven-year-old married woman of Lima who did not have any children, "despite her not taking contraceptive precautions." Her husband had undertaken a seven-month-long trip, and, shortly after his return, a kerosene stove exploded in their home. Shaken, Mrs. N fell and noticed she was bleeding from her genitals. The doctor who admitted her found "symptoms of an induced abortion" when he examined a clot that came out of Mrs. N that resembled ground meat.[53] Mrs. N's husband took this as evidence that she had cheated on him while he was away and demanded a divorce. However, Mrs. N's personal physician, R. Colareta, had a colleague analyze the clot. Upon closer inspection, the diagnosis was amended: the clot was now pronounced a uterine cyst. By then, however, the husband was upset and the wife resentful. This medical mistake had so damaged the marriage that Montoya feared a civil lawsuit against his colleague was imminent, and he used this experience as a cautionary tale for other physicians to diagnose abortions as such only with the utmost care.[54]

Out of concern for their own careers, physicians to the wealthy were careful not to identify their clients by name and went to great lengths to protect them from scandal. This helped ensure the ongoing patronage of these clients. Dr. Ismael Cáceres, for example, discussed the abortion of Mrs. "C. G. de G." in 1891. A white, wealthy married woman of twenty-two from Lima, Mrs. G. had heard that sodium silicate could produce a miscarriage when taken in repeated doses. She engineered her own abortion by having a servant purchase a large amount of the chemical. After instructing her servant to tell the pharmacist that the sodium silicate was to help cure a sudden rheumatic pain on the small toe of her right foot, Mrs. G. took the drug for two days and finally overdosed on it, experiencing pain and bleeding. Dr. Cáceres, her personal physician, was summoned to the scene. He prescribed sulfuric lemonades and a laudanum enema to prevent the miscarriage. Nevertheless, the attempt succeeded.[55] Tellingly, Dr. Cáceres did not include Mrs. G.'s confession in her medical history, nor did he report her to the police. In fact, Cáceres did not even name his wealthy client. However, he named five other women whom he suspected of inducing their own miscarriages: Fidela Reyes, a seamstress; Cecilia Barreto, a washer woman; Escolástica Zárate, a cook; María Elena Enríquez, also a cook; and Rosalía Vázquez, a street peddler. From their occupations (indeed, from the very fact that they worked for a living), we can infer that these women were not as wealthy as Mrs. G., and thus were unable to buy the discretion of a personal physician.

However, even women such as these five could protect themselves from criminal accusations by not revealing much about the circumstances that led to their miscarriages. This is exactly what one of the women Cáceres named did. To the doctor's frustration, all Fidela Reyes admitted was to feeling ill for ten days before going to the hospital. On the eleventh day, she told Cáceres that she had miscarried the night before and that she had felt less pain since then.[56] It was difficult to obtain these confessions. Physicians such as Marcelino Castellares in 1935 remembered obtaining confessions about abortion as small personal triumphs that could help doctors better diagnose future instances of pregnancy loss or write more thorough clinical histories.[57] Significantly, physicians rarely mentioned bringing criminals to the attention of the police as a goal of getting such confessions. Dr. Jesús Untiveros bombastically stated in 1946, "I have had to rectify most of the clinical histories in Wing Nine of the Maternidad [de Lima] after earning the trust of the aborting woman (which is indispensable). I have thus been able to extract declarations about the real cause [of the miscarriage]. But to get such results, one must invest so much patience, be so tenacious, and use so many persuasive means!"[58] Still, just as often, as Dr. Francisco Cabrera generously admitted in 1931, "women fooled us easily during the interview."[59]

Part of the ease with which physicians were fooled had to do with the common belief in the medical profession that "almost all women know effective contraceptives and abortifacients": from potions based on rye and celery to personal hygiene products.[60] Women also used quinine as an abortifacient, though they claimed to use it to relieve themselves of malarial symptoms.[61] P. M., a thirty-year-old woman from Huaraz, for example, with five live births and a previous miscarriage, diagnosed herself with malaria and procured quinine on her own. At the Santa Ana hospital in Lima, Dr. Beraún performed a dilation and curettage on her in 1906, after he found signs of an abortion. He concluded that P. M. had miscarried deliberately but was not able to make P. M. confirm his suspicions.[62] Of course, these tactics did not always work. The pregnant woman who asked Dr. Agustín Gavidia for quinine tablets in his Callao practice in 1904 did not have symptoms of malaria, but, and this is what gave Gavidia pause, she had five children and a previous "suspicious" miscarriage.[63]

The use of plant-derived substances to affect fertility has an even older history than the use of quinine in the Andean region. Polo de Ondegardo, a Spanish chronicler of the conquest period, refers to the use of herbs such as mallunhua to induce sterility. Hermilio Valdizán's early twentieth-century survey identified twenty-eight different plant-based abortifacients and nine other plant-based substances thought to increase the likelihood of conceiving.[64] Santiago Antúnez de Mayolo indicates that traveling naturalists such as the German Alexander von Humboldt and the French Alcide d'Orbigny had noted the use of Andean plants to induce abortion in the nineteenth century. Antúnez de Mayolo also reproduced the list of healing plants that physician Manuel Antonio Osores tested in Chota, in the northern Andes, in 1850. Some of these, like misquichilca and panisara, were used "to empty the uterus."[65] Antúnez de Mayolo added his own compilation of substances used, allegedly from time immemorial, to bring about menstruation. Other scholars have since compiled their own lists of Andean abortifacients.[66]

Social commentary about the presumed extensive local knowledge of emmenagogues in early twentieth-century Peru extended beyond scientific circles. Juan José Calle, a state attorney for Peru's Supreme Court wrote in 1924 of the "many people who, without being medical doctors, are in the business of manufacturing abortifacient medicines and potions, selling them under names that disguise their true purposes, even though they hint as to the effects they will cause."[67] In all likelihood, Calle was not only referring to plant-based potions but also to patent medicines advertised openly by pharmacies. These included Agua del Socorro, which promised to cure "irregularities" in a woman's period and return her to "health, wellness and vigor," and Cardui, "the woman's tonic," which promised to fix period delays.[68]

Despite being discussed fairly often by others, emmenagogue potions were rarely mentioned by women hospitalized after miscarrying, with exceptions such as the wealthy Mrs. G. Instead, when physicians pushed women to explain what brought them to the hospital, women often blamed sudden and traumatic external events, such as falls, abrupt movements, or emotional distress. Gavidia, for example, reported miscarriages due to moving a heavy sewing machine and to falling from a chair.[69] Two of the seven miscarriages Dr. Wenceslao Molina treated with dilation and curettage in 1896 were due to falls, according to the patients.[70] A. E., whom Dr. Beraún treated with a dilation and curettage, miscarried after she "got mad at her family."[71] Escolástica Zárate explained that her miscarriage was due to her having to lift heavy objects as part of her work as a cook. Maria Elena Enríquez claimed that her first pregnancy ended when she fell down a flight of stairs the day before her admittance to the hospital. Rosalía Vázquez said in her interview that she miscarried when she lunged to catch her baby as he was about to fall off a chair. Despite bleeding, she refused to go to the hospital for four more days. Another of her seven pregnancies ended when she watched in shock as her husband was "brutally struck." That time, the fetus was expelled after seventeen days in the hospital. Mrs. Vázquez disposed of it quietly during the night, without any investigation by medical staff.[72]

According to the puericultural tradition that dominated early twentieth-century Peruvian obstetrics, sudden and traumatic external events, pathological, physical, or mental in nature, could weaken the female body, even to the extent of making it lose its hold on a growing fetus. This is probably why some women could blame falls, physical effort, and emotional distress for their miscarriages without physicians second-guessing them. As late as 1946, physicians classified falls, physical effort, long trips, and "strong emotions" as causes of spontaneous miscarriages.[73] The fact that different women throughout twentieth-century Latin America explained their miscarriages in similar ways is important.[74] It points to a form of lay understanding of the body linking sudden and traumatic external events to pregnancy loss, a knowledge that some women could strategically use to end their own pregnancies, even though this put them at risk of physical harm. The convergence between this kind of lay knowledge and puericultural ideas was beneficial for women who did not wish to confess to having an abortion, and for physicians who wanted to avoid the attention a criminal investigation would bring. Women who did not wish to explain the circumstances of their miscarriages in detail made some physicians uneasy. But how could the latter, when faced with the resolute silence of women, prove conclusively that something like a fall was more than a terrible accident?

The desire to protect their careers, the sympathy they felt for some women, and the ease with which they could be tricked or denied information, made physicians unlikely to accuse women of the crime of abortion. This unwillingness prevailed despite the fact that medical doctors often witnessed evidence of abortions and performed life-saving interventions on women following botched attempts. Considering the obstacles to making effective criminal accusations of abortion, it is not surprising that so few of them exist. This only began to change in the 1970s, with the establishment of the Department of Abortions within the police. However, even then the increased reporting of abortion had less to do with a change in physicians' attitudes than with the increased police surveillance of hospitals in Lima.

## Investigating Abortion Accusations

My review of 26,402 criminal records in five of the most populous *departamentos* (in 1940) yielded only 233 cases of abortion. Of these, only eight (one in Ayacucho, one in La Libertad, and six in Lima) resulted in sentences. Following the unlikely event of a criminal accusation, abortion investigations faced different kinds of difficulties that made assigning criminal responsibility problematic and that, at the same time, provide us with insight into the social conditions surrounding abortions.

The professional discretion of medical and legal experts was the first of these difficulties. Experts' power to influence the application of the law could and did lead to cases against presumed criminals being dropped. Dr. Enrique Blondet, for example, alerted the Trujillo police after getting Angélica Fernandes, a fourteen-year-old domestic worker, to confess why she had been hospitalized. Ms. Fernandes told Dr. Blondet that while coming home from her employers' one day in June 1920, she felt pain, miscarried on the side of a road outside Trujillo, and left the fetus there. Acting on Dr. Blondet's tip, the police found the body of Ms. Fernandes's fetus, which led to her being charged with infanticide. However, following an examination of the remains, Dr. Blondet determined that the six-month-old female fetus, despite having taken a breath of air, "was not properly developed and would have died anyway."[75] It was largely based on Dr. Blondet's report that the *fiscal*[76] cleared Ms. Fernandes of any wrongdoing.

A similar case is that of Rosa Huamán, a nineteen-year-old homemaker from Trujillo, who accused birth attendant Rosa Valderrama of hoodwinking her out of some money in 1940. The investigation revealed that Mrs. Huamán had paid Mrs. Valderrama for an abortifacient potion, at which point the latter was accused of practicing medicine illegally. In the end, however, the Trujillo *fiscal* did not pursue charges against Mrs. Valderrama. For the illegal practice of medicine to be punishable, he wrote, the culprit must "habitually devote herself to the art of curing." Yet in this case, the *fiscal* believed that Mrs. Valderrama's activities were "a frequent and socially accepted fact among poor people, who have no resources to seek professional assistance when pregnant or about to give birth." Mrs. Valderrama, the *fiscal* concluded, "does not treat diseases unknown to her, nor does she treat people unknown to her."[77] He therefore dropped all charges against her.

Both these cases highlight the power experts had to influence the application of the law, either by disregarding standards (such as breathing on one's own as a sign of independent life), as Dr. Blondet did, or by downplaying the deleteriousness of illegal activities, as the *fiscal* did in the Huamán case. The Huamán decision, in addition, illustrates an interesting assumption about the role of traditional healers such as birth attendants and *curanderos* in society. According to the *fiscal*, traditional healers steered clear of "diseases unknown" and "people unknown" to them, and their actions were "frequent and socially accepted" among those "who have no resources to seek professional assistance." A different La Libertad *fiscal* had invoked the same logic in 1937 when he desisted from pressing charges against *curandero* Alejandro Cedamanos, who allegedly caused the abortion of a woman he treated for abdominal pain. Cedamanos, in the *fiscal*'s sympathetic opinion, intervened "following a sudden illness and under difficult circumstances, as happens so often in places where professional assistance is nonexistent."[78] Tellingly, Justina Guzmán, Cedamanos's client, never said anything against the *curandero*'s care. Both the Valderrama and Cedamanos acquittals reveal an elitist view that separated "the poor" and their healers from the rest of society. As Pablo Piccato and Julia Rodríguez have shown for Mexico and Argentina, respectively, this normalization of the poor as different from the rest of society, with their own pathologies and criminal tendencies, was directly correlated with the growing influence of scientific positivism in state institutions, a process also underway in Peru in the early twentieth century.[79] Ironically, such marginalization and contempt for the poor also protected abortion providers such as Mrs. Valderrama and Mr. Cedamanos.

In the rare instances in which the state managed to make its case against abortionists and abortion seekers, judges had the last word during the sentencing phase. Of the eight sentences handed down between the 1900s and the 1970s in the five locales studied, four of them were suspended, all in Lima in the 1970s. Judges took into account the fact that all the abortion seekers were women who survived life-threatening infections, were poor, had children, and had never before attempted to have an abortion.[80] Some of the abortion providers also produced witnesses to their "good behavior and honorability."[81] Such vouching swayed judges into agreeing that "the personal qualities of the accused and their lack of criminal records indicate that it is unlikely they will commit crimes again."[82] Still, the discretion of judges was such that predicting a sentence could be difficult. Antonio Mendoza, for example, inserted a plastic tube in Eva Salazar's uterus in 1977, which caused an appalling infection that resulted, ultimately, in the surgical removal of Ms. Salazar's uterus, both fallopian tubes, and ovaries. Mr. Mendoza had admitted performing a similar abortion in 1962, had committed a sexual assault in 1974, and was being sued by his wife in Cuzco for alimony payments.[83] Who could have foreseen that such a man's sentence would be suspended? All Mendoza, and the other guilty parties in the suspended sentence cases, had to do was pay a fine between 2,000 and 5,000 Soles, agree to never commit another crime, and not change their domiciles for a few years without notifying the judiciary. Like physicians and *fiscales*, judges too played an important role in adjudicating criminal responsibility.

A second kind of obstacle to the assigning of criminal responsibility in abortion cases concerns the difficulties investigators had gathering evidence. The accusations against Eudosia Mendoza in the village of San Damián, in Lima, and Felícita Cisneros in the town of Lauricocha, Ayacucho, for example, were substantially weakened because the remains of their allegedly aborted fetuses were too decayed to be examined.[84] Compounding the lack of evidence was the small number of investigators. Justice of the peace Gabriel Lira, who accused Mendoza in 1901, had been forced to deputize two local farmers and a silversmith to assist him because he did not have a staff to conduct the investigation. Another resource-strapped *fiscal*, who investigated the abortion of Teófila Gavilán in San Miguel, Ayacucho, complained in 1942, six years after the initial accusation, of having to juggle 200 cases on his own.[85] Not surprisingly, some investigations took so many years that the crimes could no longer be prosecuted.[86]

Investigators also faced difficulties when attempting to find witnesses to corroborate complainants' accounts. This is what happened when Jacinto

Huaynacho, of Sandía, Puno, was accused of giving his lover, Rufina Ballena, some abortifacient pills in 1977. Although the affair with the married Mr. Huaynacho came to light, there were no witnesses to Ms. Ballena's taking any abortifacients.[87] Even if there were witnesses, sometimes investigators were not able to maximize their value as accusers. Celia Jara, for example, was accused by "several witnesses" of retaining the services of a skilled male Bolivian abortionist in Trujillo, La Libertad, in 1940. In a display of unorthodox investigative skills, the police did not indicate the number or the names of the witnesses, nor how they figured out the man was Bolivian or an abortionist, nor his mysterious whereabouts, and the *fiscal* had to withdraw the accusation against Ms. Jara.[88] Likewise, Dr. Hildebrando Ortiz treated Ofelina Espejo in his private Trujillo practice in 1926 for a miscarriage without bothering to ask what Ms. Espejo had done to herself or even confirming the pregnancy. As Dr. Ortiz admitted later, he simply took Ms. Espejo's mother's word about her daughter's pregnancy and ingestion of an abortifacient and prescribed a painkiller for Ms. Espejo.[89]

These cases highlight the budgetary and technical competence constraints the Peruvian police and judiciary faced throughout the twentieth century, as well as the lack of interest of physicians, particularly those in private practice, in reporting suspected abortions. In the absence of funds, trained personnel, and health professional cooperation, gathering criminal evidence of abortions became difficult. Moreover, the 1901 case against Eudosia Mendoza reveals that the very meaning of criminal responsibility could be contested. Ms. Mendoza's father, Anselmo, declared that he kept his daughter's miscarriage secret because "no one was guilty," since "the creature had been born dead" due to the strain his daughter suffered while "lifting a heavy thing." Moreover, Mr. Mendoza buried the fetus immediately in a field because "the creature had not been baptized."[90] Mr. Mendoza's actions illustrate another documented belief in rural areas of Andean countries: that an unbaptized dead fetus may become, if not disposed of rapidly, a particular threat against the woman who expelled it from her womb and against her living children. The aggressiveness of the unbaptized unborn is unabated until their burial ends their liminal status as beings that belong neither to this world nor to the world of spirits.[91] Rather than an attempt to hide criminal evidence from investigators, Mr. Mendoza's quiet and quick burial of the unbaptized fetus might have been motivated by his concern to shield his daughter from future harm. Over seventy years later, in the rural community of Chucaripo, Puno, Catalina Machaca similarly defended her partner Ignacio Quecara's decision to burn the unbaptized fetus she miscarried, as its continued presence might bring forth hail "and other natural phenomena that can harm people and cattle."[92]

Criminal responsibility could also be contested by men and women who explained pregnancy losses as accidental or involuntary. Women, for example, invoked the link between physical stress and miscarriage. Like Eudosia Mendoza, Angélica Fernandes stated in 1920 that her miscarriage was the result of a fall from a donkey and of her working "on things that forced me to strain myself" at her employers' house.[93] Magdalena Nuñez in Puno in 1943 and Silvia Manchego and Mercedes Díaz in Lima in 1975 and 1979, respectively, also blamed falls and physical or mental trauma for their miscarriages.[94] Men too resorted to strain as an explanation for miscarriage. Manuel Díaz, a thirty-three-year-old peddler accused of causing his wife Felícita Rebaza's miscarriage through a beating in Trujillo in 1940, suggested that the beating had had nothing to do with the miscarriage. In his defense, he offered two alternative and not mutually exclusive explanations. First, he claimed that Mrs. Rebaza had made too much effort carrying a pail full of water to play with her neighbors. Second, Mr. Díaz told investigators that Mrs. Rebaza had grown frustrated because she had not been able to eat pork around the time of her miscarriage, despite craving it.[95] Ismael Ramón, another husband accused of causing his wife's miscarriage through a beating, successfully cast doubt on the charge by arguing that the birth had been difficult, and that his wife, Filomena, miscarried because birth attendant Maximina de la Vega arrived too late to be of any help.[96]

Mr. Ramón's testimony is indicative of the high regard in which the knowledge of a traditional birth attendant could be held. These birth attendants also wielded their specialized knowledge as a weapon to deflect accusations. Ruling out a pregnancy, Rosa Valderrama, for example, concluded that Rosa Huamán's "period was just suspended, her stomach aches made it evident." In January 1940, she had given Mrs. Huamán a culantrillo potion, "brewed to regularize a woman's menstrual period," over several days successfully. She had not demanded payment, as that would have cheapened the value of her work, but did accept "a gift" of money as a show of respect from Mrs. Huamán's family.[97] The skill and experience of birth attendants varied, as did those of allopathic experts. An established practitioner with thirty years of experience, Mrs. Valderrama could hardly be compared with someone like María Gutierrez, a Lima street peddler who provided abortions on the sly in the mid-1970s. Claiming to have been moved by Gladys Castillo's "begging and tears," Gutierrez inserted a plastic tube in the latter's uterus and gave her intramuscular injections of terramycin (an antibiotic) and foliculin (a female hormone). The intervention landed Ms. Castillo at the Maternidad de Lima hospital with a systemic infection she was lucky to survive. Ms. Gutierrez ultimately admitted her deed and pleaded mercy: "I have been jailed because I did not know how to cause an abortion correctly, as it is the first time I attempted one."[98]

The social networks within which abortion seekers met abortion providers also muddled criminal evidence. In 1940, Rosa Huamán, for example, quietly discussed her plight with Rosa Valderrama through a common friend in a store managed by Vicente Wong, Mrs. Huamán's husband. Mr. Wong later identified Ms. Valderrama as a skilled *curandera* and confirmed that she acted "for the good of my wife."[99] Likewise, Willi Urday ran into a wall of silence, in the form of his in-laws, when he tried to coax the name of whoever performed an abortion on his wife, Silvia Manchego, in 1975. The police investigation led them to seamstress Amparo Burgos, a neighbor of Mrs. Manchego's classmate, who dismissed Mr. Urday's concerns by insisting she had simply unblocked Mrs. Manchego's menstrual delay with a Camay soap enema. How could such a thing be harmful, Ms. Burgos taunted, when it is "the same soap I use to wash my face?"[100] These cases illustrate well how networks of family and friends provided quiet introductions, money, and support for women who sought abortions, containing the stigma and shame of abortion within an intimate social sphere. These same networks of silence, however, also protected abortion providers, including those who failed in catastrophic ways. Genara Umiña died in Lima in 1979, Rufina Ballena in Puno in 1977, and Fredesvinda Lara in Piura in 1959, all due to postabortion infections. No one was ever brought to justice for their deaths.[101]

A final factor hampering the investigation of criminal abortions was the complex interpersonal relations that gave rise to abortion accusations, into which government agents were unable or unwilling to delve. Some of these interpersonal relations reveal explosive degrees of socially tolerated violence by men against women, particularly in rural areas. In Ayacucho between 1920 and 1965, for example, thirteen of the seventeen documented cases of miscarriage resulted, according to the female accusers, from beatings at the hands of their spouses. The same occurred in thirteen out of twenty miscarriage cases in Puno between 1919 and 1975. Drunken domestic disputes over money and household duties were common denominators. Not one of these accusations led to a conviction. In fairness, the paucity of witnesses to assaults, as well as the conditions under which forensic technicians performed exams of women and miscarried fetuses, made it hard to clearly establish criminal responsibility.

These considerations aside, justice was stacked against some female plaintiffs so badly disabled that they could not make formal accusations until after healing somewhat, by which time, as a *fiscal* explained in a 1930 acquittal in Ayacucho, it had become "difficult to link a miscarriage to the trauma suffered."[102] Even more unfairly, some *fiscales* minimized the brutality of assaults by calling plaintiff's complaints "notorious exaggerations" over "a few bruises," and "simple fights without dire consequences."[103] The Peruvian judiciary's systematic failure to condemn violence against women contributed to the normalization of such violence within marriage, leading some men to consider their sexual jealousy and aggressive expectation of female obedience as perfectly legitimate. According to Filomena Ramón in 1904, for example, Ismael Ramón, upon noticing a bruise on his wife's arm, became convinced of her infidelity, saying, "someone hit you like I don't. Who was it?" A beating, and subsequent miscarriage, followed Mrs. Ramón's refusal to name the real or imagined lover. Although he contested having caused the miscarriage, Mr. Ramón did not deny the beating or his motives.[104] Likewise, Felícita Rebaza accused her husband, Manuel Díaz, of beating her to the point of miscarrying in 1940. Mrs. Rebaza had been playing with her neighbors in Trujillo. When Mr. Díaz arrived, drunk and belligerent, he ordered Mrs. Rebaza back in the house immediately. When she refused, he got mad and beat her. Manuel Díaz did not deny to the police he had been drunk or nasty to his wife, stating defiantly that he "shoved her to stop her from playing."[105]

At times, complex interpersonal relations manifested themselves as wars of words between accusers and accused, with courts as stages and a judicial audience ignorant of the circumstances that gave rise to these conflicts. Sara Sevilla in Lima in 1913, Blanca Alvarado in Trujillo in 1938, Tomasa Hidalgo in Piura in 1943, and Helen Kramer in 1946 all claimed their male partners had coerced them into getting abortions, which the men denied.[106] Ms. Sevilla leveraged her plight and family connections into a shotgun wedding with César Málaga, who later tried to annul the marriage. Ms. Alvarado wanted only for Remberto Acevedo to reimburse her for the expenses she incurred while convalescing after the abortion attempt. Ms. Hidalgo ultimately recanted and admitted that she wanted to make trouble for Luis Vignolo because one of her brothers had a feud with him. As for Helen Kramer, she simply could not wait to part from Carlos Dogni. She divorced the wealthy socialite and began proceedings for an annulment to get as far away as possible from his anti-Semitic mother (Kramer was Jewish). Dogni died in 1997, at eighty-seven years of age, famous for the surfing parties he threw for the

Lima upper crust, his family links to patrons of the arts, and his cultivated bachelorhood.[107]

The dynamics of spouses' quarreling gave rise, on occasion, to surprising reversals on the part of women. Mery Carbajal and Maximiana Zorrilla miscarried following beatings at the hands of their spouses in Puno in 1952 and in Lircay, Ayacucho, in 1924. Both pressed charges but later dropped their complaints. Mrs. Zorrilla even turned on her mother, Gregoria Chávez, who had nursed Mrs. Zorrilla back to health and provided crucial information to the police, blaming Mrs. Chávez for the "involuntary mistake" of accusing Mrs. Zorrilla's husband.[108] Even more bewildering was Hortensia Noriega's return to the home she shared with Cristóbal Mendizábal, the man whose abuse led to her miscarriage and who "made me dig my own grave, while threatening to kill me with the revolver I am enclosing."[109] Mrs. Noriega indeed turned a revolver over to the ecclesiastic authorities who ran the Casa del Buen Pastor, where she took shelter. One day later, after reconciling with her husband, Mrs. Noriega asked the Sacred Hearts Catholic congregation to give Mr. Mendizábal his gun back. Yet another woman, Julia Izquierdo, took remarkable steps on behalf of her husband, José Aguilar. In February 1901, just outside of Salaverry, on Peru's northern coast, Mr. Aguilar beat Ms. Izquierdo, stopping only when three of her female friends held him back. As a result of her injuries, said the medical report, Mrs. Izquierdo miscarried. "I have had illicit relations with my aggressor," admitted Mrs. Izquierdo, "and we have had many children, including the one he made me abort." The miscarriage worsened Mr. Aguilar's criminal responsibility for the assault, and justice was swift. By January 1902, Mr. Aguilar had been in jail for almost one year. Shortly after, Mrs. Izquierdo wrote to the judge begging for mercy for her husband. The injuries he inflicted "have not resulted in any long-lasting problem," she said, and "he has always been good to me. . . . He was simply not himself that time because of the effects of alcohol. . . . One year in jail is enough to punish him."[110]

Given the nature of the assault, the presence of witnesses, and the medical report to substantiate the miscarriage, Aguilar could have served the sixteen to twenty-four months of jail time his crime deserved, according to the 1862 penal code. It is unclear whether Mrs. Izquierdo's plea helped her husband. However, this case and others make it plain that there was often more going on in the domestic realm than abuse and asymmetrical power relations. Only the satisfaction of women's demands through channels besides those documented in the archives and the endurance of other ties (economic interdependence, mutual affection) can explain the paradox of reconciliation and of an official conviction being challenged by the victim of a beating who also had to subject herself to the embarrassment of publicly admitting to having "illicit relations" with her aggressor.

To summarize, then, the analysis of these cases confirms previous historiography that shows a substantial amount of expert influence in the application of penalties against those accused of the crime of abortion. Scholars such as Kristin Ruggiero and Beatriz Urías Horcasitas, for example, have discussed how Argentinian and Mexican courts, respectively, often showed mercy toward "honorable women" accused of committing abortions and infanticides.[111] The Peruvian cases indicate that the mercy of the court was not the only way in which an abortion accusation could be weakened. Professional discretion in the interpretation of the law, lack of physical evidence or witnesses, the protection provided by an abortion seeker's social network, credible alternative explanations for a miscarriage, the costs involved in conducting an investigation, and the difficulties parsing mutual recriminations between spouses all made the application of criminal laws messier than any penal code could anticipate.

These cases also reveal the diverse origins of abortion accusations. Physicians who treated hospitalized women were one source, but not the only one. The inquiries of local authorities also led to accusations, as did the rumors and gossip of neighbors, women's complaints about their husbands' abusive behavior, and even women's disatisfaction as consumers with the quality of the abortifacients they bought. Finally, these cases showcase the limited investigative capacity of Peruvian law enforcement and judicial institutions well into the 1970s, exemplified by their inability to reach witnesses and find evidence. This hampered the judiciary's power to sustain cases.

However, these investigative shortcomings did not dissuade women from making accusations or from responding to their husbands' actions. As Laura Gotkowitz has argued, courts were public forums where social identities were formed and contested.[112] What these records show are not simply women's attempts to obtain specific outcomes (a conviction for an abusive husband, for example), but, more broadly, women strategically seeking a day in court to negotiate for more power and status relative to their partners. Court accusations were apt vehicles to accomplish this, although other aspects of marital strife were probably too complex for any court to sort out perfectly. This can explain why some women, such as Mrs. Izquierdo, Mrs. Zorrilla, Mrs. Carbajal, and Mrs. Noriega ultimately chose to return home to their husbands, give them second chances, and even forgive them.

## Eighty Years of Abortion

There is much more to abortion than the victimization of women. For instance, physicians working in hospitals acted, formally, as gatekeepers and information providers for the state. But, as I have shown, they did not report everything they suspected about abortion to the authorities. Their silence was the result of both compassion and a self-interested desire to avoid legal and financial problems. Although some physicians sought out punishment for abortion, especially after the legalization of therapeutic abortion, others were more interested in its prevention than in serving as agents of punishment. Peruvian physicians, influenced by French puericulture, treated pregnancy as a complex phenomenon that could be negatively affected by pathologies, the environment, and a person's disposition. Lay people also articulated explanations for pregnancy losses based on the relationship between strain and miscarriage. The convergence between these forms of lay and expert knowledge is another reason for the paucity of abortion accusations.

Women accused of having abortions rarely confessed, whether out of fear of punishment or because they honestly did not try to end their pregnancies on purpose. Those who ended up in the hospital, as we have seen, rarely confessed their intention to provoke an abortion. Instead, they lied, fell back on lay theories about the body, or simply did not say a thing. There is a form of power at work here, a subaltern kind of power that denies access to the "truth" or at least to a confession. Authority figures such as physicians may have made demands on women who had abortions, but they were often thwarted in practice. As much as physicians' irregular recording of medical histories, these women's tactics are reasons why there are no accurate numbers on abortions or infanticides throughout the twentieth century.

Some of the criminal cases presented here have a clear gender violence component, one the Peruvian judiciary tacitly and unfairly endorsed by failing to act on it. However, even when the pregnancy losses occurred as a result of violence of men against women, abortion was not the main injury women complained about. Instead, they focused on the abuse they suffered at the hands of their male partners. Women's accusations about abortion were means for them to limit patriarchal authority in everyday life, against odds that included the social acceptance of male violence against women as normal. As Steve Stern has shown through the Mexican case, physical punishment by husbands of wives who challenged their authority was common in other parts of Latin America.[113] Women gambled that the public demonstration of bodily signs such as bruises and lost pregnancies would play in their favor were they able to reach authorities such as the police or physicians. After all, men were supposed to dominate their families hegemonically and not coercively. Resorting to physical abuse was a dishonorable sign of a man's incompetence to maintain order and control in his relations with women. Men, for their part, could also articulate explanations for women's miscarriages that exonerated the men from the crime of causing a miscarriage, even if they did not deny other charges that women brought against them, including battery.

Women were quite capable of procuring abortions for themselves, relying on their social networks, which included their lovers, to obtain abortifacients and meet abortion providers. Women also produced the dangerous circumstances that led to miscarriages, such as falling down on purpose. Even when they found themselves recovering in a hospital bed, women resisted the attempts of medical authorities to produce a narrative of the events that caused their miscarriages. As stated earlier, there is power in denying information to authority figures. But there is also a darker side to this story. In a time and place in which access to contraceptives was severely limited, abortion was one of the few means Peruvians could use to prevent births. Yet, many women who obtained abortions or caused their own miscarriages wound up endangering their own lives in the process, a grotesque form of gendered injustice that the use of birth control methods was designed to end.

## CHAPTER FOUR

# Contraception Crucible

## Health Workers Encounter Family Planning

Cheap and effective birth control was in short supply in early twentieth-century Latin America. Physicians rarely discussed its availability or relevance to people's lives.[1] Condoms and abortion were the only commonly used means to limit the quantity of offspring, though the prevalence of the latter inspired both public condemnation as well as ineffective repression, as we saw in the previous chapter. Only a handful of strident activists favored the use of involuntary sterilization for people deemed feeble-minded, gathering little public support.[2] In 1930s Peru, however, health workers, overwhelmingly members of the rising urban middle class, began to voice their anxieties over the dangers of the unsanitary living conditions and habits of new immigrants from rural areas and brazenly advocated fertility limitation for this population. Moreover, by the 1960s, health workers' longstanding belief in the dangers of abortion to women's health contributed to the acceptance of new and more effective contraceptives.

A combination of the noxious devaluation of recent immigrants and benign concern with maternal health prompted a change between the 1930s and the 1960s, as Peruvian health personnel began to embrace, haltingly and selectively, the value of smaller families for all. With similar transformations occurring elsewhere in Latin America at the time, it is important to understand what made Peru distinctive in this regard.[3] Under what circumstances did local physicians, nurses, midwives, and social workers first encounter the use of birth control? What did they do to advance and limit the use of contraception? How did they interact with birth control users? The answers to these questions not only shed light on the actions and mindsets of people on the forefront of a momentous development, the normalization of fertility control in the developing world, but are rather urgent given the paucity of written documentation this ebbing first generation of family planning workers has left.

Between the early 1960s and 1970s, these health workers became confident providers of family planning services. Through training and research experiences, they acquired the conviction that birth control would save women's lives and help familial economies. Not surprisingly, they favored the use of new contraceptives, IUDs in particular in Peru, which were not only effective but also reinforced expert control. The consent of their patients, the unwillingness to question each other's decisions, and Peru's inchoate regulatory framework set the stage for health workers' systematic inability to reflect on how they could respond to users' dissatisfaction, and even for the occurrence of egregious cases of abuse. At its best, then, family planning services offered throughout the 1960s and 1970s were based on an authoritarian provider-led model that simultaneously delivered the intended results of protecting women's health while never empowering users to question the terms on which care was delivered.

## Contraception and the Prevention of Harm

The Peruvian public health establishment became institutionally stronger during the recession-prone 1930s. In 1935, General Oscar Benavides created the Ministry of Public Health, Labor, and Social Welfare, building on the Office of Public Sanitation, which had existed since the early 1900s.[4] Subsequent administrations between 1940 and 1960 increased the number of hospitals, health centers, and rural health posts. During this period, the preventive medicine model as practiced and promoted in centers such as Johns Hopkins and Harvard held special sway for new generations of health workers and authorities. Students were as eager to complete specialty courses in Baltimore and Boston as half a century earlier they had been to do so in Paris. In 1942, the U.S.-funded Inter-American Cooperative Service for Public Health (SCISP, after its initials in Spanish), working from within the Ministry of Public Health, started providing training and funds for Peruvian health officers to deal with issues such as malaria, water sanitation, and obstetric care.

The popularity of preventive medicine was on the rise not only in Peru. Sponsored by the Pan-American Health Organization (PAHO), the First Pan-American Congress on Medical Education (Lima, 1951) emphasized the importance of understanding how social dynamics affected the course of health problems. Laboratories and hospital wards were no longer, the congress's organizers proclaimed, the only places where one could learn to become a physician. Two subsequent PAHO conferences on medical education (Viña del Mar, Chile, 1955, and Tehuacán, Mexico, 1956) underscored the importance of community health, holistic approaches to health (encompassing prevention, curing, and rehabilitation), and the integration of biological, psychological, and social aspects of healing.[5]

The new orientation toward prevention contributed to the greater notice health workers and social scientists took of the links between phenomena such as high fertility, migration, maternal morbidity and mortality, familial stress, and children's delinquency. Experts who analyzed the relationship between large families and poverty took note of how children were hired out as domestic workers by their own parents, the ways in which a lack of parental guidance contributed to children's criminality, the crowded housing and unhygienic conditions of the new urban slums, and even how the nutritiousness of breast milk diminished after numerous pregnancies.[6] The same experts connected the growth of urban slums to higher crime rates and the increasing rates of maternal mortality to the fact that the existing public health infrastructure simply could not care well for the growing population.[7]

The idea of voluntarily limiting the size of one's family matured in this period (see figure 5).[8] Large families, it seemed, were not conducive to financial stability or domestic harmony and began to be associated instead with poverty, parental frustration, and suffering, particularly for the least wealthy.[9] Saturnino Huillca, leader of the Peasant Federation of Cuzco since the 1940s, for example, recalled the arrival of each of his ten children as events that only added to his and his wife's sorrow. "And in the same way some of them died," he added.[10] Less mournful, but sardonically bitter nonetheless, was textile worker Martín Parodi, whose 1945 poem "Superpoblación" ("Overpopulation") seized on the indignities and inconveniences of material scarcity:

> With the demographic explosion you will have to wait in line;
> To be born, you will have to wait in line;
> To die, you will have to wait in line;
> To be buried, you will have to wait in line;
> To wait in line, you will have to wait in line.[11]

The first estimates of maternal mortality in Lima emerged in this context. The rate for the period between 1947 and 1952 was approximately 446 deaths per 100,000 births at the Maternidad de Lima, then the most technically advanced obstetrics hospital in Peru.[12] Aware of the newly available data, even hardened opponents of the regulation of family size began to change their minds. Dr. Carlos Enrique Paz Soldán, chair of hygiene at San Marcos University, for example, still believed that Peru required a larger population

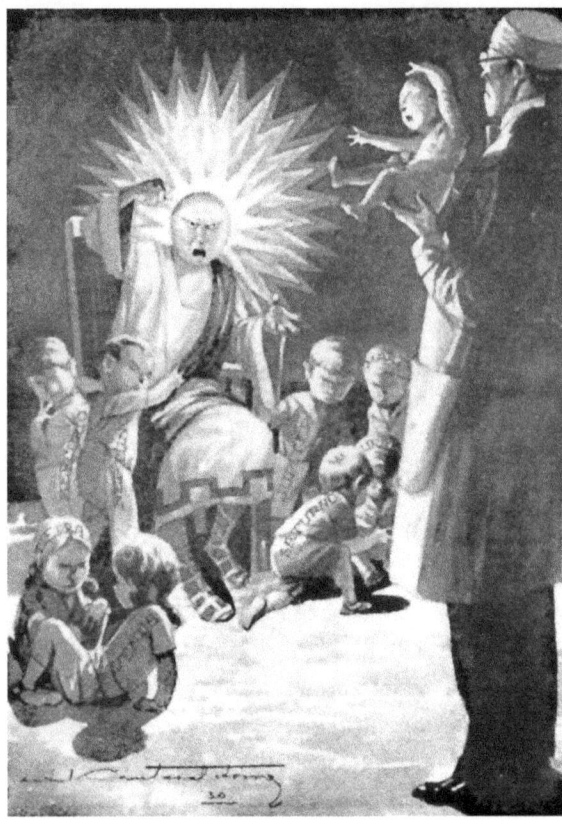

Figure 5. "The New Planet." An angry sun, surrounded by eight planets already, exclaims "Darn! What a calamity! Another damn kid to feed!" as a physician brings him Pluto, his new son, discovered in 1930. José Alcántara La Torre, *Variedades* 25, 1150 (March 19, 1930): 3.

throughout most of its territory, but he also pondered how migration from the interior to the coastal cities would strain services in education, housing, health, and food procurement.[13] Caught between two seemingly contradictory imperatives, Paz Soldán discarded his blanket condemnation of birth control and even found some support for it in the Bible: "How can one condemn it outright without first heeding the clamor of the Book of Ecclesiastes: 'I turned and saw the injustices committed under the sun, the tears of the innocents without solace; defenseless against the violence of others, shunned from all relief. And I envied the dead more than the living. And I held as fortunate not this nor that one, but the unborn, who have not seen the evils committed under the sun'?"[14]

Paz Soldán's comments are indicative of a broader trend among health workers. As Dr. Antonio Quintanilla put it in 1956, low agricultural productivity, industrial inefficiency, "and perhaps a high birth rate" negatively affected families' ability to feed their children well, which in turn caused malnutrition and disease.[15] Physicians doubted that a reduced birth rate alone could sustain Peru's long-term economic welfare. Nonetheless, they started to favor a slow decrease in birth rates over time through voluntary birth control used mainly by couples that could not materially provide for numerous children. It was these same physicians who first promoted interparity intervals (of two to three years) in the interest of maternal health for all women.[16] During this period, birth control ought to be practiced through the rhythm method, physicians counseled, since condoms, coitus interruptus, and vaginal douching were purportedly less effective and less sexually satisfying.[17]

The possibility of regulating family sizes through the rhythm method had generated enthusiasm among Peruvian physicians. A 1934 editorial in *La Reforma Médica* called it "the most transcendental biological and socioeconomic discovery of the century."[18] However, few physicians took up the idea of teaching or otherwise disseminating the method to the lay public. The high popularity of condoms, in contrast, had less to do with clinician approval. Men and women bought them in pharmacies and on the street as early as the 1880s, as contraceptives and means of protection against sexually transmitted infections.[19] Still, the condom's association with prostitution made it distasteful as a contraceptive by monogamous couples. Some psychiatrists even classified "coitus condomatus" by husband and wife as a sexual perversion, alongside homosexuality, necrophilia, and bestiality, one that was especially harmful to women, since the deposit of sperm allegedly played a role in the health of the uterus.[20]

Academic medical experts blamed condom-wearing men for the country's inability to increase its population; they also called married couples that used condoms "refined egotists" who put pleasure ahead of the national interest.[21] The ubiquity of the condom trade eventually led to a backlash. In April 1940, the Ministry of Public Health passed Resolution 920, banning the street sale of condoms. According to the ministry, the transactions had reached "alarming proportions," with hawkers offering their wares to passers-by "without regard to their sex, age, and social condition," which constituted "an affront to morality and respectability."[22] In the early 1950s, the government of General Manuel Odría ratcheted up the anticondom offensive. Article 203 of the Customs Code banned the import of condoms as contraceptives, a witless initiative that guaranteed their brisk sales as disease-prevention devices and legitimized the advertisements of condoms as prophylactics in pharmaceutical journals.[23]

Between the 1930s and the late 1950s, the increasingly salient link between poverty, the acceleration of migration, high fertility, maternal morbidity and mortality, and delinquency led health workers to soften their stance on fertility regulation. In their view, poverty caused criminality and ill health and exacerbated problems such as induced abortions among the new urban dwellers. The new professional stance favoring preventive clinical interventions encouraged health professionals to see fertility limitation as one way to ward off individual suffering and societal harm. These attitude changes occurred in the context of the 1930s recessions and the fiscal austerity regime of Manuel Prado in the late 1950s, caused in part by the economic slowdown that followed the Korean War. President Prado dealt with the crisis by reducing public spending, freezing salary and wage increases, and raising the price of basic foodstuffs.[24] Having several dependents would have been trying under these conditions for anyone but the wealthiest. The increasingly visible material squalor notwithstanding, physicians and public health experts did not stop reflecting on the need to populate other parts of Peru, particularly the eastern Amazon region.[25] Clinical workers brought to bear these complex social, clinical, and ethical outlooks when they began to consider the role birth control would play for their careers, their patients, and their country.

## "No One Did Anything": Family Planning Comes to Health Workers' Attention[26]

For the generation of health workers who came of age in the early 1960s, neither local universities nor hospitals had been institutions that welcomed training or even discussion about the limitation of offspring. Nevertheless, beneath the young professionals' and students' acquiescence to the status quo lurked an itch to intervene clinically in the lives of others, not only for the sake of preventing disease but in hopes of improving women's lives and countering the entropic effects of poverty on families.

There were limits to health workers' enthusiasm, though. Early 1960s physicians, midwives, and social workers did not commonly consider family planning for men, or for the well-off and educated. In fact, the ideal birth control user was the one social worker Teresa Giunta indignantly described: a hard-drinking immigrant widow in a peri-urban shantytown who wanted contraceptive advice, with seven children from different partners already and a physically abusive partner who had an incestuous relationship with his teenage stepdaughter. Health workers such as Giunta hoped that helping such women learn to manage their fertility would enable them to spend more time with their children and learn a trade, as well as to become less dependent on their husbands.[27]

While recently immigrated women living in poverty somewhere in the periphery of Lima were ideal targets for birth control advice and interventions, Dr. Luis Fernández, chair of obstetrics at the Trujillo General Hospital in 1963, reminds us that more fortunate Peruvians were not: "A millionaire can have ten children. I don't see why we should get in his way."[28] The concern with stagnant or declining population sizes in rural areas also contributed to the circumscription of family planning services to urban areas. Sex, racial, geographic, and class distinctions were at the heart of health workers' determination of what populations suffered from an "unmet need for contraception."[29]

Given the paucity of technical, educational, and institutional support for contraception in the 1950s, it is not surprising that health workers' nascent desire to help out was often expressed in low-key ways, such as advice sessions to women about spacing their pregnancies.[30] These efforts progressively mutated into impatient critiques of patients, peers, and the very organizations within which health workers labored. According to Dr. Victor Díaz, who graduated from medical school in 1953, "nothing was ever going to be solved through education. People just don't come to meetings."[31] Frustration led physicians and midwives to bully their female patients with "I told you so" exhortations the next time they became pregnant and also to impress their junior colleagues with shocking cases: "One thing that affected me much was when a physician once called me to see a patient with an incomplete abortion. It smelled badly and all, but he wanted to show me what happened when women did not use birth control."[32]

The most entrepreneurial young gynecologists interested in family planning capitalized on their leadership positions within national professional associations, universities, and hospitals to hand-pick curious and ambitious students and turn them into apprentices, often offering the carrot of prestigious international training fellowships. Dr. Abraham Ludmir, for example, established the first residency program in gynecology at San Bartolomé Hospital in Lima in 1961. Early on, his residents received training in family planning methods in Chile, the South American mecca of contraception research.[33] Dr. Rodolfo Gonzáles Enders, director of one of the clinics of the Peruvian Association for Family Protection, the largest network of birth control clinics in Peru, and Dr. Carlos Muñoz Torcello, chair of gynecology at the Archbishop Loayza Hospital, also recommended their best employees for training-abroad opportunities.[34]

Most health workers and students selected for additional training were honored by the attention their work attracted, eager to learn something that might be helpful to patients, and delighted by the employment opportunities their new knowledge could afford them. An enthusiastic Dr. Doris Chang recalled that, "as a young one, I was up for anything."[35] Yet, some feared that training in contraception could violate their Catholic principles and sought the counsel of ecclesiastic advisers. Dr. Delia Moreno's priest advised her to "learn, but not to put in practice what was learned."[36] Such reluctant physicians embraced an engineered distinction between "family planning," which they equated with the legitimate aspiration of all families to rationally and compassionately determine the number of offspring by preventing conceptions, and *control de la natalidad* (the literal translation of "birth control") as an abusive imposition from the United States to limit population growth by forcing individuals to use abortifacient methods. Family planning was all right, *control de la natalidad* was not. To this day, the latter term remains a pejorative way to refer to the use of contraceptives in Peru.[37]

Early encounters with family planning not only occurred through foreign fellowships but also through local training and research. The Instituto Marcelino and its founder, Dr. Alfredo Larrañaga, illustrate this well. Larrañaga had worked at St. Luke's Presbyterian Hospital in Chicago after graduating from San Marcos University in the mid-1950s, and returned to Peru in 1961. By that time, hormonal contraceptives, G. D. Searle's Enovid and Schering's Anovlar in particular, had begun to be sold in Peru.[38] Manufacturers advertised them as "pregnancy protectors" that required prescriptions, although pharmacies rarely asked for such paperwork.[39] The marketability of hormonal contraceptives stimulated pharmaceutical research. In 1966, Schering began human trials for a new injectable hormonal contraceptive at the Huando hacienda, in the highlands of Lima, with help from Dr. Larrañaga.[40]

Schering was satisfied with the trial and in 1968 funded Larrañaga's own birth control clinic and research center, the Instituto Marcelino (IM), in Lima. The IM thrived in the late 1960s and early 1970s. Pharmaceutical firms such as Schering, Wyeth, and Warner-Lambert became its main source of funding. The IM tested compounds these companies were developing, such as once-a-month pills, male contraceptives, postcoital pills, and injectable long-term hormonal contraceptives, mainly on low-income women from urban areas in Lima: "You have no idea all that we studied," Larrañaga boasted.[41] At the same time, the relative obscurity in which the IM operated and the lack of transparency regarding its recruitment practices created resentment among government officers and other health workers who believed "women were being used as guinea pigs" and worried about the IM drugs' side effects.[42]

In addition to contract research on hormonal contraceptives, the IM also provided family planning services on demand, including IUD fittings and infertility consultations, which provided a secondary source of income. During its heyday in the early 1970s, between sixty and a hundred women visited the IM every day.[43] Over time, the IM staff grew to seven physicians who also worked in various state hospitals. In addition, Larrañaga was a member of the medical faculty at San Marcos University. These academic and hospital connections allowed medical and midwifery students to acquire some practical experience with family planning, as they rotated at the IM and attended talks sponsored by its corporate partners.[44] One of these students, Dr. Augusto Chávez, gratefully described his IM education as strategic, as without its hands-on approach, "we would have been nothing."[45]

Foreign and local training and research thus framed the first forays of Peruvian health workers into the family planning field. These early clinical interventions converged with the conduction of surveys about what men and women knew and felt about their fertility, and what they did to regulate it. Carried out in dozens of countries beginning in the late 1940s, these fertility surveys were modeled on corporate marketing research pioneered in the United States.[46] Researchers routinely asked about frequency of intercourse, birth control methods used, reasons why people had stopped using a particular method, and even the number of abortions a woman had had. Such inquiries about popular knowledge, attitudes, and practices (also called "KAP studies") provided a baseline of descriptive statistics but also had a political aim: to persuade experts and policymakers that, with public support behind smaller families, there was little risk in embracing and sponsoring birth control technologies and policies. As noted demographer Frank Notestein, director of the Population Council (1959–68), pithily put it, "probably the best way to make progress in a dangerous field is to sponsor 'research' rather than 'action.' Who can be against 'truth'?"[47]

Sociologist Joseph Mayone Stycos had risen as one of the foremost KAP survey experts in the Americas since the late 1940s, having conducted this kind of research previously in Puerto Rico and Jamaica.[48] In 1960, he became the first to conduct a KAP study in Peru, with the help of a local marketing consultant, Carlos Uriarte, and a cadre of students from the Faculty of Social Work at San Marcos University.[49] On his heels came Marie-Françoise Hall, a Harvard-trained physician affiliated with Johns Hopkins's Department of International Health, who also engaged Uriarte's and the Faculty of Social Work's services.[50] Hall was not only a foreigner but also a woman and a mother following her husband, Tom, also a physician, while he conducted a manpower survey for Peru's Ministry of Health. Yet, her status as an outsider to the local medical circle emboldened rather than hindered her from delving into the touchy subject of sexuality. After all, "I did not have much to lose," she reflected, "it was my first venture. If I had failed, I would have tagged back on to my husband and gotten back to the States."[51] Moreover, unlike Stycos's work, Hall's caught the attention of *Caretas*, one of the most popular weekly magazines in Peru, which fed a nascent media interest in contraception.[52]

Entrepreneurial young physicians eager to extend the reach of family planning saw an opportunity, this time to take advantage of the national spotlight survey research garnered. They encouraged students to emulate the KAP methodology elsewhere. Dr. Mariano Bedoya, chair of the Obstetrics Department at San Marcos University, for example, supervised at least three KAP studies in Lima submitted as medical theses. Dr. Luis Fernández, chair of the Obstetrics Department in the Trujillo National Hospital, did the same for a graduating nurse.[53] Unlike Hall and Stycos, however, who sampled high- and low-income urban populations in their surveys, Peruvians focused exclusively on urban poor women. While in Peru, Hall never realized the extent to which local health workers emulated her work while adapting it to their preconceived notions of who needed contraception the most.

Local fertility surveys confirmed suspicions that induced abortions were as common an occurrence in Peru as they were elsewhere in Latin America.[54] Critics, however, took these results with a grain of salt.[55] They claimed that KAP reports presented answers as if respondents had thought about fertility enough to have formed definitive and unchanging opinions about family size that they would be willing to share with a stranger. This was an unrealistic expectation given the novelty of the very idea of using contraceptives to limit fertility. Most problematically, KAP surveys inferred actual practice from mere reported statements. KAP studies, critics argued, were above all marketing exercises to best position a product before decision makers reluctant to sacrifice their political capital for a new cause.

Even with these shortcomings, fertility surveys provided some evidence that women were interested in managing their fertility more effectively. The possibility of an actual demand for family planning justified the scattered investments health workers had been making training themselves, hectoring patients and colleagues, and decrying the organizational and legal strictures within which they worked. The sentiment among these early 1960s health workers that fertility regulation broke with previous obstetric practice, and that their old teachers and new patients lacked crucial knowledge, emboldened them to claim family planning as their province, as a new so-ciomedical field of action for them to lead, one with the potential to change the nation, families, and individuals for the better.

## "Nice Clinic, Now What?": Providing Family Planning Services[56]

In the mid-1950s, as health workers complained about the state of maternal health, urban poverty, high parity, shoddily provided abortions, and short interparity intervals, contraceptive use was not widespread. In addition to condoms and the rhythm method, douching, withdrawal, and herbal remedies were the less costly alternatives. Peruvians with means additionally availed themselves of diaphragms, spermicidal tablets and foams, and diverse forms of sterilization, though physicians also performed the latter on unsuspecting women who never consented to the surgeries.

Following the 1933 Constitution's explicit criminalization of disabling injuries, the Peruvian Medical College's Ethics Committee declared that sterilizations caused bodily injuries that disabled the reproductive function, and therefore ruled against the performance of these surgeries unless a future pregnancy posed a grave risk to a woman's health.[57] This self-censorship by the most important professional organization of physicians made it difficult to conduct sterilizations even upon patient request. In contrast, U.S. obstetricians, the main referents for Peruvian ones at the time, had been performing sterilizations since the early 1900s. As J. Whitridge Williams, obstetrics chief at the Johns Hopkins University Hospital, explained, "if the patient is intelligent, the decision should be left to her or her family; whereas with the ignorant it is incumbent upon the physician to do what he thinks is best under the circumstances. Personally, I should be unwilling to sterilize a patient at the first operation, unless she comes from a district where proper operative help might not be available in a future pregnancy. On the other hand, if she is weak-minded or diseased and is liable to require repeated Caesarean sections the operation is perfectly justifiable."[58]

Various U.S. and British obstetrics texts in the first half of the twentieth century recommended obtaining patients' permission before the surgery, as well as performing sterilizations after the third cesarean due to the increased (though small) risk of spontaneous rupture through the uterine cicatrix.[59] By 1950, however, the popular *Williams Obstetrics*, attuned to the ebbing popularity of eugenics, began to downplay feeble-mindedness as a rationale for sterilization and instead emphasized "great multiparity" (defined as eight or more viable deliveries) as a new reason why physicians should sterilize women.[60]

The earliest reports of surgical sterilization in Peru date from 1953. Dr. Landauro Valentini, for example, insisted on consulting with at least three medical colleagues, as well as confirming the patient's understanding that the operation would end her childbearing possibilities, before proceeding.[61] Similarly, Dr. Victor Díaz, who sterilized female patients during his internship year at the Maternidad de Lima in 1953, would only perform the surgeries on women who had had three previous cesareans, and only after speaking with the women and their husbands, "otherwise you would always have a big problem."[62] With guidelines in place emphasizing the risk more than three cesarean operations posed, as well as the need to obtain a patient's consent, several other hospitals began to offer surgical sterilizations by the mid-1960s, including the Maternidad de Lima, Loayza Hospital, Almenara Hospital, San Bartolomé Hospital, Rebagliatti Hospital (all in Lima), the San Juan Hospital in Marcona, Ica, and the Hospital Nacional in Trujillo.[63]

Homogeneous recommendations aside, however, physicians' experiences sterilizing women were diverse. Some declined to operate, despite the risks future pregnancies could carry, when a woman's older children had passed away and she faced the prospect of remaining childless.[64] Others were even firmer in their antisterilization stance. Dr. Delia Moreno, for example, admitted that "temporary birth control, yes, but definitive measures, such as tubal ligations, I did not like. [If anyone asked me for that] I would suggest alternatives."[65] Even those physicians who only occasionally sterilized patients were at risk of being shamed by their own colleagues for not standing up for their Catholic principles, as happened to Dr. Luis Fernández in Trujillo. In contrast, others found the courage to continue providing this option to women when they witnessed how individual Catholic authorities begged for the operation for their relatives, even when those relatives did not fit the risk profile hospitals preferred.[66]

There were physicians who, on the other hand, adopted a disturbing approach to sterilization. "I have sterilized thousands of women without their husbands' permission, nor theirs," Dr. Miguel Exebio stated defiantly, though perhaps exaggerating. "Say, a woman with sixteen children went into labor. I'd say, 'get her to the operating room.' There was no other way. I would do a cesarean and tie her tubes. Years later some have come back to say 'doctor, after that operation I never got pregnant again. What did you do to me?' 'I don't remember,' I'd say. What was I going to tell them? 'I tied your tubes'?"[67] A minority among physicians, they cast their unaccountable decisions in the language of service to the community, to the nation that could ill afford the growth of the wrong kind of population: the poor and uneducated. "You had to act thinking about the future of that poor woman, her children, and society. What kind of children would these people raise?" Dr. Ramiro Yanque asked me.[68] In any event, such professionals comforted themselves, a sterilization now was better than an abortion later.

It is easy to see how these views could and did lead to abuse, but it is also important to note how women themselves might collude with physicians in order to get sterilized, by emphasizing how difficult and risky their pregnancies were. When a physician deemed that a future pregnancy could endanger a woman's health, she could become eligible for the operation. Following their historical analysis of the ratio of caesarean surgeries to vaginal births in the early 1970s, Dr. Elmer Chávez and Dr. Carlos Bachmann became convinced that their colleagues at the Maternidad de Lima exaggerated the need for caesarean surgeries in order to have an opportunity to perform sterilizations with the complicity of women. The researchers also indicated that their colleagues seldom reported having performed these surgeries, in order to protect their patients' privacy.[69]

Still, sterilizations were not the most common medical intervention available to Peruvians. Between the mid-1950s and the mid-1960s, the appearance of hormonal birth control, and especially intrauterine devices, profoundly altered the contraceptive market. International birth control organizations fastened on the intrauterine device (IUD) as a most promising "solution" for the problem of rapid population growth in developing countries. Though coiled silver or gold wire models had been available since the late 1920s, new IUDs came to market in the late 1950s.[70] These second generation IUDs, made of flexible plastic instead of metal, were effective and cheaper than hormonal contraceptives. Like birth control pills, spermicidal foams, and cervical caps, IUDs placed the responsibility for family planning on women. Unlike other contraceptives, however, IUDs did not require any action by the user once fitted.

IUDs gave more control to medical workers over women's reproductive choices because the insertion and removal of these contraceptives required special skills and tools, and because, in Peru, physicians and midwives were the only ones licensed to prescribe IUDs. In addition to reinforcing physicians' and midwives' authority, in itself a valued outcome for health professionals, the diffusion of IUDs also converged with the goal of international birth control organizations of arresting rapid population growth in parts of the developing world. As Alan Guttmacher, chief of obstetrics and gynecology at Mount Sinai Hospital and president of the International Planned Parenthood Federation, warned, what those countries needed was less "birth control for the individual" and more "birth control for a nation."[71] Faith in the IUD was such that Population Council vice president Bernard Berelson believed that "from several standpoints, it may be best to provide a cafeteria choice—'here are all the recommended methods, select the one most suitable to you'—but at the same time to stress the desirability of the IUD."[72]

Latin America had its share of prominent IUD promoters, most notably Dr. Jaime Zipper, from the Obstetrics and Gynecology Department of the Barros Luco Hospital in Santiago, Chile. In the early 1960s, he and his colleague Hernán Sanhueza invented a simple and cheap IUD, consisting of a two-meter-long thread of sterilized nylon coiled into a ring of approximately 25mm in diameter.[73] The physicians believed the low cost of their device made it an appropriate technology for use in low-income areas and began publicizing it as a means to prevent both the human and hospitalization costs of induced abortions as well as "a technique of great value for the safe control of mass population growth." Zipper's stance against lay people choosing contraceptives was more extreme than Guttmacher's or Berelson's. In his opinion, "the medical profession rather than the patient must ultimately decide on the efficiency of any procedure in the light of all the relevant factors, and accommodate one or several techniques to the specific conditions of a country."[74]

In the early 1960s, Peruvian health workers were hardly in a position to dictate the use of IUDs to the general population. For starters, some, such as Dr. Delia Moreno, started offering family planning services only grudgingly, when ordered to do so by superiors in the Ministry of Health hospital where she worked.[75] People such as Dr. Hugo Calle, who considered IUDs, including Zipper's nylon rings, "magnificent contraceptives," were rare.[76] The few who admitted that these novel, untested technologies might be beneficial faced the challenge of persuading skeptical colleagues and female patients to heed their advice. These clinicians began turning routine interactions into opportunities to talk up family planning. They also started referring to women who consented to using birth control as "users" instead of "patients." As Dr. Hugo Oblitas explained, birth control "was not clinically necessary," and therefore "demand had to be generated, by tagging it to cancer screenings, gynecology exams, and sex education lectures. We had to market ourselves to generate users."[77] Carlos Bachmann, of the Maternidad de Lima, even took it upon himself to provide instruction on contraceptive methods for women who had just given birth or were recovering from an attempted abortion. He reported that "most" of his patients had no knowledge of birth control methods and that, after his "informational lecture," about 60 percent of them "chose" to have an IUD fitted.[78]

As elsewhere in Latin America, researchers and even the popular press highlighted the role family planning could play in the prevention of induced abortions, which not only endangered women's lives but also taxed the human and technical resources of hospitals.[79] The Bravo Chico Hospital in Lima's Barrios Altos, in response to its reported high rate of hospitalization following abortion, established a family planning program in 1966 that aimed to turn approximately 8,000 female outpatients into "users." "Women will choose the contraceptives," the hospital affirmed, "however, medical criteria will prevail ultimately, and IUDs will be prioritized, given the cultural and economic characteristics of the population, the IUDs' low cost, their greater acceptance, and superior clinical and demographic results."[80] In 1969, the Hospital Docente del Rimac adopted a different, yet still authoritarian, policy, refusing to issue either postabortion care discharge papers or an infant's birth certificate until the patient had listened to an improvised family planning lecture. With the policy in place, recalled midwife Luisa Parra, the hospital's family planning program went from zero to twenty-five consultations per day within two years.[81]

For most hospitals, however, family planning was merely one service among many they provided. Often, it was not the most frequently or competently offered, with short clinic hours and reluctant providers.[82] Private family planning clinics emerged in this context, including the IM and the Catholic Church Responsible Parenthood program, to be discussed in chapter 6. The largest and most notorious of these providers were those the International Planned Parenthood Federation funded.[83] The IPPF's Western Hemisphere Region arm began sponsoring birth control clinics in Latin America and the Caribbean in 1954, and the Peruvian Association for Family Protection (Asociación Peruana de Protección Familiar, APPF) became its first grantee in 1967. While the APPF's business office was located in the posh Lima district of San Isidro, its first clinics were located in the low-income neighborhoods of Callao, San Miguel, Rimac, Breña, Surquillo, El Agustino, and Barrios Altos. By 1970 the APPF had three clinics outside of Lima, in Ica, Huancayo, and Chimbote.[84] Between its establishment in 1967 and 1970, the APPF reported that 4,032 women had been fitted with IUDs; 3,673 were put on the pill; 1,898 had received injectable contraceptives; and 120 had received some other form of birth control.[85]

In 1973, the IPPF began to fund its largest venture yet in Peru, a training and clinical program at the Arzobispo Loayza Hospital in Lima, euphemistically known as "Studies in Human Fertility." The program provided instruction and practical experience opportunities for health care workers and medical students in counseling techniques, physical exams, Pap smear tests, and the use of all contraceptive methods available except for sterilization. Between November 1973 and January 1976 the hospital received approximately US$44,000 for this task. Almost 90 percent of these funds were earmarked for instructors' salaries and administrative fees. IUDs were the most used method: between February and October 1974, 90 percent of all 509 birth control users had been fitted with such devices.[86] Foreign donors' predilection for the IUD was such that it discouraged skeptical physicians from seeking funds to investigate alternative contraceptive means. As Dr. Walter Llaque, an endocrinologist who directed a natural birth control clinic in Trujillo between 1968 and 1980, recalled, "they liked the easy way out. If you did not insert IUDs, there was no money for you."[87]

Ironically, the year 1973, which marked the beginning of the IPPF's program at the Arzobispo Loayza Hospital, was also the year of the demise of the APPF. A left-leaning wing of the military, alienated by President Fernando Belaúnde's inability to overcome congressional opposition and his unwillingness to take on the powerful landed elite to implement a promised agrarian reform, ousted him in a coup in 1968. Led by General Juan Velasco Alvarado, this faction instituted the "Revolutionary Government of the Armed Forces" (1968–75). Velasco's distrust for U.S.-funded activities in Peru extended from oil extraction to landholding and included family planning as well. In December 1973, Velasco accused the APPF of receiving financial support from an organization, the IPPF, whose goals "do not match the humanist ideals of the Revolutionary Government of the Armed Forces" and whose very presence in Peru constituted "an affront to morality and decency."[88]

With the APPF's closure determined at the highest and most inscrutable political level, there was little the IPPF could do to help its ailing grantee. Instead, it began to channel more financial, material, and technical aid to the newer "Studies in Human Fertility" program at the Arzobispo Loayza Hospital. IPPF grants officer John Robbins even recommended upgrading that program's priority level; "let's keep the flag flying," he urged his colleagues.[89] It is not entirely clear why Velasco singled out the APPF for obliteration. Its fifteen clinics made it the most prominent family planning organization in the country, but the APPF was not the only organization that received foreign funding: the Instituto Marcelino and the Catholic Church's Responsible Parenthood Program also received U.S. funds. At the very least, Velasco's actions showed the extent of the naïveté of U.S. experts who believed anti-Americanism in Latin America extended only to U.S. government agencies. Private agencies with U.S. ties were not inconspicuous and could also be tarred with the "Ugly American" brush with ease.[90]

Regardless of the reason for Velasco's attack on the APPF, its violent end was a defining event for workers in the family planning sector. Some, like anthropologist Dr. Carmen Delgado de Thays, APPF education director, and social worker Emperatriz Matallana abandoned the field entirely and faced financial and career insecurity for a while.[91] A few were determined not to let their patients go without care and increased family planning activities in the hospitals in which they worked and in their private practices, even stealing contraceptive supplies from the shut-down APPF storage.[92] Some, like midwife Luisa Parra, opened up private practices directly in response to the perceived injustice Velasco committed. Adding insult to injury, Parra then had to endure the threats of physicians who believed she was encroaching on their professional jurisdiction.[93] Even those not affiliated with the APPF felt the sting of the governmental rebuke and lowered the profile of their family planning activities, fearing "fifth columnists, people from inside the profession who might tell others what we were doing."[94] Persecuted, antagonized, yet still defiant, family planning workers came to dislike Velasco's regime in the 1970s. At the same time, they held on tightly to the image they carved for themselves in the early 1960s, as pioneers making bold choices for the good of their nation and their patients, even as they struggled to turn those patients into users.

## "People Loved You for This" vs. "My Wife is Not a Bad Woman":[95] Reaching the Most Important Stakeholders

The expansion of family planning services in the late 1960s led to a number of benefits for professionals and organizations. The opportunities came not only in the form of employment for physicians, midwives, family educators, and even anthropologists, but also in the form of generous program grants and paid trips to learn the latest contraceptive and sex education techniques.[96] Of course, workers and administrators welcomed the perks. Just as important, reaching more people meant greater contact with Peruvians who had little experience with the very idea of limiting fertility. Health workers' actions and aspirations, when analyzed alongside those of actual and potential contraception users, reveal just how much of a source of pleasure and frustration family planning work could be, and what expectations birth control users had of such personnel and the technologies and services they peddled.

Most family planning workers were very pleased with the respect, and even affection, women expressed toward them, and they returned the feelings empathically. "I'd see lights in small houses," a volunteer recalled, "and start thinking, 'a man and a woman there feel the same things I do, they share the same aspirations and problems I have.'"[97] Emboldened, they organized clinics in crime-ridden neighborhoods with confidence: "They knew us over in the Barracones del Callao," Dr. Helí Cancino bragged about his work in the famously tough neighborhood, "nothing ever happened to us there. People looked out for us, on the contrary." Such regard cemented the conviction of the earliest converts, such as Dr. Alfredo Larrañaga, that users would not be deterred by government or religious injunctions against birth control: "people will do what they want," he scoffed, "the rest is bunk." Still, it was not only popularity they craved, as Dr. Nazario Carrasco remembered, but also professional growth. The demand for birth control pushed workers to hone their skills, "say, if I used to insert thirty IUDs in two hours, I started aiming to insert sixty in two hours."[98]

These workers were also in an excellent position to apply their superior clinical skills to midwifery, obstetrics, and gynecology private practices. In fact, because of the lack of professional and governmental oversight of private practices relative to public hospital services, physicians and midwives were freer to discuss and utilize birth control in those settings, although with a smaller number of people (i.e., patients who could afford private consultations) Private practice also provided opportunities to teach colleagues and students about the use of birth control. Each of the nineteen physicians and midwives I interviewed had a private practice in the 1960s. Combining that with work in hospitals and NGOs was the only way to make ends meet, and sometimes even that was not enough. Their status as paying customers emboldened private patients to ask for illegal and expensive medical services, particularly abortions. Most physicians, such as Dr. Doris Chang, publicly frowned upon the practice: "When they came to me with the cake already baked, asking me for a, you know, then no. Anything before, nothing after. [Patients] try to tempt you most often with that. If I had wanted yachts and planes, I would have been doing [abortions] for a while now."[99] Just as tellingly, no clinician ever accused a colleague of performing abortions, despite the fact that most claimed to know someone who made a living that way.

Many users trusted health workers' technical competence when it came to family planning and defended their authority in matters of choosing birth control methods, especially for people other than themselves. Teresa Pareja, director of the National Institute for Statistics in the late 1970s observed, for example, that buying birth control in pharmacies without a prescription "could be bad, not only for the woman who uses it, but also for the future. Who knows how her children might turn out? Much medical control is required. Still, family planning is a must, especially for certain social groups. It is not convenient for them to have so many children."[100]

The faith health personnel had in IUDs found echoes among users as well, as showgirl Teresa Dávila's testimony suggests: "I used to be on the pill, but not any more because it is bad for you. It uses up your *foliculina*, and ages us before our time, with wrinkles appearing. I much prefer an IUD. Those never give trouble, and when you want to have a child, you just have one, just like that." Women also expressed gratitude for health workers' advocacy on their behalf. Peasant leader Victoria, for example, wished to use birth control, citing the difficulties of combining her work with the care of her children. She quite welcomed her physician lecturing her reluctant husband: "He said to my husband, 'Why don't you have your wife use birth control? [*¿Por qué tu no haces controlar a tu señora?*] Here's a prescription I made out for her four years ago. Now she is in danger. She was hospitalized fifteen days without giving birth, and we had to do a cesarean.' Thanks to that, it's been now eight years that I have been on the pill."[101]

Alongside the stories of satisfied, well-supported, and vindicated users, however, are those of others: the unreachable, the unsatisfied dropouts, and the outright opponents. Women who failed to keep their appointments for IUD fittings and follow-up interviews especially vexed clinicians and led them to devise ways to find those unreachable women. Since the availability of contraceptive services spread mainly by word of mouth, Peruvian family planning workers, like their counterparts throughout Latin America, curried the favor of local opinion leaders and community organizations.[102] Social worker María Montero, for example, point blank asked long-term residents of El Agustino for clues to find the women who missed their appointments for IUD fittings.[103]

Efforts to enlist community support did not succeed without effort. In the early 1970s, for example, a group of nursing students from San Marcos University worked in the El Planeta shantytown of Lima, delivering talks on first aid, children's health, and nutrition, as well as on flower arranging, rug making, weaving, and bottle decoration. When the students attempted to persuade the leaders of the communal assembly of the importance of disseminating information about family planning, the latter began to bargain with the students. Many of the most influential assembly members worked during the nighttime, and they did not wish to spend their days persuading their neighbors to use birth control, at least not without proper compensation. The students, assembly members claimed, "wanted something without giving anything back." After a heated discussion, the assembly voted to help the students, by a slim margin of two votes in the twenty-six-person governing body.[104]

Even after IUD insertion and a successful follow-up interview, problems could emerge. Rarely, IUDs simply failed to prevent a pregnancy. Carlos García, sales chief for Schering Pharmaceuticals in Peru, recalled with irony seeing the Copper T IUD his employer manufactured being expelled during his own daughter's birth.[105] More frequent were the side effects of IUD use, including bleeding and headaches, which some researchers minimized as "discomforts" that went away over time. These "discomforts" were so severe for some women that they opted to have their IUDs removed at hospitals, or even attempted to remove the devices on their own. Not surprisingly, few of these women could be counted on to continue using the recommended method.[106] Perhaps most damagingly to the reputation of the IUD, dissatisfied users shared their negative experiences with other women, discouraging them.

The quiet rejection of contraception by dissatisfied users contrasted with the open and hostile opposition demonstrated by certain women and, especially, the husbands of female users.[107] Family planning workers anticipated some of these reactions and took proactive measure, such as asking women to have a signed consent form from their husbands, especially before IUD insertions. Not all women adhered to the recommendation, of course: some refused; some faked their husbands' signatures; and some did not have husbands. Health workers were rarely strict about enforcing the need for consent letters. As Dr. Jorge Ascenzo coyly admitted, "you know all rules have exceptions."[108] What some did do was ask women not to reveal their new status as users to their husbands. Keeping the secret was not always possible, and, on occasion, men beat their wives once they found out: "[Men] would ask [women] 'why did you do this? You are trying to cheat on me! [¡eres una mañosa!]' We would tell [women] 'it was your choice! You have so many children already, and you cannot support them. So why did you tell him? Once you decided, you should have kept your mouth shut.' We then had to remove the IUD, or else they would have been beaten to death."[109]

Sexual jealousy was the most common reason for men's violent outbursts. Nevertheless, some men were also genuinely concerned for the physical safety of their birth control–using partners, as well as for the sexual looseness contraception might encourage. Some men approached the family planning clinics with their children, attempting to shame providers and to blame them for the strife they had caused in the men's home lives.[110] "Only bad women want birth control. . . . My wife is not a bad woman," some men lamented as they sought an explanation as to why health workers had thus violated and corrupted their wives.[111] Family planning workers reported little success confronting or persuading angry men on behalf of female users in the face of such negative reactions, which the workers recalled with a mix of pity and revulsion.

## Who, Why, How

Historically contextualized accounts encompassing the experiences and emotions of the first Latin American family planning workers are still rare.[112] In a way, this is understandable in a field that is only beginning to attract attention. At the same time, the features of the Peruvian case indicate the emergence of broad outlines useful for future comparisons across the region. The first of these features is the protean nature of the workforce involved in birth control activities between the 1950s and 1970s. Physicians, medical students, biomedical researchers, social scientists, pharmaceutical company representatives, nurses, social workers, hacienda owners, and volunteers: all part of a wide-ranging and loosely coordinated group. The field was rife with opportunity for entrepreneurial individuals and organizations to receive training, equipment, educational and promotional materials, travel opportunities, networking prospects, cash, and the less tangible but no less important appreciation of patients-turned-users.

Of course, those working in this field rarely mentioned profit and career advancement as reasons that motivated them. Instead, they stressed the sacrifices they made to persuade colleagues and lay people of the value of family planning to protect women's lives from risky pregnancies and abortions and to prevent families and communities from sinking further into poverty. On the other hand, it is also true that the services provided, from the IUD on down to advice sessions, reinforced health workers' authority. While this mode of action helped protect women's health, it seldom empowered users to take charge of their reproductive decisions, much less question some of the model's possible perversions and limitations, such as the emergence of instances of abuse by physicians, the exclusion of men as users of birth control, the targeting of the poor, and the dismissal of iatrogenic problems as simple discomforts.

Although opportunities for professional advancement existed, promoting birth control use was also riddled with pitfalls. Institutional and state support was tenuous. Stirring interest among health workers took time and money. Interfacing with local and foreign stakeholders and canvassing communities to let people know of the availability of what were radically new and unfamiliar services required a tremendous effort by many. Making women keep their appointments for IUD insertions was a task in itself. Countering the stories disseminated by dissatisfied IUD users was difficult. Persuading leaders in organized communities required careful negotiation skills that birth control advocates sometimes lacked. Compensating for setbacks such as the closing of the APPF reveals how flexible local advocates and their foreign allies had to be.

Considering this picture, it is difficult to think of birth control as something that Latin American family planning workers could simply impose on the general population. The wide-ranging initiatives supported by the governments of Chile and Colombia in the 1960s were far from the rule in the region.[113] What we witnessed in Peru and other parts of Latin America between the 1950s and 1970s, instead, was the development of vast, complex, and fragile local family planning establishments that managed, despite great odds and flaws, to convince many women and men of the value of having fewer children. Governments did not automatically warm up to these social phenomena. The history of governmental participation in contraceptive matters continues in the next chapter.

## CHAPTER FIVE

# The Government Steps In (and Out)

*Family Planning and Population Policymaking*

Teasing out the historical distinctiveness of population policy formulation is a fruitful way to address the aspirations and interests of different societies, and different groups within those societies. As I argued in chapter 1, Latin American republics' attempts to understand and control the size, composition, and geographical movements of their populations can be traced to the late eighteenth century. These attempts gathered momentum in the early twentieth century with increasingly efficient state agencies and the imperative to build up the "right kind" of population. The twentieth century also added new technical possibilities to regulate fertility, and the post–World War II period brought to life institutions such as the United Nations (UN) and the World Health Organization (WHO), whose legitimacy contemporary Latin American governments accepted inasmuch as these organizations recognized Latin Americans as valid interlocutors.

As they had before, Latin American policymakers in the mid-twentieth century continued asking themselves how, for example, could the management of population characteristics help a nation become wealthier? How could it protect the lives of women and infants? How did it affect phenomena such as migration and the provision of social services? Who should be technically and politically responsible for the implementation of these policies? What national resources should they receive? Yet, the mid-twentieth century availability of programs and technologies to manage fertility added a new twist to the story, one that can help us better understand the extent to which population limitation fit the agendas of governments in the developing world.

The focus of this chapter is the interactions between Peruvian, Latin American, and U.S. agents and ideas, which led to the consideration, for the first time in Peruvian history, of family planning as an aspect of national policy. Latin American governments in the mid-twentieth century saw family planning policies through the lens of their aspirations to greater socioeconomic development and improved health for women and children. The integration of family planning alongside other, more established objectives such as the management of migration, the improvement of sanitation and education, the reduction of poverty, the creation of employment, and the increase of agricultural and industrial productivity did not lend itself to any simple reconciliation. U.S. organizations and their Latin American allies were staunch proponents of the notion that family planning was consistent with the goal of national development. Such commonality of purpose belied the fact that pro–birth control institutions also competed among themselves, as their visions of family planning policymaking were not identical. Moreover, the transition from a civilian to a military government in Peru in 1968 gives us the opportunity to appreciate the continuities and changes between two very different forms of political regimes.

## Global Population Studies

Mid-twentieth-century population policy development in Latin America partook of a broader conversation about the relations between existing resources and the possibilities for "Third World" nations' progress. The 1945 charter of the United Nations Organization called for the establishment of a Population Commission within the UN's Economic and Social Council. Frank Notestein, then a demographer at Princeton University, became the first UN population adviser, and the Peruvian Alberto Arca Parró became the first president of the Population Commission. The commission's role was to advise the UN council on matters such as changes in the size and structure of population, the interplay of demographic factors and economic and social ones, and policies designed to influence the size and structure of population.[1] In addition to the Population Commission, the UN established the Economic Commission for Latin America (ECLA) in 1948, which encouraged a more systematic collection of population data.[2] Underlying ECLA's thirst for demographic knowledge was the understanding that population increases, decreases, and movements were intimately linked to phenomena in the politicoeconomic sphere, including individual incomes, natural resource consumption, industrial productivity, and governmental stability.[3]

Consistent with the belief in the link between population changes and economic and social development, in 1949 the UN determined to help the governments of member countries elaborate population policies. Most requests for help were for conducting censuses, for the training of statisticians, and for the funding of regional seminars on demography, rather than for population-limitation assistance. A few years later, the UN began cooperating with local institutions for the further production of demographic knowledge. Accordingly, the Population Commission helped create regional demographic training and research centers in Chembur, India (1956), Santiago, Chile (1957), and Cairo, Egypt (1963).[4] The UN regional center in Santiago, named the Centro Latino Americano de Demografía (CELADE), played a crucial role in the dissemination of new knowledge about population trends and in the training of Latin American demographers at a time when university and governmental research in Latin America in this field was negligible and uncoordinated.[5]

Besides advanced training, CELADE also provided technical assistance. In the late 1950s, the United Nations launched its Population Census Program. Thanks to this initiative, 157 countries carried out comprehensive national censuses between 1958 and 1963. Peru benefited from CELADE's help in the performance of its Sixth National Population Census in 1961.[6] According to this census, the country's population had grown to over 10 million people, up from 7 million in 1940.[7] National authorities were transparent in their admission that Peru's demographic growth had been explosive. The introduction of antibiotics and DDT in the 1950s had, according to the National Institute of Planning, halved mortality rates, which previously had been grievously high, especially among malnourished infants when exposed to common infectious diseases such as tuberculosis, smallpox, malaria, and poliomyelitis. Total mortality rates dropped from 27.1 per 1,000 in 1940 to 15.4 per 1,000 in 1961, with life expectancy increasing from thirty-six years in 1940 to fifty-one in 1961, and birth rates increasing slightly from 44 per 1,000 in 1940 to 45.4 in 1961. Given these figures, the future rapid growth of the Peruvian population was guaranteed, a pattern repeated in virtually all of Latin America.[8]

In addition to training and technical assistance, CELADE disseminated research produced mainly in the United States. Importantly, some U.S. scholars and activists in the 1940s and 1950s had begun to treat population growth as a threat to the collective well-being of humanity.[9] In 1945, Princeton University's Frank Notestein predicted that food scarcity would become more likely once the world's population grew past 3 billion. Environmentalist William Vogt, future director of the Planned Parenthood Federation of America, warned of the need for humans to take better care of the planet's supply of natural resources. Economist Richard Nelson formulated his theory of the "low-level equilibrium trap," in which economic development was hampered despite modest increases in the gross domestic product because per capita income was outstripped by population growth. Demographers Ansley Coale and Edgar Hoover argued that an increase in the number of young people in a developing country negatively affected the country's chances of cultivating its own industrial base, because the young required expenditures in health and education, money that would not be available, at least in the short term, for technology acquisition and capital investments. Institutions such as the Population Council, the International Planned Parenthood Federation (IPPF), and the Population Crisis Committee advocated against population growth in developing countries and enthusiastically promoted the massive use of new contraceptive technologies, particularly hormonal drugs and the intrauterine device.[10]

## The Center for the Study of Population and Development

Several elements came together in early 1960s Peru that led to cautious governmental overtures in favor of family planning, including funding from foreign agencies, the availability of new contraceptives, greater emphasis on the governmental planning function, and the legitimacy conferred to demographic and fertility research by entities such as the UN. Cornell University sociologist Joseph Stycos, working as an adviser to the Population Council, was among the first to encourage, unsuccessfully, greater family planning involvement on the part of the Peruvian government. His presence in Peru at the time was no coincidence. Cornell attained a prominent place in the national research scene when it took on the Vicos Project in 1952. The project's goal, to modernize an impoverished rural area in the central Andes, led to short- and long-term sojourns of a sizable contingent of U.S. social scientists in Peru until 1966, when the project ended.[11]

Following an IPPF family planning "Seminar for Latin American Leaders" in New York in 1963, Stycos contacted a few of the Peruvian attendees. Banking on the organizers' view that the seminar had succeeded in making the Ministry of Health "very interested in family planning," Stycos meant to ask influential Peruvian physicians to support a plan for a Population Council–funded conference on limiting population growth.[12] During two trips to Peru in February and April 1964, Stycos met with Dr. David Tejada de Rivero, the Ministry of Health's director of planning, Senator Alberto Arca Parró, the architect of the 1940 census, and Minister of Health Javier Arias Stella. These men favored the idea of a conference such as the one the Population Council proposed to capitalize on the recent publication of the 1961 census results, as long as it remained an experts-and-bureaucrats-only affair, thus limiting the political exposure of a topic Peruvian politicians considered "very delicate."[13]

Despite having left with the impression that the conference would be convened, Stycos was disappointed to see that his Peruvian allies had made no progress toward that goal months after his departure. In fact, while the Population Council managed to carry out similar conferences in Mexico and Colombia in the interim, the Peruvians had simply stopped responding to Stycos's letters.[14] Meanwhile, Dr. Carlos Muñoz Torcello, a gynecologist and close adviser to President Fernando Belaúnde (his cousin by marriage, to boot), had been discussing population growth matters with an old mentor from Johns Hopkins University, gynecologist Nicholas Eastman. An adviser to the Ford Foundation, Eastman pointed out the potential convergence between Belaúnde's cautiousness and the Ford Foundation's own approach, which privileged the conduction of social science research before making national policy recommendations.[15] Quickly, Eastman brought Peru to the attention of Oscar "Bud" Harkavy, the Ford Foundation's population programs director. Eastman warned Harkavy that Peruvians were not ready "to establish clinics in every corner with intra-uterine devices and pills available for all comers," but that they were willing to set up a Division of Demography at the Ministry of Health. Moreover, engaging prestigious professionals such as Dr. Muñoz Torcello and Minister Arias Stella "would be a feather in our caps," as Eastman put it.[16]

This meeting of the minds led to the drafting of a proposal from Minister Arias Stella, submitted to the Ford Foundation by October 1964. The Program for Studies on Population Dynamics portrayed Peru as beset by an uneven geographic distribution of its population, shortages of housing, food, and health services, "social instability," and high rates of criminal abortion. Rapid population growth might play a role in these problems, but what relations between them might exist still needed to be made explicit to be of help to policymakers. The program would be managed through the Public Health Special Service, a semiautonomous agency with ties to the Ministry of Health created in 1962 to succeed the U.S.-funded Inter-American Cooperative Service in Public Health. Though most robustly linked to the public health establishment, the program would be supervised by a board with members drawn from the central government, the National Institute of Planning, and medical schools.[17]

Stung by the sudden turn of events, Stycos attributed the Ford Foundation's getting the upper hand in Peru to Eastman's being "in Lima at the right time."[18] This was an oversimplification: Peruvian leaders generally shied away from the Population Council's more aggressive emphasis on the promotion of contraception as the main ingredient of a governmental approach to the undeniable fact of rapid population growth. They gravitated instead toward the view, exemplified by the Ford approach, that the causes and consequences of population changes were related to complex socioeconomic phenomena, and concluded they still had much to learn about these phenomena.[19] The Program for Studies on Population Dynamics was renamed the Centro de Estudios de Población y Desarollo (Center for the Study of Population and Development, CEPD) and established by presidential decree in December 1964.

The promotion of birth control was not a part of the CEPD's original mandate. The founding charter of the CEPD only stated that "the close relationship between demographic growth and economic development should be systematically studied in order to formulate programs of action with which to face the problems of population and socioeconomic development, as has been consistently recommended by the General Assembly of the United Nations under the auspices of its Economic and Social Council." In addition to conducting and disseminating demographic research, the CEPD was to train population specialists and serve as liaison between the Peruvian government and foreign agencies interested in population issues.[20] Senator Alberto Arca Parró and Dr. Carlos Muñoz Torcello became the CEPD's president and vice president, respectively. The board also included Minister of Labor Frank Griffiths Escardó, and Numa León de Vivero, of the National Institute of Planning (INP).[21] In order to fund its activities, the CEPD reached out to the Ford Foundation, the Population Council, and the U.S. Agency for International Development (USAID). Ford personnel who read the Peruvian proposal were impressed by its breadth and commitment to seeing population issues as another aspect of national policymaking instead of seeking to quickly implement a population-limitation program, the kind that, in the foundation's eyes, was "gradually fashioning the substance of demography and population policy into a kind of animal husbandry."[22]

The Ford Foundation was the CEPD's main benefactor in its fragile first year, awarding it a grant for US$282,000 to cover salaries, research, training fellowships, and fees for foreign technical advisers.[23] Part of the CEPD's fragility stemmed from the fact that Congress would have to approve appropriations for it once foreign funding ended in 1968. With Congress controlled by the opposition APRA party, the CEPD was a likely candidate to become a pawn of political rivalries from its inception. Another source of organizational weakness was the fear the CEPD created among officers in other government agencies, particularly within the Office of Statistics and the Census, the National School of Public Health, and the Ministry of Education, who worried the CEPD might duplicate their work and wondered, not without reason, why some of Ford's generous funding had not reached them.[24]

Against this tense background of promise and peril, the CEPD organized its first conference in December 1965 south of Lima, in the town of Paracas. The meeting gathered seventy-four guests from the Organization of American States, CELADE, the Food and Agriculture Organization, the Pan-American Health Organization, the USAID, the Ford Foundation, the Population Council, and several ministries. CEPD director Alberto Arca Parró opened the meeting with an explosive admission: Latin America could not match its population growth with corresponding levels of economic and social development. President Belaúnde concurred, admitting that "the demographic explosion is a reality," and calling on all government sectors to brace for further population growth.[25] Foreign observers' reactions to the CEPD's maiden event were positive. Ozzie Simmons, director of the Institute of Behavioral Science at the University of Colorado and Ford-appointed adviser to the CEPD, was impressed by the quality of the information shared, by the opening of channels of communication between people in strategic positions, and by the good press coverage of the conference. Frank Notestein, now president of the Population Council, congratulated Arca Parró by telling him that "as we have seen in other countries, this initial breaking of the ice is often the most difficult accomplishment, but usually leads to an increase in action and interest."[26]

Despite the CEPD's broad mandate for demographic research, it was clear to those present at the Paracas seminar that family planning projects were a priority for the new agency's leaders. With the conference over, Raúl Vargas, a sociologist working for the WHO in Buenos Aires, stepped down as executive director, and José Donayre, an endocrinologist from Cayetano Heredia University, who had trained with Gregory Pincus at the Worcester Foundation, took on the job.[27] Ozzie Simmons's parting advice to Donayre, the CEPD's president, and the board was to "encourage and plan action programs in family planning" by launching a series of birth control pilot programs, which "can reveal much about the feasibility, operation, and effectiveness of methods of family planning," and by carrying out surveys of knowledge, attitudes, and practices regarding contraception and abortion among "all sorts of decision makers and gatekeepers."[28]

The CEPD took this advice and moved family planning in a muscular new direction with the assistance of a new partner, the USAID. Until the mid-1960s, the U.S. government had been reluctant to support population limitation in developing countries. Early recommendations to do so for the sake of accelerating economic development and neutralizing communist inroads, such as the recommendations made by the Draper Committee in 1958, were sidelined by both the Eisenhower and Kennedy administrations.[29] When Joseph Stycos began knocking on Peruvian doors asking for support for a population conference, the officers at the USAID Lima office struck him as lacking initiative. "If Washington expected something out of them," he complained, "they would have to specify it and give it high priority."[30]

The first overt sign of change was President Lyndon Johnson's State of the Union address on January 4, 1965. At that time, Johnson vowed to "seek new ways to use our knowledge to help deal with the explosion in world population and the growing scarcity in world resources." Shortly after that, the USAID sent a policy directive to directors in all countries, indicating that "AID would entertain requests for technical, commodity, and local currency assistance in support of family planning programs initiated by host governments."[31] More specifically, in 1966, Jonathan Fine of the USAID Latin America Bureau in Washington began to circulate, informally and confidentially, a working paper on population, promising recipients that it would become official U.S. policy "somewhere down the pike." It started by accusing multilateral aid agencies and Latin American governments, except those of Chile, Honduras, and Colombia, of being "slow to move from resolution to action," but also acknowledged the role the USAID ought to play persuading Latin American governments to submit requests for assistance, as well as its need to tailor interventions to the peculiarities of each country in the region. Regardless of the country strategies pursued, the USAID's main goals should be, according to Fine, to "create a climate of opinion" and "the network of services" that would extend "the knowledge and means of family limitation to all Latin American families."[32]

From 1966 on, the USAID could be found sponsoring, quietly but relentlessly, most family planning initiatives throughout the developing world. Its funds for these activities rose steadily, from US$10 million to nearly US$125 million between 1965 and 1972.[33] Such a shift was also responsible for the support the United States gave to the establishment of a new United Nations division, the Trust Fund for Population Activities, within the World Health Organization, and to the Pan-American Health Organization, which led to dramatic reversals of longstanding policies against the promotion of birth control on the part of the latter two organizations.[34] Between 1966 and 1968, the USAID also awarded some US$413,000 to Peru's CEPD, surpassing the

Ford Foundation's grants, and Jonathan Fine, recently appointed to the Peru USAID office, became an adviser to the CEPD alongside University of Florida sociologist John Saunders, representing the Ford Foundation. Meanwhile, the Peruvian government's share neared US$70,000, with smaller amounts provided by the Population Council, American Friends Service Committee, and the Pathfinder Fund.[35] Given the financial and technical contributions the U.S. government made to the CEPD, the latter's claim to be "free from any kind of political pressure" was, at best, naïve and, at worst, disingenuous.[36]

By mid-1968, the CEPD had held a Conference on Population and the Family, an International Seminar on Physiology of Reproduction and Advances in Fertility Regulation, and a Conference on the Family, Childhood, and Youth in National Development. Its small staff conducted research on a variety of topics, including women's attitudes toward gestation, the effect of iodine on reproduction, and the incidence of abortion, by itself and in collaboration with the National Institute of Planning, Cayetano Heredia University, the Catholic University, the Ministry of Health, the Pan-American Sanitary Bureau, the Instituto Indigenista, and the Ministry of Labor. The CEPD had also sent fifty-nine experts to short demography courses at CELADE in Chile and funded seven master's and doctoral scholarships abroad and eighteen local baccalaureate undergraduate thesis students. It also produced two promotional films, *Dos Familias* and *Datos Explosivos*.[37] Given the novelty of population studies in Latin America, the CEPD's productivity in the 1960s was remarkable.

Yet, a significant amount of executive director José Donayre's time and energy in this period was devoted to the set up of a series of pilot birth control operations in Lima:[38] the ambulatory clinics of the Christian Family Movement, the Pamplona Alta maternal and child health clinic, the IUD program at the Hospital de Enfermedades Neoplásicas, and the family planning clinics at the Bravo Chico Hospital in El Agustino and at the Preventive Medicine Center in Breña.[39] Whereas the Ford Foundation and the Population Council declined to fund these clinics, the USAID agreed to do so, and approvingly compared Peru's "logarithmic phase of increase in family planning activities" to Colombia's.[40]

The lessons learned through the CEPD pilot clinics became one of the pillars of the Family Planning, Genital Cancer Screening, and Abortion Prevention Project, a nationwide program the Ministry of Health approved in early 1968 to make family planning a routine part of maternal and child care services in all Ministry of Health facilities. The second pillar was the sweeping convergence supporting family planning as an aspect of Latin American socioeconomic policymaking in the late 1960s. The first meeting of Latin American government officers with the goal of establishing region-wide population policies had taken place in Caracas, Venezuela, in September 1967.[41] The Caracas Report made it clear that population policies focusing mainly on the provision of birth control services would not suffice. Dealing with rapid population growth would require adopting additional policies that expanded foreign trade and improved its terms. Recognizing that most Latin American governments' incomes depended on the export of primary commodities, this recommendation addressed the chronic insolvency of governments and the difficulties this caused for the delivery of social services. The Caracas Report also urged the adoption of new policies to modernize and broaden educational systems, placing special emphasis on the education of women and adults who were already in the workforce, as well as the reduction of rural poverty.

It is important to note the influence of former ECLA director Raúl Prebisch on the trade, education, and rural development theses of the Caracas Report, which shone through most clearly in his short 1964 treatise *Towards a New Trade Policy for Development*. There, Prebisch had also argued for regional integration as a means for developing countries to leverage their bargaining power in negotiations with industrialized ones. The formation of economic blocs and the issuance of joint regional policies, such as the Caracas Report, were means to that end. And, while Prebisch continued to support ECLA's 1950s view of rapid population growth as a brake on development, he also warned that limiting it could not "in any sense be an alternative to the vigorous development policy advocated in this report."[42]

The Family Planning, Genital Cancer Screening, and Abortion Prevention Project was the result of both the experience acquired through the CEPD pilot programs in family planning and the pan–Latin American commitment to treating family planning as an element of socioeconomic policymaking. As part of the agreement, the Peruvian Ministry of Health would adapt its infrastructure and reassign and retrain the necessary human resources for the program. The USAID would pay for the remainder, approximately US$1.25 million, disbursed through agreements with the Pan-American Health Organization, the Ministry of Health, and the CEPD.[43] The project's first stage would focus on the Lima and Callao region, where eighteen Ministry of Health facilities would start providing family planning services and education within existing Maternal and Child Health units, as well as training in contraception for physicians and paramedical personnel. In a second stage, all Ministry of Health hospitals and health posts, particularly those in rural areas, would join the program. As this stage matured, it would gradually shift its emphasis away from birth control and toward preventive medicine and nutrition training for medical and paramedical personnel.[44]

The CEPD became the receiving and administrative entity for the totality of the project's funds. At first, the Ministry of Health's commission that designed the project had not considered the CEPD as the project's ideal administrative home. Instead, it had projected bestowing this responsibility on the Peruvian Association for Family Protection (APPF), a private network of birth control clinics and providers affiliated with the IPPF.[45] This original design was based on the experience of the Profamilia private program in Colombia. There were, however, several reasons why Peruvian health policymakers ultimately refused to follow the Colombian example and chose the CEPD instead. First, unlike Profamilia, the APPF was still a relatively young network, lacking the administrative resources to run a national program. Second, the CEPD had already shown it had the organizational agility to channel resources in a manner attuned to the Ministry of Health's priorities. Third, the CEPD's position as a semi-independent research institution somewhat sheltered the government from the potential charge of harboring a population-limitation agenda, a very damaging accusation to befall the Ministry of Health as President Belaúnde's term came to a close.

The ministry's decision was controversial. The Population Council acknowledged the talent of the CEPD's personnel and realized the strategic import of giving the organization this responsibility, but the council warned the minister that the CEPD would not "be able to assume the massive responsibilities of a national program," at least not without increasing its staff of four and increasing its authority to match its new duties.[46] Peter Fraenkel, the Ford Foundation's representative in Peru, suspected the Peruvian government's decision to pursue a national family planning program through the CEPD would weaken the latter's fledgling but promising research and educational initiatives and feared that, should the program fail, "the Center is likely to go down with it."[47] More critically still, William Moore, a Ford Foundation consultant, believed Minister Arias Stella was treating the CEPD "as a funnel through which USAID money can be diverted into the Ministry of Health for use, supposedly, to develop a controversial family planning program in an election year." Moore ominously predicted that, "should political or religious lightning strike," it would be "almost certain that the Center will be burned to a crisp and not unlikely that the Ministry of Health will also get a considerable jolt." Minister Arias Stella condescendingly told Moore that he "sounded just like Peter Fraenkel."[48]

Not all within the Ford Foundation were as negative as Fraenkel or Moore. John Saunders, the Ford Foundation–appointed adviser to the CEPD, believed that PAHO's approval and technical support of the project bode well for it, especially after the ministry reduced the number of family planning clinics it projected to open from eighteen to less than half that, so as to focus on the quality of the services provided and reduce the visibility of the USAID's funding.[49] Meanwhile, William Dentzer Jr., USAID director in Peru, did not hide his delight, believing that "recent developments in Peru give every indication that population dynamics and family planning will be a program area not merely of promise in the period 1968–1970, but of fulfillment."[50] Despite all these preparations, anxiety, and enthusiasm, the program was never implemented. The "Revolutionary Government of the Armed Forces" took care of that.

## Planning Families the Army Way

The military strongman has been a recurring character in the political life of republican Latin America. In Peru, none of these strongmen achieved the intellectual or organizational sophistication of the reformist military leaders of the 1950s. The changes began during the regime of General Manuel Odría, who became president following a coup against President José Luis Bustamante y Rivero in 1948. It had been during Bustamante's presidency that officers such as Minister of War José del Carmen Marín began to envision the creation of an advanced training institute similar to the war colleges of Spain and France, both of which trained Marín.

Peru enjoyed a brief economic bonanza during Odría's rule thanks to the development of the local fishmeal industry and the discovery of copper in the south. In addition, the Korean War (1950–53) increased foreign demand for Peruvian goods. In 1950, Odría reinvented himself as a civilian candidate for the presidential race, which he won while running unopposed. As president, Odría further liberalized the trade controls that favored mining and agricultural corporations. Deliberately cutting back the governmental planning function, Odría did not even honor Peru's international commitment to conduct a census in 1950.[51] Odría also passed a number of laws in the early 1950s that decreased taxes for military personnel who had large families, increased the salaries of public health personnel and teachers with many children, and made being married and having a large family prerequisites for those seeking to buy homes in the newly created housing projects of Risso, in Lima.[52] The early 1950s were also significant because officers such as José del Carmen Marín, sidelined from executive posts because of their allegiance to the deposed Bustamante, went on to establish the Center for Advanced Military Studies (CAEM) within the Ministry of War. The CAEM's mission was to train officers destined for high command posts to think in terms of long-term strategies of national security through a curriculum that included social science education. CAEM's doctrine was based on the view of war as something that required the utilization of all human and material resources of the nation.

Concretely, CAEM promoted the idea that strategic natural resources such as oil, minerals, and fisheries ought to be in the hands of the Peruvian government and not be dominated by foreign corporations. In addition, CAEM supported the creation of a national strategic planning institute, along with the conduction of regional development projects to better secure frontier areas and relieve rural poverty. CAEM's slogan, "no defense without development," described well its philosophy. The center adopted a critical attitude toward governmental neglect of rural areas and the abuses heaped on the poor by Peru's powerful because this created resentment, exacerbated conflicts, and turned the people against agents of the state, such as the military. CAEM's reformist perspective gradually became hegemonic among Peru's military officers and even popular among political actors opposed to Odría. Just as important, CAEM fashioned a new image for Peru's military as the nation's foremost development agent: patriotic and competent.[53]

The military played a crucial role during the contested 1962 elections. Surprisingly, the APRA party's Victor Raúl Haya de la Torre had made a deal with his past nemesis, former dictator Manuel Odría.[54] With rumors of fraud thickening, the military intervened. A coup removed President Manuel Prado from office in July 1962, and General Ricardo Pérez Godoy established a governing junta. It was that regime (1962–63) that began to implement the reforms CAEM had been demanding for over a decade. The junta created the National System for Economic and Social Planning and its main technical body, the Instituto Nacional de Planificación (INP).[55] The fact that this was one of the few actions the military government took before calling for new elections is indicative of the high regard Peru's military elite had for national strategic planning, and of the extent of CAEM's influence over this elite.

Fernando Belaúnde, whose Acción Popular party had lost to APRA in 1962, won the 1963 election. His administration continued supporting the newly minted INP and created the CEPD. Though not in power, military officers kept watchful eyes over the country's political direction and became increasingly disappointed with the elected civilians. Despite the infrastructure-building boom of the early 1960s, peasant and leftist guerrilla uprisings checked Belaúnde's presidency. The violent repression of the uprisings not only discredited the president but also the military, which retreated into a position that was increasingly critical of the social inequalities that had given rise to the uprisings in the first place. In addition, almost from the beginning of his administration, Belaúnde had had to deal with the fact that APRA and the supporters of former president Manuel Odría mounted an effective opposition in Congress, which, among other things, limited the CEPD's budget and scope of action.[56]

The tipping point was Belaúnde's inability to prevail upon the International Petroleum Company (a subsidiary of the Rockefeller-controlled Standard Oil) in negotiations over the profits generated by the oil fields on Peru's northern coast. Alienated, a wing of the military, led by General Juan Velasco Alvarado, stepped back into the limelight and ousted Belaúnde in October 1968. With celerity, Velasco nationalized the disputed oil fields. Then, he set out to organize his grandest project, his most controversial one, and the one that failed most spectacularly: the agrarian reform, which aimed to redistribute the country's arable land, 76 percent of which was in the hands of just 0.5 percent of all landowners.[57]

The coup led to several immediate changes at the CEPD. Its president, Alberto Arca Parró, and vice president, Carlos Muñoz Torcello, quit in protest. José Donayre stayed on as executive director, but the USAID's Jonathan Fine stepped down as adviser, leaving only the Ford Foundation's John Saunders in that role. The new government's attitude toward the population policy crafted by the previous government remained unknown until Donayre submitted the proposal for the Family Planning, Genital Cancer Screening, and Abortion Prevention Project, renamed the Plan to Extend and Improve the Maternal and Child Health Program, to the new health minister, the CAEM-trained Major Eduardo Montero Rojas. In his reply, Major Montero praised the project's goals of reducing maternal and child mortality and morbidity, curbing abortion rates, and improving women's and infants' nutrition, but he ruled out family planning. The CEPD's plan "must only include actions related to sex education, and sanitary education for maternal and child health, eliminating completely any reference to family planning or any method of birth control, which must not be mentioned, much less used."[58] Montero's categorical decision was followed by a January 1969 order from the cabinet to shut down all the pilot family planning clinics the CEPD had set up.[59]

If Donayre held any hopes for the resuscitation of the family planning program, they were dashed in the next few months. Dr. David Tejada de

Rivero, second-in-command at the Ministry of Health, reviewed the government's stagnating policies regarding population. As a result, the USAID was allowed to continue supporting private family planning programs, such as the APPF, the Instituto Marcelino, and the Christian Family Movement clinics. In Tejada's view, however, the CEPD needed to change the image of "an anti-natalist, population control organization" that it had acquired because of its USAID-sponsored birth control projects.[60] Tejada's plan contemplated a scaled-down version of the original, focusing on the provision of oral contraceptives within Ministry of Health facilities in the city of Lima. Private family planning providers were free to set up or maintain their operations outside of the capital, as well as to use a broader range of contraceptives. The CEPD's new role would be to monitor the quality of family planning services available nationwide. Its other educational and population research functions remained unchanged. The Ministry of Health would also designate a larger number of representatives to the CEPD's board, thus diminishing the executive director's power.[61]

John Saunders tried to reassure the disappointed Donayre by pointing out that evaluation and training had been, by original design, the areas in which the CEPD could best contribute to an official family planning policy. In addition, the ministry modifications of the CEPD's initial project created an "opportunity to place renewed emphasis on socioeconomic studies." Donayre's failure to act on the latter request began to strain the CEPD's relation with the Ford Foundation.[62] A year into Velasco's rule, Ford auditors squarely blamed the formerly esteemed CEPD executive director for the center's loss of momentum as a producer of population insights for policymakers. The auditors thought that Donayre, with input from John Saunders, elected education fellowship awardees with little more than a rubberstamp from the CEPD board and later failed to use the awardees' talents, that the institution's research program was ad hoc and incoherent, that the staff Donayre hired added little technical prestige to the CEPD's image, that there was no way of knowing how influential all the workshops and talks the CEPD sponsored had been with attendees, and that nobody of importance read the *Boletín CEPD*.[63]

The Ford Foundation's audit concluded that the CEPD never coalesced into a distinctive enterprise and remained merely "the pieces of a foundation, mostly in the form of sponsored studies and scattered fellowship holders, unharnessed by either the Center or the decision-makers to program objectives."[64] Donayre, not surprisingly, had started to look forward to leaving the CEPD. In fact, the very continuity of the center was now in question.

In late 1970, the Cabinet squashed the possibility, favored by Donayre, of the CEPD being absorbed by a proposed new Ministry of Planning.[65] Shortly after, Donayre took a post in the Latin American Division of the UN's Fund for Population Activities (UNFPA) and helped promote Dr. Federico Moncloa, an old colleague of his from Cayetano Heredia University, as his replacement.

Moncloa was a savvy choice as executive director. He was amenable to working within the strictures of a more active board and, given his sympathy toward Velasco's reforms, he was "less objectionable to public officials and intellectuals" than Donayre was.[66] The CEPD's self-assigned mission for the 1970s was to strengthen the competence of public sector agencies in population matters. To this end, the CEPD proposed to continue subsidizing baccalaureate theses as well as graduate study fellowships. In addition, the CEPD would strive to find internships for recent graduates and recently returned fellows within governmental and academic institutions. Returning fellows would also become eligible to submit fundable research proposals to the CEPD. Among the new research the CEPD began to conduct was the production of monthly unemployment statistics for the Ministry of Labor, a priority area for Velasco. The Peruvian government, the USAID, the Ford Foundation, and the Population Council funded the reinvigorated CEPD mission.[67]

Unfortunately, the obstacles the CEPD board placed before Moncloa became too burdensome. Especially frustrating was his inability to hire and retain high-caliber demographers Roque García Frias, Alicia Unger, Alván Zarate, and Krishna Roy. A defeated Moncloa resigned in April 1972 to become the medical director of Merck Sharpe & Dohme Peru.[68] His replacement, Dr. Arnaldo Cano, chief of army psychological evaluations, did not arrive for months. In the interim, the publication of the *Boletín CEPD* became erratic, and the graduate fellowships program stopped.[69] External observers were disappointed with Cano's poor understanding of CEPD operations and with his lack of initiative in putting the funds at his disposal to good use.[70] Compounding matters was the government's dismissive attitude toward the CEPD, demonstrated by its delay in appointing not only Cano but also delegates to the organization's board. The kiss of death came in 1972, when the government froze the CEPD's budget at a time of rising inflation.

Amid staff desertions and generalized low morale, the government's first population agency agonized until its final demise in 1975, when the Ford Foundation, its first and last supporter, declined to renew its financial aid. After ten years together, Ford officers self-critically admitted they had given the CEPD too many responsibilities and leeway as a producer of research on population and family planning, when in actuality it might have been a more sustainable enterprise with more circumscribed duties as a promoter of research conducted by others. They saved their harshest judgment, however, not for themselves, or for the Ministry of Health, but for the USAID, whose "plethora of money and paucity of judgment" seduced Donayre into building an overly ambitious family planning program, in the process irrevocably impairing the CEPD's credibility before an important group of government officials and professionals, and even tarnishing the Ford Foundation's very reputation.[71]

## Family Planning Politics after the CEPD

The USAID and the UNFPA had stopped supporting the CEPD in 1973, long before its final hour.[72] It had already become clear to them that family planning had a low priority for the military government. Contraceptives, for one, were not part of the Ministry of Health's Basic Medicines program, which meant those interested in obtaining birth control would have to pay full price or be referred to an APPF, Instituto Marcelino, or Christian Family Movement clinic. Wariness of the U.S. government's history of supporting population limitation through the promotion of family planning was only one of the reasons for Velasco's antipathy toward contraception. The idea of Latin America as an underpopulated area with vast regions still to colonize and riches to exploit had been popular among Latin American intellectuals since the eighteenth century.[73] Military personnel that considered Peru's borders unsecured had an additional reason to mistrust population limitation. In fact, Velasco was so worried that Peruvians living in frontier zones would register their children as something other than Peruvians when they could not find a civil registration office nearby that he eased the procedure and gave municipalities the power to conduct these registrations.[74]

Peru's National Development Plan of 1971–75 contained no explicit discussion of population pressures in relation to development. Although it acknowledged shortages of employment opportunities, schools, and physicians, the plan did not consider population growth a cause or contributing factor to any of these shortages. Moreover, although it reported demographic data such as the rate of population growth, mortality rates, and current and projected economically active population rates, the plan did not concern itself with other important indicators such as fertility rates, projections of future population size, and projections of future school-age population. The plan was optimistic about Peru's economic development prospects, stating that the government's agrarian reform would increase productive capacity to such an extent that "it will permit the living standards of the majority of poor people of the country to rise without extreme sacrifices by the middle class."[75]

Scuttled as a component of a national development plan, family planning was still a carefully regulated aspect of Velasco's reform of Peruvian maternal and child health services. The country's health expenses had been growing for the previous twenty years by the time of Velasco's coup, from US$4.2 million in 1945, to US$23.6 million in 1956, to US$68.3 million in 1968, or about 6 percent of the national GDP.[76] However, committed as he was to underwriting the costs of the agrarian reform, Velasco reduced the health sector's proportion of the national budget. By 1971, the Ministry of Health was assigned only 3.7 percent of the GDP. This allowed the ministry to run its 335 hospitals, 388 health centers, and 936 rural sanitary posts. In addition, there were 7,818 physicians, 3,722 nurses, and 13,200 nurse assistants in the public sector, most of whom worked in Lima. More specifically for the maternal and child health subsector, there were about 2,900 beds available in public obstetrics/gynecology units, as well as 591 gynecologists, 994 university-trained midwives, and 340 pediatricians.[77] Velasco tried to increase the accessibility of health services through, for example, the law of Civil Service for Medical Graduates (SECIGRA), and the transfer of the charitable Beneficence Society hospitals to the authority of the Ministry of Health.[78]

Reforms to the maternal and child health subsector started with a new Sanitary Code, promulgated in 1969, that defined women's health needs as exclusively related to pregnancy, motherhood, and the postpartum period.[79] Velasco's main vehicle for the implementation of maternal and child health reforms was the Institute of Neonatology and Maternal-Infant Protection (INPROMI), created in 1971.[80] Again, regional coordination had played a role in the formulation of Peru's national objectives. The meeting of American Chiefs of State of Punta del Este (Uruguay) of 1967 had committed all attendees to strengthening their maternal and child health programs. These agreements were reaffirmed in subsequent meetings of Health Ministers of the Americas in 1968 (in Buenos Aires) and in 1972 (in Santiago), sponsored by the Pan-American Health Organization.[81] It was a significant step, as maternal and child health then became a PAHO priority area, on a par with the control of infectious diseases, the most important item in PAHO's agenda throughout the 1950s.[82]

To Velasco, improving maternal and child health not only fulfilled his international commitments but was also a lever for economic development and the political consolidation of his regime. "Making people aware of their right to health," INPROMI declared, "will make them more willing to organize politically to demand health services. As their demands are progressively addressed, productivity will increase."[83] Velasco did not just hope for healthier citizens. He looked forward to politically inspired and mobilizable citizens who readily acknowledged the benefits the Revolutionary Government of the Armed Forces wrought, particularly in areas where the agrarian reform was under way.

There was indeed much to demand from Peru's health services. The nation's maternal mortality rate in 1973 neared 24.5 per 1,000 infants born alive. Hemorrhages, toxemias, lack of hygiene during interventions, and induced abortion explained, in that order, most of the mortality observed. In terms of children's health, over 30 percent of all deaths in Peru occurred among children younger than one year of age. Preventable diseases such as diarrhea, respiratory infections, poliomyelitis, measles, diphtheria, tetanus, and tuberculosis accounted for most of these fatalities. Still, according to INPROMI, "the real underlying factor" for such high mortality rates was poverty, expressed as a series of widespread social ills including unemployment, illiteracy, inadequate health services, insufficient housing, and bad sanitation.[84] Like the CEPD, INPROMI was a semiautonomous agency with links to the Ministry of Health, receiving financial support from the USAID and UNFPA and technical support from the PAHO. In its heyday, it numbered about 300 employees, mainly physicians and nurses at the Children's Hospital in Lima. Its main role was to design guidelines to be implemented throughout Ministry of Health facilities. The closeness of INPROMI's three directors, physicians Luis Suarez, René Cervantes, and Antonio Meza Cuadra, to General Velasco was decidedly an asset. While the CEPD lingered on starved of funds, the INPROMI's budget was increased sixfold from 1971 to 1973.[85]

One of the problems INPROMI wished to address immediately was the low frequency of pre- and postnatal checkups. The number of women who had access to and used these services varied by region. In urban areas such as Lima, some 34.6 percent of pregnant and parturient women had regular checkups, whereas in rural areas near Huancavelica, for example, the number dropped to a mere 1.3 percent. INPROMI's goal was to extend checkups to at least 60 percent of all pregnant and parturient women by the end of the 1970s, with each woman meeting a physician at least four times during her pregnancy.[86] The assumption was that frequent clinical encounters could prevent potentially fatal complications that might emerge during a pregnancy. In addition, such encounters could be opportunities to impart notions about healthy lifestyles for women and infants, particularly the importance of vaccination and hygienic habits.[87]

It was also through this emphasis on pre- and postnatal clinical checkups that INPROMI revived the notion of family planning as part of a national policy. INPROMI's limited forays into family planning took PAHO's technical advice regarding contraception seriously. Dr. Abraham Horwitz, PAHO director from 1958 to 1974, had originally decided to focus his attention on the continental problems of malaria, scarcity of trained medical personnel, high infant mortality, low availability of water for human and industrial use, poor sanitation, and weak national health institutions, with the ultimate goal of contributing, through improved health, to the economic development of all American nations.[88] Preventing maternal mortality was not one of PAHO's early goals under Horwitz. It was thanks to pressure from the United States in the mid-1960s that PAHO's priorities began to shift. Yet, Horwitz remained unconvinced after three PAHO conferences on population dynamics that the liberalization of birth control would be more effective than curbing infectious diseases, training more clinicians, and improving general sanitation as a means to curb maternal mortality rates.[89]

Moreover, beyond the relevance of maternal health, Horwitz was well aware of the USAID's efforts to push population limitation onto the political agendas of developing countries through networking with professionals such as the ones who attended the PAHO conferences. Opponents of family planning, he feared, could construe this as a kind of indirect assault on national sovereignty that would lead to a backlash against maternal and child health units that provided birth control information and contraceptives. Horwitz challenged the 1967 conference attendees by insisting that the power of government experts in matters of contraceptive technologies ought to have limits, since there existed "great gaps in knowledge upon which judgment and decision must be founded." Speaking directly to the U.S. government officers in the audience, Horwitz acknowledged the existence of theses linking population growth and underdevelopment, but insisted on "the non-universality of any particular thesis" and the need for reproductive choices to be left up to "individual families." Ultimately, Horwitz believed, PAHO's actions as a regional WHO office must not exceed the WHO's mandate to provide family planning information only (1) if governments requested it; (2) if such programs aimed to ameliorate the health of women and children; and (3) if these programs did not interfere with health care systems' curing and preventive work.[90]

As Horwitz knew, INPROMI leaders were keen to preserve the substance and image of Peruvian sovereignty in health matters, and they resented the aggressive attitude of the United States in the field of family planning, which they believed threatened to turn state-supported maternal and infant health programs into fronts for the distribution of contraceptives.[91] Consequently, INPROMI's family planning component was watered down and subordinated to the provision of government-sanctioned health education for women in the context of the clinical checkup. Following a delivery, the attending clinician could, if he deemed it appropriate, "suggest an appropriate inter-parity interval"[92] to the new mother and let her know "about the availability of contraceptives by prescription" and of the contraceptive effect of prolonged breastfeeding.[93] This type of intervention was meant to "prevent the risks involved in frequent pregnancies and in pregnancies among very young women, and, especially, to prevent induced illegal abortions."[94]

Despite the curtailment of governmental contraceptive services, both the USAID and UNFPA continued to provide financial assistance to INPROMI.[95] Moreover, INPROMI was open to the possibility of collaborating with organizations that provided birth control services, including the APPF, in order to fulfill its mission of preventing the risks inherent in teen pregnancies, short interparity intervals, and induced abortion. Institutions such as APPF, partnering with INPROMI in Ministry of Health hospitals, however, were forbidden from providing direct contraceptive services and took charge only of patient and family education, health care provider training, research, and preparation of pedagogical materials.[96] Even maintaining this low level of family planning offerings, however, was not a priority for Velasco, who decided in 1974 to make all pregnancy, labor, and postpartum care free of charge in all Ministry of Health facilities. With the predictable rapid rise in demand for these services, the ministry's capacity to provide them suffered, particularly in Lima.[97] As a result, services deemed less politically expedient, such as family planning, became rarer in the public sector.

Toward mid-1973, the USAID announced it would stop supporting all of its population-related activities in Peru. Direct collaboration between the USAID and the Peruvian government on these issues resumed only in 1979, through Primary Health and Population Project 219, to provide family planning services in Ica, in south central Peru.[98] By then, the Second Phase of the Revolutionary Government of the Armed Forces, led by General Francisco Morales Bermúdez, had already convened a congressional assembly to draft a new constitution, after quietly removing General Velasco from office in

1975, backpedaling on the latter's cherished but failing agrarian reform project, and overseeing a transition to civilian rule in 1980.

A less publicized accomplishment of Morales Bermúdez's administration was his convening of the commission that drafted the Guidelines for Population Policy in 1976, to which I will return in the epilogue. The legitimacy this document conferred to family planning as an aspect of state development policies was key for the 1979 creation of the Division of Maternal and Child Health within the Ministry of Health. With this, the government finally embraced the need to institutionalize maternal and child health as a function of the central government, instead of one run from satellite organizations such as the CEPD or INPROMI. The government of President Fernando Belaúnde, elected in 1980, began providing some family planning services in state hospitals and promulgated the National Population Law in 1985, which went into effect only two years later, executed as the National Population Program.[99]

## The Local and the Regional in Population Policymaking

The earliest historiography of family planning in Latin America tends to focus on how foreign agents, mainly from the United States, carved a niche for family planning in a hostile territory dominated by the Catholic Church, conservative military forces, and left-leaning nationalists, all of whom allegedly deplored birth control as an imperialist tool.[100] This downplays the crucial participation of local agents institutionalizing birth control in their own countries, something that more recent scholarship has started to address, and which this chapter does for the Peruvian case.[101] In addition, somewhere between the stimulating focus on the peculiarities of each Latin American nation and the undeniable influence of U.S. ideas and money on post–World War II population policies, there is a vast, underexplored, and rich territory of inquiry that we have only begun to consider, one that emphasizes the common features of the region in response to the conundrum of determining the place of birth control programs within national development strategies.

Even before the U.S. government became interested in funding family planning worldwide, a number of organizations existed with that goal in mind, and, although linked by similar ideas and personal connections, they also competed to expand their programs in Latin America. The Ford Foundation, with its emphasis on social science research, was more successful persuading the Peruvian political elite than was the Population Council, which privileged more direct interventions. Competition persisted after the U.S. government entered the fray, most emblematically between the USAID's pressure to fund birth control as an element of maternal and child health services and PAHO's reluctance to do this. The contest was as much about bragging rights as it was about advancing different visions of the role of birth control in the political life of the developing world. Should research about the need and applicability of contraception policies take primacy over action? Would too great a focus on contraception detract from the provision of other important services? How much should policymakers know before making decisions on these vital issues? Nations such as Colombia, Chile, and Honduras answered these questions differently than Peru or Argentina did, yet all Latin American countries faced a similar set of problems charting paths toward greater socioeconomic development.

The emergence of the above questions depended on the previous establishment of a link between state-directed strategic planning and national development. Could governments really navigate the complex path toward socioeconomic improvements? Institutions such as the UN's Economic and Social Council, its Population Commission, CELADE, the Alliance for Progress, and, in the Peruvian case, CAEM and the INP, answered in the affirmative. Two significant points of convergence, relevant for all of Latin America, were the emphasis on training the first generation of Latin American demographers and the diffusion of the idea that underplanned population growth and migrations could hold a nation's progress back. Again, the responses of regional leaders to the latter realization varied and evolved over time.

As they had since the eighteenth century, Latin American governments in the mid-twentieth century treated population policies as intersectorial tools to manage migration, improve education and health, reduce poverty and urban chaos, increase employment and incomes, and expand agricultural and industrial productivity. Reducing birth rates through the mass promotion of birth control, a new possibility in the early 1960s, was not welcomed without problem as a governmental goal. The Latin American health officers who met in Caracas (1967), Buenos Aires (1968), and Santiago (1972) were in agreement that the goal of lowering birth rates was to be subordinated to broader development aims, even if population control could help accomplish these aims. In this context, the Pan-American Health Organization was not only a channel for funds and technical expertise but also a conduit for mutual support and legitimacy for countries that did not jump on the family planning bandwagon as quickly as the USAID wished. PAHO's position of respect for national sovereignty, rooted in its WHO-derived mandate, led it to clash with the USAID in the early 1970s over the extent to which maternal and child health services ought to promote family planning. The role of such a transnational foil to the pretensions of the United States during this period has gone relatively unnoticed by scholars who focus on the United States' success in promoting population limitation in countries such as India.[102]

Of course, regardless of these lofty stated aims, population policies with family planning components affected some more than others in practice. For one, the architects of these policies in Peru continued the Lima-centric tradition of initiating pilot programs in the capital, justifying their decision because of the city's size and the convenience of monitoring it but hardly considering what needs might have existed for these services outside of Lima. In addition, both the victories and the setbacks of governmental family planning initiatives reflected mainly the role of the executive, as this government branch was the institution most responsible for all family planning programs. President Belaúnde created the CEPD, and General Velasco the INPROMI. The participation of other institutions in this area, such as Congress, the Catholic Church, or civil society organizations, was negligible during the Belaúnde years and nonexistent during the Velasco administration. Bilateral and multilateral aid organizations, such as the PAHO and the USAID, in almost constant communication with the Peruvian executive, were far more influential policymakers than Peruvian citizens were.

At the same time, there were important differences between the civilian and military regimes of 1960s Peru. By design, the CEPD conceived of family planning as only one, and not the most important, activity among the many in which the state should be engaged in order to promote development. Yet in practice, the CEPD's first leaders gave birth control pilot programs a preeminent place and ended up designing an ambitious national family planning program with USAID money. When the military staged the 1968 coup, the CEPD's family planning activities ended abruptly. Velasco resented the power the United States had over Peruvian resources. With the United States funding the CEPD's family planning work, the whole enterprise became tainted by association. Perhaps more decisively, family planning had a low political priority for Velasco, who believed his agrarian reform would lead to radical social improvements, including lower fertility rates. Neglected by the executive, the CEPD was never able to adapt to the exigencies of the new political elite, whose position toward population matters, at first, had been consistent with the CEPD's founding charter of research.

As Velasco's regime wore on, however, even its initial position of openness to considering the links between population and development changed.

Most crucially, Velasco's National Development Plan of 1971–75 ignored this topic altogether. Ironically, just as Velasco's line against family planning hardened, he rolled out the first agency exclusively devoted to maternal and child health, a subsector that, by 1971, had become ground zero for the provision of contraception services and education throughout Latin America. The notion that access to birth control might help promote women's health, let alone be a woman's right, was alien to Velasco.[103] His vision of birth control was based on a long-held understanding of fertility regulation as inconsistent with an individual rights model, a model that gained traction elsewhere in the 1970s, including the United States. As a result of the increasingly sclerotic position of Velasco regarding population and family planning issues, the government squandered an opportunity to become an effective locus for the public debate of the links between birth control, health, and national development. With the governmental failure to think and act, it would be an invigorated group of Peruvian intellectuals, including those in the Catholic Church, who took on this role in the 1970s, as the next chapter will show.

## CHAPTER SIX

# Priests and Pills

## Catholic Birth Control in Peru

The restricted use of anovulatories does not infringe on the terms of the Encyclical.
—Juan Landázuri, archbishop of Lima (1955–90) and cardinal (1962–90)

How did the Catholic Church respond to the conundrum of rapid demographic growth in the second half of the twentieth century? This chapter analyzes a program sponsored by the Catholic Church of Peru that combined the provision of contraceptive pills with health exams, sexual education, and responsible parenthood training for couples in poor urban areas. This program was based on the belief by church authorities that the Catholic faith was compatible with the regulation of fertility. In addition, these authorities emphasized that Peru's environment of material poverty had deleterious effects on the quality of family life and on the upbringing of children. Faced with such an environment, the Peruvian Catholic Church focused on providing family planning services to the neediest in its flock, becoming, in practice, an ally of U.S. birth control organizations and a critic of local conservative Catholics.

At the same time, Catholic leaders were reluctant to treat fertility control as a prerogative of individuals (women or men), emphasizing instead its family, community, and transnational dimensions. Time and again, these leaders pointed to cultural and economic factors such as sexism, lack of education, and uneven terms of foreign trade as causing individuals' reproductive irresponsibility. It was a cycle of unfairness begetting unfairness, as the church elite saw it, with wealthy countries oppressing poor ones, and the richer in poor countries oppressing the most marginal. It was the desire for solidarity between nations, between poor and well-off families, and between men and women, that galvanized the 1960s Peruvian Catholic Church in pursuit of a means to give men and women more control over their fertility.

The family based on a heterosexual marriage is still the model that the Catholic Church upholds as the ideal unit in which children ought to be raised, and in which decisions regarding offspring size ought to be made.[1] This insistence on the heterosexual household as the proper locus for fertility is key.[2] The longstanding importance of heterosexual marriage for the Catholic Church, as a sacrament, a source of companionship, and the context for having and raising children, has put the church at odds with those writing from a tradition that equates family planning with individual choices. Historian Linda Gordon, for example, called birth control "an individual human right" and the process leading up to its public acceptance a "struggle for self-determination by women," while criticizing the Catholic opposition to birth control methods as stemming from "anti-sexual and anti-woman attitudes."[3] At the heart of this position is the belief that the respect for human rights can only be guaranteed by secular authorities, with religion playing a role that is counterproductive to the satisfaction of rights, including sexual and reproductive ones.[4] The above argument has long underlay the separation of church and state in Western democracies. Some, such as sociologist Kingsley Davis, have gone as far as to cast Catholicism as an institution that "clashes with the liberalism, individualism, freedom, mobility, and sovereignty of the democratic nation."[5] In the United States, scholars have often interpreted the Catholic Church's position against most birth control methods as an intrusion in the realm of civic life.[6] Epidemiologist Phyllis Piotrow, for example, blamed the "inflexibility of the Catholic Church" for the U.S. government's inability to widely promote the use of birth control methods in the 1960s.[7]

However, U.S. history cannot be invoked to explain the history of Catholicism elsewhere. The range of attitudes toward family planning among the Catholic priesthood varied widely in the twentieth century between and within places such as Ecuador, Mexico, Ireland, and Québec, from overt support to banishment from the church for parishioners using birth control methods.[8] Likewise, the attitudes of Catholics worldwide regarding the control of their fertility has tended to be favorable, particularly among the wealthier and better educated, regardless of church opposition.[9]

The Catholic Church in Latin America played, particularly during the 1960s and 1970s, a more complex role than U.S. writers have heretofore assumed in debates about the acceptability of contraception. As Stycos, Hall, and Sobrinho have pointed out, during this period the Catholic Church was not as opposed to discussing the problems brought on by rapid population growth as leftist activists and nationalist military officers in the region were.[10] Instead, Latin American Catholic authorities and intellectuals insisted time and again on the importance of educating parents-to-be on their duties to their potential children. This "responsible parenthood" included providing children with material goods, an education, and spiritual values. These tasks did not exclude "restricted or limited procreation in view of the total responsibilities of parenthood."[11]

The promotion of the idea of responsible parenthood led to the Peruvian Catholic Church's support for the limitation of fertility by married couples. That this resulted in the ecclesiastic embrace of a technology such as the contraceptive pill is consistent with a pragmatic attitude by Peruvian lay Catholics, clerics, and theologians. Lay Catholic activism, with roots in the early twentieth century in Peru, intersected with the U.S. lay Catholic movement that turned its financial, missionary, and technical attention to the developing world in the late 1950s. The Peruvian Catholic family planning program of the 1960s was one of the products of this convergence.

## Catholic Activism in Peru

Peru had been a Catholic country, with substantial manifestations of popular religiosity and devotion, since the Colonial period. However, the first widespread lay Catholic movement, with the explicit aim of not only living one's faith but also promoting Catholic beliefs and driving them into the heart of political and social institutions, began only with the Eucharistic Congress of 1935, which gave rise to the Acción Católica Peruana (ACP) the same year.[12] Led by Bishops Mariano Holguín in Arequipa, in southern Peru, and Pedro Pascual Farfán, in Lima, the ACP began publishing journals such as *Acción Católica Peruana* and *Sígueme* in the 1930s and 1940s and establishing sections for women, workers, and youth.[13]

From early on in its history, the ACP was deeply concerned with the social conditions that affected the patriarchal family model. The most important of these were the availability of civil divorces and employment for women.[14] The ACP advocated a clear divide between men's and women's realms of action and between their moral, intellectual, and physical capabilities. Hardliners such as Fr. Manuel Noriega insisted that men were most adept at managing a family's public affairs since they were "willful, logical, unforgiving, strong, courageous, independent, and bold." Conversely, he praised women's skills in running a family's private matters because women were by nature, "pious, intuitive, patient, forgiving, gracious, docile, and resigned to their fate." The equality of men and women was, therefore, nothing but "socialist pap."[15] Nevertheless, several members of the ACP had been concerned with the subject of women earning incomes since the early 1930s. To them, it was not a problem with a quick and easy solution. Reluctantly, ACP members admitted that extending political, economic, and civil rights to women might improve their lot enough that they would not feel obliged to abandon their main role as domestic administrators.[16]

The ACP's promotion of civil rights and social safety nets was part of a broader Catholic drive to spread the Catholic social doctrine. Social doctrine documents were different from most other pronouncements of the Catholic Church in their level of public engagement. These documents urged social and political reforms rather than formal or doctrinal modifications. Tellingly, some of these documents were addressed to "all men of good will," and not just to Catholics.[17] The first among these social doctrine documents was Pope Leo XIII's 1891 *Rerum Novarum* encyclical, which laid out the rights and responsibilities of capital and labor to each other and to the broader community, followed by Pius XI's 1931 *Quadragesimo Anno*, which condemned corporate greed and the unaccountability of political and economic power.[18]

Shortly before *Quadragesimo Anno*, Pope Pius XI issued the *Castii Connubii* encyclical. This was the first Catholic statement concerning the use of contraception by married couples. *Castii Connubii* condemned abortion and eugenics laws that prevented marriage for those deemed unfit. More important for this discussion, *Castii Connubii* maintained that, although procreation was the main purpose of sexual relations within marriage, "the cultivating of mutual love and the quieting of concupiscence" were its secondary ends, even if sex sometimes did not lead to procreation, due to "natural reasons either of time or of certain defects."[19] By sanctioning these "natural reasons" and "defects," the Catholic Church for the first time allowed nonprocreative sex. Moreover, the encyclical placed great emphasis on the spiritual education of children and considered it irresponsible for parents to have more children than they could care for and educate.[20] *Castii Connubii* also partook of the spirit of the Catholic social doctrine. If families were too poor to care for their children, it argued, governments should intervene on their behalf: "Those who have the care of the State and of the public good cannot neglect the needs of married people and their families, without bringing great harm upon the State and on the common welfare. Hence, in making the laws and in disposing of public funds they must do their utmost to relieve the needs of the poor, considering such a task as one of the most important of their administrative duties."[21]

Despite these developments, the Peruvian Catholic Church's first formal pronouncement regarding fertility limitation emerged many years after *Castii Connubi*, in 1947. At that time, Cardinal Juan Gualberto Guevara named and condemned the "enemies of the Christian home": divorce, "Malthusianism" (the use of contraceptives), abortion, and the sterilization of the feeble-minded.[22] However, the church tempered its objections to contraception following Pope Pius XII's support for the rhythm method of birth control in 1951.[23] In 1954, during the Fifth National Eucharistic and Marian Congress, the Peruvian lay Catholic movement publicly embraced Pius XII's position. The congress attracted a group of Catholic physicians, who organized a satellite conference. During this meeting, Dr. Froilán Villamón upheld the value of the rhythm method and reviled the use of contraceptives including chemical or surgical sterilization, coitus interruptus, spermicidal substances, and barrier methods. He also vilified abortions when not performed by a physician to save a woman's life, as well as the existence of birth control organizations. Still, Villamón recognized that often people did not wish to have children because they could not support them financially. Because of that, he reasoned, and in line with the Catholic social doctrine, reducing contraceptive use would only be accomplished through policies to improve wages and the quality of life of the poor, and through the guidance of physicians.[24]

By the 1950s, transnational actors and their local allies were already sowing the seeds of what would become population-limitation campaigns in developing nations. Catholics the world over were concerned about the allegedly excessive freedom that new contraceptive technologies placed in the hands of individuals, as well as with contraceptives' side effects. More distinctly for Latin America, Catholic leaders worried about the possibility that governments, under financial pressure from foreign agencies, would use their power to indiscriminately push birth control on people, such as the poor, who had little opportunity to reflect on what it would mean for their lives.[25]

In response to these concerns, Pope John XXIII set up a Pontifical Commission on Population, Family and Birth in 1963, as Vatican Council II was in session, to advise the pope about the effects of contraception on the lives of Catholics. Vatican Council II, a meeting of bishops from around the world, was in session from 1962 to 1965. The topic that occupied this reunion was the manner in which the church ought to engage with Catholics' changing expectations, particularly those arising from the maintenance and deepening of social injustices. It was the defining moment of John XXIII's papacy, one that, in accordance with the social doctrine tradition, had been and would continue to be critical of the widening socioeconomic gaps between rich and poor nations, nuclear proliferation, and the violation of human rights.[26]

The Pontifical Commission on Population, Family and Birth's original membership was limited to social scientists and theologians; but in 1965, after John XXIII passed away, the new pope Paul VI saw fit to include physicians and Catholic couples in the commission as well. The new members included Patrick and Patricia Crowley of Chicago, the presiding couple of the U.S. Christian Family Movement (CFM). By the early 1960s, the CFM was the world's largest organization of Catholic married couples, hence the relevance of the Crowleys' participation. Contrary to the Vatican's demand for secrecy, the Crowleys actively sought out the opinions of fellow CFM members regarding the use of periodic abstinence methods of birth control and shared the results of their inquiries with the commission. For several members of this group, that survey was their first chance to hear how difficult Catholic couples found the practice of periodic abstinence, and how much these couples yearned for alternatives.[27]

Despite some indications that the Pontifical Commission might endorse the use of contraceptives, Paul VI's July 1968 encyclical *De Humanae Vitae* restated the injunction against birth control methods, while demanding that couples have only those children they could raise lovingly and provide for.[28] To understand the reception of the encyclical in Peru, we must refer to the politically engaged Catholic laity in the country. The fulfillment of the Catholic social doctrine was of great import to the Peruvian Catholic Church following World War II.[29] The disapproval of the excesses of capitalism in the form of a preferential option for the poor, most poignantly articulated by Pedro Arrupe, SJ, the general of the Jesuit Order, was one of its manifestations. This was at the heart of the critique elaborated by liberation theologians, who adopted some tenets of dependency theory to affirm that poverty in Latin America was tied to capitalist expansion, which rendered the so-called peripheral nations chronically underdeveloped as wealthier capitalist countries drained resources and surplus capital away from them and toward the capitalist centers.[30]

In March 1968, a group of Peruvian priests issued a declaration denouncing the chronic conditions of injustice that "tormented the country." In particular, the priests criticized the unequal system of land tenure, the poor quality of education, the lack of regard for workers' rights, and "the large imperialist consortia" that controlled Peru's natural resources "under conditions that harm the nation's interests and dignity."[31] The declaration is significant because it was supported by Cardinal Juan Landázuri Ricketts and by priests who later became involved in the church's family planning program, Enrique Bartra and Luis Bambarén, then auxiliary archbishop of Lima.[32]

A month earlier, the Peruvian Bishops Conference had acknowledged that rapid demographic growth was a social problem. Moreover, the bishops shared "the anguish of numerous families whose homes and conjugal lives are seriously troubled" by having too many children. Nevertheless, they also indicated that birth control programs alone should not take the place of development initiatives. In fact, the bishops claimed that demographic growth could become beneficial for the country if accompanied by a rational exploitation of its natural resources and educational improvements. In addition, the bishops reviled the potential for foreign aid to become contingent on the implementation of population-limitation campaigns and rejected any attempt to limit population growth if it affected the ability of parents to make free decisions about the size of their families.[33] The Jesuit Enrique Bartra had criticized population-limitation initiatives in Peru in 1965 and instead argued for the "intensification of institutional, social and mental changes in the Peruvian population" to make better use of the nation's natural resources.[34]

How did this politically charged Catholic Peruvian environment react to *Humanae Vitae*? Not surprisingly, as Leo Alting von Geusau has documented, Western economists and demographers, as well as the mostly U.S.-based population-limitation establishment, criticized Paul VI's encyclical. A few Peruvian medical professionals and newspapers voiced their disagreement too. An editorial in *Acción* on August 7, 1968, accused the pope of wanting "a society composed of poor families, horrified by the fear of a new conception, a world of misery and malnourishment." A psychiatrist warned that "limit[ing] sex relations to infertile periods would have psychotic effects." Interestingly, groups of Chilean, Brazilian, and Peruvian theologians made pronouncements indicating that "the Encyclical could be fallible as a matter of fact, and that the personal conscience of the married couple was the final authority on the subject."[35] For the most part, however, Peruvian priests and theologians remained silent, at least at first.

The Second General Conference of Latin American Bishops took place in Medellín, Colombia, in September 1968. Paul VI addressed the bishops at the opening of the conference and defended what had become his most divisive encyclical. *Humanae Vitae*, he held, did not endorse a "blind race towards overpopulation" or diminish the responsibilities of couples toward their children. In addition, Paul VI said that the encyclical did not forbid "an honest and reasonable limitation of births, or legitimate medical therapies, or the progress of scientific research."[36] In the end, the Latin American bishops endorsed *Humanae Vitae* and, in line with the social doctrinal developments accumulating since the nineteenth century, the conclusions of Vatican Council II, and the liberation theology critique, they added a series of reflections. First, the bishops acknowledged the shift from rural to urban societies in Latin America, along with changes in family structure away from patriarchal families toward families with greater emotional intimacy and a more even distribution of responsibilities. Second, the bishops denounced that the process of development had led to material abundance for a few families, greater insecurity for others, and economic marginality for the rest. Third, even though population growth was not the only important demographic variable to consider, the bishops indicated that population growth in Latin America exacerbated economic, social, and ethical problems such as low marriage rates, single-parent families, out-of-wedlock births, and housing shortages.[37]

Faced with this situation, the Medellín bishops expressed their solidarity with families burdened with too many children, while calling for educational reforms to instill a sense of responsible parenthood among the young and more compassion toward struggling families. The situation of poverty and neglect in which many Latin American families lived, the bishops suggested, constituted an act of violence that was inherently sinful. According to the bishops, the injustices to correct in Latin America had a transnational dimension, related to the terms of foreign trade that made raw materials cheaper than manufactured products. Because of that, the producers of raw materials, such as most Latin American countries, remained subordinated to industrialized nations that produced more manufactured items. At the same time, the bishops accused, foreign companies operating in Latin American countries often used subterfuge to evade taxes and send most of their dividends abroad without reinvesting them in the region.[38]

Thus, by the late 1960s the Peruvian Catholic Church affirmed that population growth caused unjust suffering for many families. Yet the church also posed two challenges. To modernization theorists, who believed in the power of industrialization to overcome, eventually, the social dislocations it caused, the church responded by endorsing the critique of dependency theory: industrialization exacerbated social inequalities instead of reducing them. The church warned advocates of population control campaigns that such efforts risked trampling the right of couples to make free decisions about their fertility. These views were remarkably consistent with those of the political elite that seized power by force in 1968. But how could this convergence translate into action on the part of the church?

## Dr. Kerrins and His Mission to Peru

Dr. Joseph Kerrins was greatly responsible for the early stage of the Peruvian Catholic Church's family planning program. Born in 1928, Kerrins had been a New England Catholic almost his whole life. He attended Providence College, run by the Dominican order, and, after serving in the U.S. Coast Guard, enrolled at Tufts University Medical School, graduating in 1954. By the early 1960s, Kerrins and his wife, Helen, were active in organizations such as the Christian Family Movement and the Anti-Defamation League. In addition, Kerrins started the Family Life Clinic and Marriage Institute to teach the rhythm method to Catholic couples in Attleboro, Massachusetts, where he was the chief of obstetrics and gynecology at Sturdy Memorial Hospital.[39]

Though aware that missionary work would mean giving up his lucrative practice, Kerrins increasingly saw such activism as an extension of his volunteer work in New England. In 1966 he contacted the Association for International Development (AID), a Catholic charity based in Patterson, New Jersey. Since its foundation in the early 1960s, AID-Patterson had specialized in supporting Catholic professionals seeking to do volunteer work in the developing world. In this respect, AID-Patterson had four main functions: (1) it ran training sessions so volunteers could learn about the challenges of living and working abroad; (2) it helped raise funds to provide for the living expenses of the volunteers; (3) it provided the volunteers with a network of local supporters who could assist them as they settled; and (4) it coordinated with the Catholic authorities in the communities where the volunteers would work. India and African and Latin American countries were some of the destinations of AID-Patterson volunteers.[40] The profile of the AID-Patterson volunteer was that of a man between twenty-one and forty-five years of age and ready to work anywhere in the world "for the fulfillment of God's Design in human society."[41]

U.S. Catholics had begun to organize volunteer corps for service overseas after Pope John XXIII's 1961 request for lay volunteers to assist local churches in poor countries. To the U.S. volunteers, this was not only a chance to assuage an acute priest shortage but also an opportunity "to help combat the Communist menace" through good works that would earn them new allies.[42] Their zeal was awesome, and their paternalistic attitude intense. As George Wolf, of the National Catholic Welfare Council put it, "you ask how might these young Americans be received? I might say, who cares, when we look at it in the light of whether St. Francis Xavier was wanted in Japan. . . . The important thing is that Christ wants us in these places. . . . Americans cannot show their love of these people through our local State Department people, through our dollars, through our films on horror, sex, etc. We can only do it in the real form that a parent has for his child—through personal contact, suffering, joys and the like."[43]

Part of the reason for the convergence between anticommunism and the activism of U.S. Catholics lay in the Cold War. Pope John XXIII's call for volunteers coincided with John F. Kennedy's creation of the Alliance for Progress in 1961. Not only did the Alliance for Progress exclude the newly Soviet-aligned Cuba, it also called for U.S. Catholic volunteer agencies to play a role in the delivery of Alliance for Progress aid to Latin America. The National Catholic Welfare Conference became one of the largest voluntary overseas relief agencies in the United States when Kennedy advised that the U.S. International Cooperation Administration and its foreign aid missions use the services of voluntary agencies to carry out the country's foreign aid program.[44] Thus, for U.S. volunteers, the pope's demand to assist churches in the so-called Third World was in line with their nation's demand to steer the poor away from communism. As Gerald Mische, cofounder and assistant director of AID-Patterson, put it, "Christianity must come up with a positive solution to the socioeconomic problems of the people in Latin America or the Church will be left out of the picture."[45]

Although local Catholic authorities had a say in determining how to use the talents of the AID-Patterson volunteers, soon the highly skilled, motivated, and zealous U.S. volunteers began to bristle under the control of the Latin American Catholic authorities. AID-Patterson did not wish to be "just another local priest helper operation."[46] As a result, the organization increasingly encouraged the volunteers to find projects that best suited their dispositions and skills before committing to volunteer work. To help them with this, AID-Patterson began to sponsor a summer training program at Seton Hall University in 1962.[47] Here, potential volunteers learned about non-Western cultures, languages, and societies from personalities such as anthropologist Margaret Mead.[48] When Dr. Joseph Kerrins and his family moved to Lima, they received help from Sal Piazza, an AID-Patterson volunteer who was working for the American Institute for Free Labor Development, the international arm of the AFL-CIO, which promoted the formation of nonsocialist trade unions.[49]

It was through AID-Patterson that Kerrins met Father John Coss, a Catholic priest in the order of the Sons of Mary. The Sons of Mary first went to Peru in April 1961, also in response to the need "to combat the Communism that was rampant at that time."[50] Peruvian Cardinal Juan Landázuri asked the Sons of Mary to take over the parish of Santa Magdalena Sofía Barat in the Lima neighborhood of El Agustino. Coss was named parish priest in October 1965 and found himself back in the United States and meeting Kerrins in the summer of 1966.

During a preliminary trip to Peru later that year, Kerrins met Brother Francisco Tanega, another Sons of Mary priest and a medical doctor from the Philippines. Tanega ran clinics in several poor neighborhoods in Lima between 1961 and 1969. Speaking of the female patients in those clinics, Kerrins recalled that "there seemed to be no doubt in their minds they wanted me to help them to stop having so many babies."[51] Brother Tanega, Father Coss, Father Roger Reedy (another Sons of Mary priest), and Joseph Kerrins then designed a program that would permit birth limitation within acceptable Catholic teachings. The contraceptive pill, effective, noninvasive, and, in 1967, deemed likely by the pope's Pontifical Commission on Population, Family and Birth to become a part of the Catholic family planning toolbox, seemed like a good choice at the time.[52]

The contraceptive pill did not form a physical barrier between the sperm and ovum, as other birth control methods did (including condoms, spermicidal jellies and foams, cervical caps, and diaphragms). Rather, the hormones in the pill interrupted the maturation of ova in the ovaries. This was not the only remarkable chemical feature of the pill. Some Catholic physicians used oral contraceptives to make ovulation cycles more predictable among women who wanted to use the rhythm method. These physicians believed that a woman's spontaneous infertile period was similar to the pill-induced infertile period, because both were caused by hormonal fluctuations. The only clinical and moral difference was, in their view, the longer duration and higher predictability of the pill-induced infertile period.[53] Kerrins himself had used G. D. Searle's Ovulen since 1964 in his private practice for this very purpose.[54]

More important, in line with the longstanding Catholic concern for family integrity, Kerrins and the Sons of Mary believed that the ultimate goal of the program should be to improve marriages and make better Catholic families, and they did not think contraception alone could accomplish that. Therefore, they devised an educational component for the program. As members of the Christian Family Movement in Massachusetts, Joseph and Helen Kerrins had conducted seminars to coach married couples toward the improvement of conjugal love, sexuality, communication, and their relationship to their children. The seminars consisted of eleven sessions on these different subjects, and the Kerrinses suggested using their seminar curriculum as the blueprint for the educational program.[55]

Father Coss and Brother Tanega submitted a proposal to Cardinal Juan Landázuri outlining the clinical and educational components of the program and emphasizing that the pills (conspicuously referred to as "anovulatories"

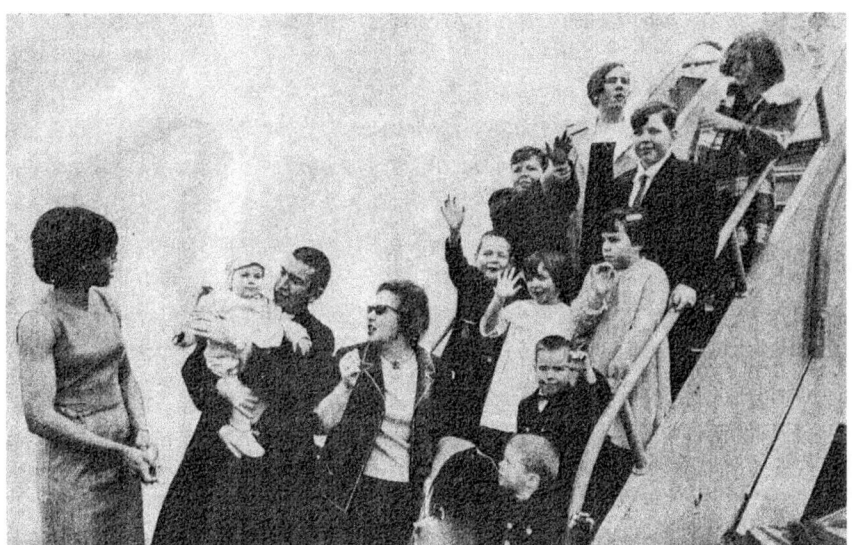

Figure 6. Joe and Helen Kerrins with their ten children boarding an airplane to Lima, February 1967. Courtesy of Dr. Joseph and Mrs. Helen Kerrins.

instead of "contraceptives") would be provided for a period of eighteen to twenty-four months at the most. This period was based on the observations Tanega had made about how long low-income urban women breastfed their infants and on the belief that breastfeeding women should be fully dedicated to nurturing an infant. The corollary of that belief was that it was morally legitimate to prevent a new conception during the lactation period. Cardinal Landázuri gave his permission for this program to operate in El Agustino, although he labeled the program as experimental at first.[56]

The months leading to the departure of Joe and Helen Kerrins generated a significant amount of planning headaches for the couple. At the same time, their willingness to help the poor and sacrifice the comforts of suburban life made them newsworthy (see figure 6). The *Attleboro Sun* designated reporters to cover life in Peru for the Kerrinses and their ten children.[57] In September 1966 Joe and Helen took an exploratory trip to Lima and firmed up their commitment to spend eighteen months working among impoverished *barriada* dwellers in the city.[58]

Migration from rural to urban areas had accelerated throughout Latin America since the 1930s. New arrivals in Lima, however, often had to contend with housing costs that were out of their reach, when housing was available at all. Even for city residents, housing conditions deteriorated for almost everyone but the well-off, and poor tenants rarely succeeded in making owners and authorities act on the rising problems of uncollected garbage, delinquency, and malfunctioning municipal services such as water, sewage, and electricity. The decision of where to settle, for new arrivals, and of where to resettle, for fed-up urban dwellers, was not easy. A substantial amount of strategizing and leadership was required to locate vacant space, negotiate with the owners before or after settlers had taken over the space, and then try to organize communities to lobby for the extension of city services to newly colonized spaces.[59] The aspect of these communities in formation in the 1960s, known then and now as *barriadas* or *pueblos jóvenes*, was for outsiders one of rampant chaos made worse by poverty. El Agustino was one such *pueblo joven*.[60]

Joe Kerrins's range of reactions to life in El Agustino varied widely, from annoyance at the "horde of dirty, lean kids in rags" who followed him when he worked, to optimism following his first successes: "I'm swamped. The poor in the barriada of Agustino seem to be very anxious to do something to try to limit the size of their families."[61] Most notable among Kerrins's reactions was his critique of wealth inequalities within Peru and between Peru and the United States: "If your neighbor has an abundance of bread and you have none, you have a right to some of his. . . . Everywhere we look we see dogs, walls and barred windows to prevent the poor from taking any of the possessions of the rich. One wonders what the poor, not just in Peru but in the world, will do when they finally find out how much we have in the States. Will we be able to build high enough walls and strong enough bars for our windows and train enough ferocious dogs?"[62]

Signing off his letters to friends in the United States as "yours in a prayer of action,"[63] Kerrins rolled up his sleeves and got to work. The Rules Committee of the Peruvian Faculty of Medicine gave him a broadly worded temporary permit to assist in "sanitary work, health posts, nutrition clinics and other problems that directly affect the inhabitants of the barriada of El Agustino."[64] Likewise, Kerrins bore a letter of support and introduction from the bishop of Fall River, Massachusetts.[65] Significantly, though, Kerrins did not have the support of the U.S. government, even though the latter was already funding the Peruvian government's fledgling family planning clinics, as we saw in the previous chapter. Instead, Jonathan Fine, the human resource development officer of the USAID in Peru, told Kerrins that "although it may be too late for you to reconsider your plans for coming to Peru," he still hoped Kerrins would "realize how politically sensitive family planning programs were, and how dangerous it was for American citizens to become openly identified with such work." Fine urged Kerrins to keep in close contact, as the Peruvian press routinely "misinterpreted the motives of those working in this field and raised the false specter of 'Yankee Imperialism.'"[66]

On any given day, Kerrins would drive to pick up his assistants and then head for the clinic. He set up his equipment in the parish's function room, using a private area as the exam room and a desk to welcome patients. The clinic provided a range of gynecology services, including screenings for cervical cancer and tuberculosis, in addition to the pill. A social worker would note each woman's name, address, number of pregnancies, children living and dead, age, and reason for coming. Then Kerrins would take her medical history and give her a physical exam. If she wanted to be on the pill, the physician showed her how to take it and discussed possible side effects. The social worker would repeat the instructions before giving her the first month's supply. If breastfeeding, the social worker would also give the user a supplement of minerals and vitamins. Then the user made an appointment for the following week, in case any problems arose. Finally, the social worker gave the user a consent form that the user's husband was obligated to sign, and that the user was expected to bring to her next appointment. Kerrins estimated that the early team of volunteers saw an average of forty women seeking the pill every day. The work took about five hours, including travel time.[67]

Soon, priests from other parishes began to approach Kerrins and the Sons of Mary to ask that similar clinics be established in their parishes. By June 1967 there were four more clinics in *pueblos jóvenes*: one in Dos de Mayo, another in El Montón, and two in Comas. The early adopters were parishes managed by foreign priests, in particular those belonging to the Oblate, Columban, and St. James missionary orders.[68] The workload became too burdensome for a group of volunteers, and Kerrins applied for and received a grant of US$5,000 from Peru's Center for the Study of Population and Development (CEPD) to hire two social workers and a nurse to assist him. Kerrins himself did not benefit from this grant. AID-Patterson paid him a living allowance during his time in Peru. By August, some of the clinics were so popular they had to be open twice a week, and Kerrins received a US$6,000 grant from the Pathfinder Fund.[69]

By 1965 the pill had become a very profitable drug in the United States, pleasing its creator, G. D. Searle.[70] Not surprisingly, other pharmaceutical companies attempted to bring to market a contraceptive pill of their own. Warner-Lambert was one of these companies, and it had one product in need of human trials. This pill was a combination of quinestrol, an estrogen that was stored in and released progressively from fatty tissue and that, as a result, had a long-lasting effect, and quingestanol acetate, a progestagen. The novelty of the formula consisted in the fact that it needed to be taken only once a month to have a contraceptive effect.[71] The substance, known as "Q1-Q2," was simultaneously tested in Mexico, Chile, and Peru, and its advocates baldly promoted it as a solution to the problem of rapid population growth in the Third World.[72] Warner-Lambert approached Kerrins in August 1967, during the program's fastest period of expansion, and thus its period of greatest financial need, and offered him a US$10,000 grant, in addition to the medication itself, for free, in exchange for a report of its acceptability among the urban poor, and Kerrins accepted.[73]

Accepting Warner-Lambert's help turned out to be a costly bargain for Kerrins. His advocacy of methods other than periodic abstinence had already raised eyebrows among members of Peru's lay Catholic movement. Warner-Lambert's offer turned these doubters into enemies. To them, Kerrins was no well-meaning Catholic volunteer, but the employee of a U.S. corporation that profited by preventing Peruvians from being born.[74] Ironically, these critics came mainly from the Peruvian Christian Family Movement (MFC), among whom Kerrins had his closest allies when he began the educational component of the program in August 1967. As in the United States, Peru's MFC was made up mostly of middle-class Catholic married couples who promoted not social activism but an inward-looking reflection about the quality of one's married life and the maintenance of traditional gender roles of men in the public sphere and women in the domestic one.[75] Yet, a few couples in the MFC were persuaded by Kerrins's position and by the support of the Catholic hierarchy for this program. These couples translated the Kerrinses' curriculum from English into Spanish. After taking the course themselves, these MFC couples in turn began conducting the workshops on conjugal love and responsible parenthood in parishes in *pueblos jóvenes*. Their experience teaching about conjugal love in an environment of material squalor and violence was both challenging and inspiring; some made friends with the couples they met in the workshops and with the priests who hosted them.[76]

In late 1967 the program faced a crisis. It revolved around whether or not Cardinal Landázuri had given appropriate consent to open additional clinics besides the experimental one in El Agustino. During the course of the controversy, it became known that Kerrins was being supported by Warner-Lambert. "The Cardinal exploded!!!" Kerrins wrote.[77] Believing Landázuri to be "very nationalistic and anti-gringo," Kerrins rushed to assure him that it had never been Kerrins's intention to offend the church.[78] Kerrins also emphasized the importance of his educational initiatives and offered to close all the clinics to appease the cardinal.[79] Mastering his own irritation over the scandal, Landázuri commissioned Enrique Bartra, a Jesuit theologian, to evaluate the moral appropriateness of the program in order to decide whether or not to phase out the clinics. By early 1968, with Bartra appointed as the cardinal's representative to the management of the program, the crisis was over. At that time, approximately 699 women were taking oral contraceptives in eight parish clinics, and by June 1968, when Kerrins departed, the number had grown to 1,200 women.[80]

Kerrins had recently returned to the United States when *Humanae Vitae* was issued. Stunned by the news, he called the pope's decision "an unjust imposition" and claimed that "the society in which the Peruvians live—uneducated, uncultured, poverty-ridden—has not attained a level of Christianity at which they could be expected to follow an edict which would worsen for them the major problem they have so recently began to combat."[81] Kerrins, however, had underestimated how committed the highest officers of the Peruvian Catholic Church were to this program.

## After *De Humanae Vitae*

Cardinal Landázuri was aware of the increase in the number of birth control clinics in Lima, sponsored by both governmental and private initiatives. Unlike these clinics, those run by the parish were committed to the promotion of Catholic values through the educational program. Moreover, as shown above, there was an important sector of the Catholic hierarchy that took seriously the legitimacy of a couple's right to determine how many children they should have. This sector was sympathetic to the continuation of the program, and it included the auxiliary archbishop of Lima, Luis Bambarén; the bishop of the province of Callao, Augusto Durand; and the Jesuits Enrique Bartra and Juan Julio Wicht.

To consolidate the program in the *pueblos jóvenes* where it already operated, the cardinal turned its administration over to the Peruvian lay Christian Family Movement, which in turn split the program into clinical and educational branches. While the latter stayed firmly under the control of the MFC, the former began to be managed by paid medical professionals. With its new structure in place, the program earned the endorsement of the National Office for the Development of Pueblos Jóvenes (ONDEPJOV). This was an agency created by General Velasco Alvarado in December 1968 to coordinate social policies for residents of *pueblos jóvenes* and to mobilize support for the regime among them. ONDEPJOV went as far as to recommend that the government's family planning policy be modeled on the Catholic Church's program, a recommendation that Velasco did not follow.[82]

Throughout the changes, the Catholic Church's program still aimed to strengthen couples and families so they could "be active and organic components of the people of God," to provide relief for "the anguish of numerous families caused by the lack of balance between demographic growth and the development of our country," to broaden the knowledge that "rational family growth leads to dignified progress for mankind," and to develop the concept of responsible parenthood. Nevertheless, in a clear allusion to the Q1-Q2 affair, the program also aimed to provide "pills that have passed all experimental stages and are authorized by Peruvian health authorities."[83]

Faced with the increasing popularity of the clinics, the leaders of the MFC sought to enlist the help of more MFC couples to deliver the educational curriculum in the *pueblos jóvenes*. This was not easy. Several leading members of the MFC had become vehemently opposed to the use of oral contraceptives after *Humanae Vitae* and were critical of the foreign funding the program received. According to them, the project had "helped the [US]AID once again enter the country and begin birth control activities for political reasons in a dangerous manner. They will even be capable of continuing support for the Educational Plan to accomplish that goal."[84] The critics were not wrong about the funding sources. The bulk of the project's financing in 1969–70 (1.4 million Soles, or approximately US$33,000) came from the CEPD, which channeled donations from the USAID. Another US$16,000 consisted of a donation from the Pathfinder Fund.[85]

By early 1970, educational program director Pedro Pazos estimated the medical program had approximately 2,500 users, and he believed this number would grow to 3,300 within six months. According to him, the program needed 111 new MFC couples to train *pueblo joven* couples, yet only 26 MFC couples had completed the course up to that point. Of those couples, only 9 worked actively in *pueblos jóvenes*.[86] Pazos's pleas for greater MFC involvement were unsuccessful, leading him to seek more administrative autonomy. As a result, two new organizations emerged between 1970 and 1971. The Programa de Apoyo Laico Familiar (PALF) took charge of clinical operations, while the Centro de Capacitación y Promoción Familiar (CCPF) focused on offering courses on responsible parenthood and leadership training for *pueblo joven* couples. By August 1970 the clinical program had over 4,000 users of the pill in fourteen parish clinics in Lima, Callao, Huacho, Ica, Ancash, and Tacna. It employed twelve obstetrician-gynecologists, a psychologist, and several nurse assistants. Meanwhile, the educational program, still lagging, had enrolled a little over 1,000 people to complete the curriculum.[87] By June 1973, there were nineteen parish clinics and over 5,500 users of the pill.[88] The PALF assured its U.S. sponsors that in one year they could have 4,480 additional users, as long as their budget was increased to 5.1 million Soles, approximately US$118,000. Harold Crow, Family Planning International assistance officer, endorsing the PALF's request, told the chief of the USAID's Family Planning Division that "in the Peruvian context, the PALF program has always impressed me."[89]

Father Enrique Bartra, the Jesuit adviser to the PALF, went from cautiously criticizing the program to enriching the theological justification for the provision of oral contraceptives for up to twenty-four months. He began by stating that women's monthly ovulating cycles were suspended after giving birth and that maintaining, and even inducing, this "natural ovarian resting period" was morally justified because there are tight biological, psychological, and spiritual links between mother and child during pregnancy that continued through the breastfeeding period. Bartra deemed these links "essential for the formation of the human being" and claimed they could be upset by the sudden arrival of another baby. Bartra also emphasized that the duration of the breastfeeding period could not be precisely determined because it was not only a biologically but also a culturally determined phenomenon. In any event, "the breastfeeding mother appears to have the right to ovarian rest during that whole period, as long as it may be."[90] Even if a woman who recently gave birth did not breastfeed, Bartra went on, she still had the right to ovarian rest, but in that case it was necessary to set limits to this period. To come up with an estimate, Bartra cited chronicles from Peru's Colonial period, the Bible, a survey conducted by the PALF in a *pueblo joven*, and even the Koran, and suggested that, in Peru, the normal rest period lasted between eighteen and twenty-four months, the same duration Kerrins and the Sons of Mary had used as a reference. Bartra also noted that many *pueblo joven* women would like to breastfeed, if only to save money on formula, but could not because of their poor health, arising from malnutrition and worsened by poor hygiene and by having given birth numerous times in unsanitary conditions. In making the theological case for the provision of oral contraceptives, Bartra simultaneously reveals a rigid view of women's roles as the natural caretakers of infants. Nowhere in his thesis are men portrayed as potential nurturers.

With Bartra as spiritual adviser, the program began to emphasize the training of couples in methods of periodic abstinence as part of the educational component so they would be ready to put those methods in practice after the twenty-four-month regime of pills. Bartra's arguments in favor of the program matched the attitude of Cardinal Landázuri himself. Father Pedro Richards, the spiritual adviser of the MFC in Latin America, wrote to Landázuri in December 1976 from Uruguay, criticizing the program and claiming that "while, throughout the continent, there are those who courageously fight for what is prescribed in *Humanae Vitae*, the Lima experiment seems subservient to the pildoristas [pill pushers]." Landázuri replied that this project had his approval and cited Bartra's work as evidence of ongoing efforts to "improve its medical aspects, according to advances in natural methods." Downplaying Richards's knowledge of Peruvian realities, Landázuri referred to him as "a priest just passing through Lima," then delivered a sharp rebuke: "As Cardinal and Bishop I strongly reject these and other expressions in your letter which, in addition to being insulting, are untrue. I cannot allow you or anyone else to doubt my fidelity to the Holy Father, the doctrine or the directives of the Church!"[91] Richards's criticism was unusual. Father Luis Bambarén, assistant archbishop of Lima and chair of the Commission on Social Action of the Peruvian Bishops' Conference, had made the program public at a meeting of Latin American Bishops in Chile in 1970. Cautious interest and not condemnation were the most common reactions from his peers, although there is no evidence yet that other bishops pursued similar projects.[92]

Despite Bartra's and Landázuri's best intentions, however, clinicians involved in the project did not always comply with the guidelines set by the MFC in 1969.[93] According to those guidelines, each parish priest had the ultimate power to decide whether a given woman was eligible to receive contraceptives in his parish. Physicians were required to notify the medical director and the parish priest if they believed there were valid reasons why a woman should stay on the pill beyond twenty-four months. Physicians also had to inform the women of their duty to participate in the educational program with their husbands. In reality, physicians were reluctant to end the supply of contraceptives under different conditions. Physicians continued providing contraceptives, for example, when a woman had been on the pill for over twenty-four months but had not yet with her husband completed the educational program, which consisted of talks given over several weeks.[94] Physicians also made exceptions when they estimated that a new pregnancy would be too risky for a woman, given her physical state. If women asked physicians for contraceptives other than the pill, physicians had no qualms about referring those women to hospital outpatient or private clinics.[95] When women who had been on the pill nevertheless became pregnant and had abortions, physicians allowed them to restart the twenty-four-month regime of oral contraceptives. Exceptions were often made to the rule that husbands had to give their written consent for their wives to go on the pill because a good number of *pueblo joven* women were not married to the fathers of their children.[96]

By the mid-1970s, the program faced a new crisis. The troubles began with a bold declaration by the Peruvian Bishops' Conference about the challenges contemporary society posed to the family. The bishops stressed that unemployment, single-parent homes, high imprisonment rates, the eroticization of everyday life (evident in movie titles and salacious newspaper cover photographs), and, most significant, the inability of parents to provide for many offspring, threatened Catholic family values. The bishops cautiously admitted the need to consider governmental population policies to address the latter point. At the same time, they refused to reduce the demographic problem to "a debate over the legitimacy of the use of contraceptives." Such reductionism, the bishops contended, was typical of the "'happy families' who live with their backs turned to the unhappiness of other families and the injustices of society."[97]

The swipe at the "happy families" angered some of the wealthier leaders of the MFC, who pointed out the existence of divisions among the Peruvian clergy. These MFC critics claimed that, since the bishops of Huancayo, Yauyos, Abancay, and Cajamarca found the Catholic family planning program unacceptable, "there is disorientation and confusion in the consciences of lay members of the Church, because priests do not speak with one voice." In addition, the critics complained that the arguments in favor of population limitation to stave off future food scarcity were weak. Peru, according to them, had "infinite unexploited riches awaiting the science and technology of the Peruvian worker to begin to be productive." Moreover, the critics believed the pill made men see women as more sexually available. Finally, they were suspicious of the support the clinical side of the program received from the International Planned Parenthood Federation (IPPF), because the MFC leaders did not know how those funds were used. With irony, the critics noted how the medical program used IPPF monies, even though General Velasco cancelled the activities of the Asociación Peruana de Protección Familiar in 1973 precisely because of its reliance on such funds.[98]

In response, Cardinal Landázuri had a meeting with his auxiliary bishops, the MFC leaders, and a group of parish priests. The meeting was favorable to the continuation of the program, and therefore Landázuri had no choice but to divest it from the MFC, although he hoped some of its members would still help out individually. Landázuri was disappointed: "I am sorry to have to make this decision, and I trust the members of the MFC will reflect on the reasons that have made me do so." The cardinal believed that, through this program, the MFC supported the archdiocese's social mission, "in accordance with the demands of our time, through an authentic and effective commitment to the poor and the oppressed."[99]

Even after this, the program continued for several years. However, after 1976 it began to decline for a set of interrelated reasons. General Velasco died in 1977, shortly after being quietly removed from power by General Francisco Morales Bermúdez. As for demographic growth, Morales Bermúdez called for a committee to draft the country's first population policy guideline in 1976, which legalized the use of all contraceptives save for sterilization. As a result, foreign donors increasingly chose to finance organizations that used a broader range of contraceptives than the Catholic program did. Still, the program continued to request funds from the IPPF at least until 1979. By then, the program had developed a financial self-sustainability plan, based on the sale of magazines and pamphlets, individual and institutional donations, charging for services to private organizations, in-kind support from the Catholic Church and volunteers, and increasing the cost of client services.[100] Moreover, the program was based in twenty-two parishes in Lima, Huancayo, Callao, Huaraz, Ica, Huarochiri, Trujillo, and La Oroya.[101] In the late 1970s, however, the Catholic Church itself began to lean more heavily on periodic abstinence methods and on responsible parenthood education instead of the promotion of the pill. As a result, the clinical program slowly wilted until its final demise sometime in the early 1990s.[102]

## Not the End

The Peruvian Catholic Church family planning program went by two names. Kerrins and the Sons of Mary dubbed it the "Responsible Parenthood Program in the Barriadas of Lima." The cardinal and the Peruvian MFC went with "Project for Conjugal and Family Promotion in Peripheral Neighborhoods." The names suggest the objectives of the program's founders and supporters: parental responsibility and the freedom to determine how many children to have, and the improvement of families as Catholic communities. The initiative was based on a longstanding commitment to the Catholic social doctrine, present since the late nineteenth century. In the 1960s, the Peruvian Catholic Church connected this commitment to the suffering caused by having too many children. However, Catholic authorities did not see fertility control only as a means to limit births, or only as an individual right. Their family planning program was part of a broader education plan to promote the duties of responsible Catholic parents for the betterment of families and the nation.

For priests, particularly those working in poor parishes on a daily basis, the most compelling aspect of the program was not its relation to U.S. funds or the discourse of nationalistic development in Latin America. Rather, it was the way the program combined a popular demand for smaller families with a duty to transform Catholics through consciousness-raising and education. To these priests, responsible parenthood meant not just conceiving children but providing moral values, material support, love, and education for those children.[103] None but an observant Catholic married couple, they believed, was so well prepared to fulfill these requirements. Likewise, no organization was entitled to decide for this couple the number of children they ought to have. The most the church could do was provide guidance so couples made this decision in a conscientious and free manner.

At the same time, this program unfolded within the context of the Cold War and a resurgence of Peruvian nationalism. Social forces such as the increasing relevance of the discourse of development, dependency theory, the nationalistic reaction to the influence of the United States and its zealous Catholic volunteers, and the introduction of new contraceptives also affected the direction and content of the program. A preference for smaller families can help explain why, from the outset, more people partook in the clinical part of the program than in the educational one. Only about one *pueblo joven* woman out of four who went on the pill also completed the educational curriculum. But it is not the only factor that explains the large discrepancy. The clinical program grew so much and so fast that volunteers alone could not run it, even during Kerrins's tenure. The program needed paid professionals and a division of labor between field clinical workers and managers. This growing workforce depended largely on foreign funds. Particularly after 1968, U.S. foreign policy regarding population growth in the developing world was oriented toward the quiet but relentless support of national governments that wanted to lower birth rates. The sheer amount of funds and resources the United States made available to those working on family planning in the 1960s and 1970s throughout Latin America was partly responsible for the greater development of the medical program relative to its educational component.

Nevertheless, these attempts to direct family planning policies and practice were not welcomed by everyone. Peruvian nationalism in the 1960s affected this story in multiple ways. There was strong criticism of the program on the part of certain members of the MFC in Lima who perceived sinister links between the promotion of family planning and the corporate greed of pharmaceutical companies, the oversexualization of women, and the economic subordination of some nations to others. The latter link was particularly relevant for General Velasco's regime. His hostility toward the IPPF's presence in Peru and his alignment with the nations that attacked the 1974 World Population Draft Plan of Action at the United Nations are representative of his conviction that population could be turned into an asset for the nation's development.[104]

A third level of analysis is also discernable, beyond the Catholic Church's insistence on both spouses' involvement in fertility decisions, and beyond the disagreements between Velasco's nationalism and the United States' population-reduction efforts. The popularity of the clinics illustrates the demand for medical and contraception services on the part of poor Peruvians. Particularly for women living in *pueblos jóvenes*, the prospect of free health services and family planning must have been alluring, as indeed the number of users suggests.

On a more practical level, it is clear that not all national Catholic churches adopted a hard line against birth control following *Humanae Vitae*, which is what some students of the Catholic Church in the United States suggest.[105] In Latin America in the 1960s, the Catholic Church was as committed to denouncing social injustice as it was to being faithful to the Vatican. In Peru, this double commitment led the church to foster an approach to family planning that did not embrace the connection between birth control and industrialization, or the connection between birth control and women's expanded autonomy from the domestic sphere. This is an important revision of the portrayal of Catholic leaders as uniformly opposed to birth control. In fact, they embraced birth control, but on different terms. Negotiating such terms required theological creativity, such as that displayed by the Sons of Mary and Enrique Bartra, along with the recognition that popular demands have legitimacy and deserve support, such as that provided by Cardinal Juan Landázuri. This also suggests that the contemporary polarization between civil society and the Catholic Church in Latin America on issues such as emergency contraception need not seem hopeless, as long as Catholic leaders in the region can, once again, tap into the well of theological creativity and courageous leadership that was one of the hallmarks of their church in the 1960s and that surely has not been extinguished despite the conservative turn of its upper management.

# Epilogue

In 1976, the military government of General Francisco Morales Bermúdez charged a Jesuit economist, two gynecologists, an Italian feminist journalist, and five bureaucrats (four local and one Argentinean from the PAHO) with crafting the basis for a subsequent population policy.[1] The resulting text, Peru's Population Policy Guideline, embraced the position of most developing countries at the UN's International Conference on Population, held in Bucharest in 1974, namely, that high birth rates were not a cause but a consequence of underdevelopment, and that attempts to set population-limitation targets were racist and driven by the will of powerful countries to violate the sovereignty of weaker ones. U.S. critics were dismayed at the World Population Plan of Action's definition of population problems as derivatives of social and economic ones, at the imputation of colonialist attitudes on the part of their country, and at the corollary that economic development was the first and foremost way to tackle population problems effectively.[2] The guideline was, and remains, the most important Peruvian manifesto on population.

The Population Policy Guideline was meant as an aspirational document, one that defined the great national shortcomings and assets and provided a vision of the country Peruvians wished they lived in. It acknowledged the gains made in lowering overall mortality rates since 1940 but devoted the bulk of its arguments to showing how longstanding unjust conditions such as illiteracy, racism, and gender inequality persisted. At the same time, echoing the demographic optimism of the 1940 census makers, the guideline affirmed that, while there might be a limit to the indefinite expansion of human population, "we have not yet reached that final natural barrier."[3] Thus, instead of setting quantitative birth-rate targets, the guideline set national qualitative goals based on strengthening families, promoting equality of rights between men and women, ensuring freedom and responsibility in parental decisions regarding family size, protecting children, and achieving national security and development. That established, the guideline acknowledged that rapid population growth worsened problems such as urban chaos and unemployment. It also acknowledged the individually painful experiences of women regarding maternal mortality and malnutrition, worsened by having too many children or by short interparity intervals. The document utterly criticized men's views of women as sexual objects, their abusive attitudes, and their lack of commitment to their families.[4]

Future population laws must, according to the guideline, entail coordination between different sectors to address housing availability, the use of technology for the production of food, the improvement of demographic data gathering, employment generation, environmental pollution, and the distribution of the population in the country's territory. However, the guideline also indicated that, even more important than the above, at least in the short-term, was the promotion of the equality of rights and responsibilities for men and women, including their right to choose fertility-limitation methods (all but abortion and sterilization were legalized). Crucially, the guideline did not cast this right as an individual right, but rather as the right and duty of a couple, a position that is still commonly accepted in Peru today.[5] The right to choose birth control methods, in turn, demanded extending access to medical services as well as popularizing knowledge about family planning methods, sexual education, and responsible parenthood, which was officially defined as the "free and informed choice by couples to decide the size of its offspring, a choice that not only must consider the partners' responsibilities towards each other, but also towards their children and society."[6]

From a policy standpoint, the guideline's implementation was a disappointment. As early as late 1976, even though family planning research and clinical services began a slow but steady rise, intersectoral collaboration within the government to foster legislative changes to improve gender equality, population distribution, sexual education, and employment opportunities proceeded more slowly or stalled.[7] Although the Ministry of Health created an Office of Health and Population in 1977 on the premise that "it is every Peruvian couple's right to determine the size of its family, in an informed and free manner," the office was chronically cash-strapped and failed to set up any national objectives.[8] Worse, the INPROMI, which had been, since the scaling back of the CEPD in 1968, the main state agency focusing on maternal and infant health, was shut down in the late 1970s. Further, although the 1979 Constitution, which ended the military government, stated in its sixth article that "the state supports responsible parenthood," the civilian governments that led Peru from 1980 on were tepid about implementing the bold reforms urged in the Guideline for Population Policy. Under newly elected president Fernando Belaúnde, the Ministry of Health began providing some family planning services in state hospitals in the 1980s. In addition, Belaúnde relaunched the CEPD as the National Council on Population (CONAPO), which drafted the first National Population Law in 1985.[9] The law, however, concerned itself only with health reforms that were not enforced until 1987, when the National Population Program was established during the presidency of Alan García.

Given this picture, it is easy to understand the frustration of the originators of the 1976 Population Policy Guideline. Jesuit Juan Julio Wicht, the guideline's main architect, lamented in 1980 that "almost nothing" had been done to address the complex problems identified in the guideline, and, in 1996, that improvements in the provision of family planning services had occurred slowly and unevenly.[10] Analysts have often asked what went wrong during the execution phase of the country's 1976 population policy. According to historian Marcos Cueto, the fits-and-starts nature of Peru's policy reveals chronic governmental difficulties to build on previous efforts, a process he has referred to as "a vocation to start over again."[11] Medical practitioners affiliated with the Peruvian Academy of Health concur, citing in addition the pusillanimous and balkanized bureaucracies at the ministries of health and education as complicit in the state's neglecting the design of strategies to address gender equality and sex education.[12]

From a historical point of view, what is most significant about the Peruvian Guideline for Population Policy is not how well or poorly it was enacted but how accurately it reflected the desires of an important swath of Latin Americans in the 1970s, as well as the extent to which it gave voice to regional concerns long predating the 1970s. It is remarkable, for example, to see the fertility-linked problems diagnosed in the early 1900s take pride of place among those the guideline tackled: women's victimization, men's irresponsibility and lack of compassion, urban chaos through unplanned growth and rural migration, and poverty. Multiple observers, from the 1890s to the 1970s, had noted how these factors blended into a cocktail of "weak" families, forsaken children, and national degeneration.

The late nineteenth century gave birth to the notion that caring for the reproductive potential of the nation was a task for all: men and women, the wealthy and the poor, white, indigenous, and African-descended Peruvians, though never on equal terms or with equal obligations. While mothers were the keystones of all initiatives, increasing the quality and the quantity of population also demanded the participation of fathers and of the medical profession. Prejudice against nonwhites ran deep then and reproduced colonial assumptions about the cultural and even biological inferiority of non-whites, but the latter too were called upon to join in the project of national aggrandizement, albeit through their submission to the nation's political leadership, and as the junior associates of whites. However, large urban areas in Latin America, where most whites lived, were not only seats of power, but also the epicenters of national anxieties. It was mainly cities that experienced both the heady new affluence of the early twentieth century as well as the concomitant challenges of rapid population growth and poverty. The very necessary production of good citizens demanded high-quality parenting under rapidly changing conditions. The prevalence of abortion was a reminder of the multiple biological, legal, and social pathologies that threatened parenthood. The Latin American citizenship that the Peruvian guideline celebrated through "responsible parenthood" was predicated on an acknowledgment of parents' rights and duties to their children and their homelands.

By the 1970s, some important changes had taken place, of course. Above all, rapid population growth was a reality, as was the existence of new contraceptives. New forces also entered Latin America's family planning debates, particularly second wave feminism and the Cold War. Cognizant of these transformations, the Peruvian guideline committee, led by a Jesuit, admitted the unfair burden that unwanted pregnancies placed on women, and fell squarely on the side of easing restrictions on family planning methods and education to alleviate poverty and human suffering. This process mirrored events elsewhere in Latin America. At the same time, it was a cautious and contested opening. For example, after a tortured debate the Peruvian guideline committee refused to legalize surgical sterilization as a contraceptive. This is symptomatic of how conflicted health workers and social reformers felt about pushing for more radical options in this field, even with governmental support. "We had already accomplished so much, and did not want to risk having the whole document rejected because of the inclusion of sterilization," reflected journalist and guideline committee member Luciana Biseo years later: "The way we saw it, we had begun from absolute zero, and yet managed to agree on important points. The rest might happen later, perhaps in a few years. Although I felt like I was betraying women, I accepted that this was not the right time to continue fighting."[13]

The Cold War also shaped the aspirations of Latin American countries in ways that set them on a collision course with those of the United States. The 1974 World Population Plan of Action defined rapid population growth as caused mainly by social and economic inequalities that needed to be remedied. This was a short-lived and mainly rhetorical moment, since most Latin American nations did include family planning as a component of their population policies in the 1960s and 1970s.[14] Nonetheless, as an act of defiance against a world power, it held great symbolic value for governments such as Peru's seeking to assure their subjects of their own potency. The guideline, in denouncing the United States' intromission in Latin American affairs, revealed itself as a product of Cold War tensions and not only a benign map of the future. It, moreover, helped perpetuate the myth of Peru as a country with vast underexploited natural riches.

There is no question that contemporary Peruvian society is less naïve about the country's natural resources and their distribution, especially in the aftermath of the bloody civil war the Shining Path waged in the 1980s. We have a more robust women's movement, new forms of political mobilization that incorporate previously marginalized populations, and new conflicts too, particularly due to environmental exploitation. Despite these changes, the Guideline for Population Policy, now over thirty years old, is still compelling as a diagnostic tool and a proposal for change. The same deep gender and racial inequalities identified in the 1970s continue to limit people's access to family planning services. The forced sterilizations scandal with which I began my story clearly shows who are still the least cared for and most vulnerable Latin Americans. It would be simplistic to call this a governmental shortcoming. Something older and more insidious is also at play in Peru's failure to revise its own norms on therapeutic abortions. Although these have been legal since 1924, there is not yet a definition of what kinds of pregnancy complications could cause a woman a "permanent and grave injury" and thus could warrant a therapeutic abortion. Karen Llantoy, a young woman, was forced to carry an anencephalic fetus to term in 2002 because of this legal ambiguity and the trepidation with which medical professionals continue to approach reproductive health.[15]

Where did things go wrong for family planning in Peru? In the mid-1960s, several private organizations provided these services for moderate prices, along with other maternal care services. Within a decade, these organizations had ceased to exist or had been greatly weakened. In their stead, the Peruvian government had taken their place or projected to take their place. To some extent, private family planning organizations actively sought out this outcome. The state's taking responsibility for something those organizations pioneered validated their efforts and sacrifices. Moreover, physicians' preoccupation with governmental approval and sponsorship has been a constant in Peru since the creation of the Office of Public Sanitation in 1903.

Governmental and health expert collaboration is important, especially to address matters such as the legal limbo of therapeutic abortions and emergency contraception and the regulation of clinical trials of new contraceptive technologies. However, there are also new opportunities for other Peruvians and their allies in Latin America and elsewhere to broaden and refresh this debate beyond the medical and governmental circles where reproductive health has lain for too long. Nongovernmental organizations created by demographers, feminists, Catholic activists, and midwives have done some of this work since 1976 and have helped showcase the persistent shortcomings of family planning services in rural areas. The proliferation of women's rights organizations such as Manuela Ramos and CLADEM is one of the hopeful signs recent Latin American history affords in the ongoing struggle for greater equality. Part of improving the quality of and access to family planning services in Peru will require the greater diffusion of the initiatives these organizations conduct, acknowledging that the Catholic Church can become, again, a strong ally for sexual and reproductive health, as well as the recognition that not all Peruvians will feel duly represented by the philosophies those different organizations embrace. This recognition may well lead to ever larger and more diverse groups of people speaking up and informing themselves about the stakes involved in the promotion of family planning. That greater complexity may be vexing for the incumbents, but it is not a bad outcome in a region still struggling with democratic institutions. To paraphrase an Argentinean physician of note, creating two, three, many Manuelas, ought to be our goal.[16]

# Notes

## Abbreviations

AAL    Archivo Arzobispal de Lima, Lima
ACP    Archivo del Congreso del Perú, Lima
AGN    Archivo General de la Nación, Lima
APL    Archivo Penal de Lima, Lima
ARA    Archivo Regional de Ayacucho, Ayacucho
ARL    Archivo Regional de La Libertad, Trujillo
ARPi   Archivo Regional de Piura, Piura
ARPu   Archivo Regional del Puno, Puno
CDT    Personal archive of Dr. Carmen Delgado de Thays,
           former APPF director of education, Lima
CENDOC Centro de Documentación de la Historia de la Mujer, Lima
CEP    Archivo de la Conferencia Episcopal Peruana
FF     Ford Foundation Papers at the Rockefeller Archive Center,
           Tarrytown, N.Y.
JMS    J. Mayone Stycos Papers, Cornell University, Ithaca, N.Y.
KP     Personal archive of Dr. Joseph Kerrins and Mrs. Helen Kerrins,
           St. Petersburg, Fla., and East Falmouth, Mass.
MFC    Archivo del Movimiento Familiar Cristiano del Perú,
           c/o Mrs. Graciela de Leidinger, Lima
MRZ    Personal archive of Dr. Miguel Ramos Zambrano,
           former APPF director, Callao
NCWC   Papers of the National Catholic Welfare Council, Catholic University of
           America, Washington, D.C.
PC     Population Council Papers at the Rockefeller Archive Center,
           Tarrytown, N.Y.
PPFA   Planned Parenthood Federation of America Archive, Sophia Smith
           Collection, Smith College, Northampton, Mass.

## Introduction

1. Fujimori, "Discurso del Presidente, 1995."

2. Peru, Amendment 155/95 (Decreto Ley 346).

3. See Peru, *Informe de la Defensoría del Pueblo* 01–98; U.S. House of Representatives Committee on International Relations, "Hearing on the Peruvian Population Control Program"; and Reyes, "No Somos Bultos."

4. See special issues of the following newspapers: *El Comercio* (July 12, 1996), *La República* (May 31, 1998), and *Expreso* (May 31, 1998).

5. UNFPA, "By Choice, Not by Chance," 106–11. The rhythm method is, in present day Peru, the means of fertility control that women use most frequently. See Rodríguez and Venturo, *¡Ampay Mujer!*

6. Klausen, *Race, Maternity and the Politics of Birth Control*; Hodges, *Contraception, Colonialism and Commerce*; and Connelly, *Fatal Misconception*.

7. Warren, *Medicine and Politics in Colonial Peru*; Rohden, *A Arte de Enganar a Natureza*; Soto Laveaga, *Jungle Laboratories*; Felitti, *La Revolución de la Píldora*; Pieper Mooney, *The Politics of Motherhood*; Zárate, *Por la Salud del Cuerpo*; Briggs, *Reproducing Empire*.

8. See, for example, Mass, *Population Target*; Hartmann, *Reproductive Rights and Wrongs*; Symonds and Carder, *The United Nations and the Population Question*; Silva Colmenares, *No . . . Mas . . . Hijos!*

9. Taft-Morales, "Peru in Brief." See also http://www.worldbank.org/en/country/peru (accessed March 1, 2013).

10. Pan American Health Organization, "Health Situation in the Americas."

11. Pan American Health Organization, "Gender, Health and Development."

12. Arana, "The Kids Left Behind."

13. Thompson, *Danger Spots in World Population*; Carr-Saunders, *World Population*; Blacker, *Voluntary Sterilization*; Landry, *La Révolution Démographique*; Notestein, "Population: The Long View." See also Teitelbaum, "Relevance of Demographic Transition Theory"; Demeny, "Social Science and Population Policy"; Caldwell, "Restatement of Demographic Transition Theory"; and Szreter, "The Idea of Demographic Transition."

14. Ariès, *Centuries of Childhood*, Coale and Watkins, *Decline of Fertility in Europe*; Reher and Iriso-Napal, "Marital Fertility and Its Determinants"; Schneider and Schneider, *Festival of the Poor*; Fischer, "Uncertain Aims and Tacit Negotiation."

15. See special issues of the *Milbank Memorial Fund Quarterly* 43 (1965) and 46 (1968). See also Kiser, "Population Trends and Public Health"; and Davis and Casis, "Urbanization in Latin America."

16. Hartmann, *Reproductive Rights and Wrongs*; Crane, "The Transnational Politics of Abortion"; Guzmán et al., *Fertility Transition in Latin America*; Yon Leau, *Hablan las Mujeres Andinas*.

17. Lipset, "Some Social Requisites of Democracy"; and Rostow, *The Stages of Economic Growth*. See also Latham, *Modernization as Ideology*.

18. Kessler and Stanley, "Human Reproduction and Family Planning"; Tucker, "Barriers to Modern Contraceptive Use"; Finkle and McIntosh, "The New Politics of Population"; Tucker, "Haiti."

19. Almeida, "Circuito Aberto."

20. Schwartz, "Midwife in Contemporary Latin America"; Shorter, *A History of Women's Bodies*; Leavitt, *Brought to Bed*; Jeffery and Jeffery, "Traditional Births Attendants"; Vargas and Naccarato, *Allá, las Antiguas Abuelas Eran Parteras*; Renne, "The Pregnancy that Doesn't Stay"; Davis-Floyd and Sargent, *Childbirth and Authoritative Knowledge*.

21. Canguilhem, *Le Normal et le Pathologique*, 186; Lock, *Encounters with Aging*.

22. Martin, *The Woman in the Body*; Ginsburg and Rapp, *Conceiving the New World Order*; Sherwin, *The Politics of Women's Health*; Ram and Jolly, *Maternities and Modernities*; Fisher, *Birth Control, Sex and Marriage*; Summers, "Intimate Colonialism"; Lock and Kaufert, *Pragmatic Women and Body Politics*; Hunt, *A Colonial Lexicon of Birth Ritual;* Inhorn, *Local Babies, Global Science*; Few, *Women Who Live Evil Lives.*

23. Mannarelli, *Limpias y Modernas*; Carrillo, "Nacimiento y Muerte de una Profesión"; Ruggiero, *Modernity in the Flesh*; Rodríguez, *Civilizing Argentina*; Agostoni, "Las Mensajeras de la Salud"; Zárate, *Dar a Luz en Chile, Siglo XIX*; Reber, "Blood, Coughs and Fever"; Stern, "Buildings, Boundaries and Blood"; Needell, "The Revolta Contra Vacina of 1904."

24. Halperín Donghi, *Historia Contemporánea de América Latina*; Abel, *Health, Hygiene and Sanitation*; Bulmer-Thomas, *The Economic History of Latin America.*

25. Hale, "Political Ideas and Ideologies in Latin America."

26. See Weismantel, *Cholas and Pishtacos*; Aguila, *Los Velos y las Pieles*; Lavrin, *Latin American Women*; Macias, "Women and the Mexican Revolution"; Guy, "Women, Peonage, and Industrialization"; Graham, *House and Street*; Chassen-López, "A Patron of Progress"; O'Phelan and Zegarra, *Mujeres, Familia y Sociedad.*

27. Bolton and Mayer, *Andean Kinship and Marriage*; Millones and Pratt, *Amor Brujo*; Ortiz Rescaniere, *La Pareja y el Mito*; Hunefeldt, *Liberalism in the Bedroom*; Dore and Molyneux, *Hidden Histories*; Caulfield, *In Defense of Honor*; Bliss, *Compromised Positions*; Rosemblatt, *Gendered Compromises*; and Hutchison "Add Gender and Stir."

28. Stevens, "Marianismo"; and Chaney, *Supermadre.*

29. Cueto, *Missionaries of Science*; Birn, *Marriage of Convenience*; Quevedo et al., *Café y Gusanos*; Cueto, *El Regreso de las Epidemias*; Zulawski, *Unequal Cures*; Palmer, *Launching Global Health*; Hochman, *A Era do Saneamento*. See also the special issue of the *Canadian Bulletin of Medical History* 25, 1 (2008).

30. For some fine examples of the links between medicine and the consolidation of state power in Latin America, see Stepan, *Beginnings of Brazilian Science*; and the essays in Hochman and Armus, *Cuidar, Controlar, Curar.*

31. David, "Abortion in Europe, 1920–91"; Brouwere, "Comparative Study of Maternal Mortality."

32. Birn, "No More Surprising than a Broken Pitcher."

33. Stepan, *Eradication.*

34. Chambi et al., *Así Nomás Nos Curamos*; Few, *Women Who Live Evil Lives*; Palmer, *From Popular Medicine to Medical Populism*; Sowell, "Contending Medical Ideologies and State Formation"; Castañeda, García, and Langer, "Ethnography of Fertility and Menstruation"; Sainz de la Maza, "Contraception in Three Chibcha Communities."

35. Kleinman, *The Illness Narratives*. See also Polanyi, *Personal Knowledge*; Good, *Medicine, Rationality and Experience.*

36. Brown and Mikkelsen, *No Safe Place*; Steven Epstein, *Impure Science.*

37. Morgan, "Imagining the Unborn."

38. Note, for example, a more nuanced parsing of these distinctions in Anderson, *Tendiendo Puentes.*

39. Johnson-Hanks, "On the Modernity of Traditional Contraception"; and Bledsoe, *Contingent Lives.*

## Chapter 1

1. "El Culto de la Raza," *La Reforma Médica* 20, 183 (March 15, 1934): 290.
2. Warren, *Medicine and Politics in Colonial Peru.*
3. Iza and Salaverry, "El Hospital Real de San Andrés."
4. Woodham, "The Influence of Hipólito Unanue"; Salaverry, "Los Orígenes del Pensamiento Médico de Hipólito Unanue."
5. Salaverry, "El Inicio de la Educación Médica Moderna en el Perú."
6. Paz Soldán, *Heredia y sus Discípulos*; Zárate, *Los Inicios de la Escuela de Medicina de Lima*; Arias Stella, "Anatomía Patológica en el Perú."
7. Pamo Reyna, "Estado Actual de las Publicaciones Periódicas Científicas Médicas del Perú."
8. Cuba, "Influencia de la Medicina Francesa en la Medicina Peruana."
9. Bustíos Romaní, "Historia de la Educación Médica, Primera Parte."
10. Contreras, *El Aprendizaje del Capitalismo*, 176.
11. See Burga and Flores Galindo, *Apogeo y Crisis de la República Aristocrática*; Bonilla, *Un Siglo a la Deriva*; and McEvoy, *La Utopía Republicana.*
12. Ugarte Taboada, "Historia de los Servicios de Emergencia de Lima y Callao"; Vidal Amat y León, *Historia de la Obstetricia y Ginecología en el Perú*; Bazul, "El Profesor Doctor Constantino T. Carvallo"; Guevara Chacabana, "Aspectos Históricos de la Enseñanza de la Pediatría"; Mariátegui, "Hermilio Valdizán y la Facultad de Medicina San Fernando."
13. *Transactions of the First Pan-American Medical Congress, 1893*; *Memorias del Segundo Congreso Médico Pan-Americano, 1896.*
14. Pamo, "Estado Actual de las Publicaciones." See also the first available issues of *La Acción Médica* (January 1927), *La Reforma Médica* (April 15, 1915); and the *Anuario de la Academia Nacional de Medicina* 1 (1952–53). *La Crónica Médica*, published until 1970, was the longest-running medical periodical in Peru.
15. See *Anales de la Academia Nacional de Medicina de Lima* 1 (1919): 1.
16. Finally created in 1935.
17. Eight medical doctors were elected to the first Congress of Peru in 1822, out of eighty-seven members of Congress. See *Reseña Histórica del Congreso*, 2008, ACP.
18. *Boletín del Ministerio de Fomento* 1, 5 (November 30, 1905), AGN.
19. *Boletín del Ministerio de Fomento* 1, 4 (1905): 62–116, AGN; and *Boletín del Ministerio de Fomento* 2, 1 (1906): 53–83, AGN. See also "¿Por Qué Se Abandona a los Niños?" *El Universal* (November 17, 1936): 7.
20. See, for example, Cañizares-Esguerra, *Nature, Empire and Nation*; Pick, *Faces of Degeneration*; and Nye, *Crime, Madness and Politics.*
21. See, for example, Borges, "Puffy, Ugly, Slothful and Inert"; Bliss, *Compromised Positions*; Sater, "The Politics of Public Health"; Blake, "The Medicalization of Nordestinos"; Ruggiero, *Modernity in the Flesh*; Stepan, *The Hour of Eugenics*; Skidmore, *Black into White*; Graham, *The Idea of Race in Latin America*; Meade,

*"Civilizing" Rio*; Palma, *Gobernar es Seleccionar*, 6–9; Suárez Findlay, *Imposing Decency*; Eraso, "Biotypology, Endocrinology and Sterilization."

22. González Prada, *Pájinas Libres*, 38; Gálvez, *Una Lima Que Se Va*; Capelo, *La Despoblación*; Lissón, *Breves Apuntes*, 80; Garland, *Reseña Industrial del Perú*, 4; Graña, *La Población del Perú*; Palma, *El Porvenir de las Razas*.

23. Rodriguez Pastor, *Hijos del Celeste Imperio*; Casalino Sen, "De Cómo los 'Chinos' Se Transformaron"; and Muñoz Cabrejo, *Diversiones Públicas en Lima*.

24. Olivares, "Sobre el Mejoramiento de la Raza," *La Unión Médica* 1, 2 (February 1, 1932): 7; Cueto, *El Regreso de las Epidemias*.

25. Arce's 1901 essay, "Provisión de Brazos para la Agricultura" ("On the Provision of Labor for Agriculture") earned him an award from Peru's National Agricultural Society and is cited in Tudela, *El Problema de la Población el el Perú*.

26. Catálogo de los Expedientes del Congreso y de la Cámara de Diputados, libro 12, legajo 6, cuaderno 1, expediente 1, "Asuntos de carácter general pendientes en la Comision Auxiliar de Gobierno: Inmigración china, prohibiéndola en el territorio de la República, 1909"; libro 12, legajo 7, cuaderno 1, expediente 26, "Asuntos de carácter general pendientes en la Comisión de Inmigración: Inmigración asiática, prohibiéndola en la República, 1916," ACP.

27. Catálogo de los Expedientes del Congreso y de la Cámara de Diputados, libro 12, legajo 4, cuaderno 1, expediente 8, "Asuntos de interés general resueltos por Diputados: Inmigración y colonización Italiana—Protección, 1906," ACP.

28. On European migration to Peru, see Bonfiglio, *La Presencia Europea en el Perú*; and Riviale, *Una Historia de la Presencia Francesa en el Perú*.

29. Julio Egoaguirre, "La Natalidad y la Mortalidad General e Infantil en el Callao," *La Acción Médica* (February 2, 1929): 5. "To govern is to populate" is attributed to Argentinian political theorist Juan Bautista Alberdi, dating from 1852. See Alberdi, *Bases y Puntos de Partida*. See also Herón Frisancho, "Mortalidad Infantil y Movimiento Demográfico," 27–28; and Quijano, *La Emergencia del Grupo Cholo*.

30. *Boletín del Ministerio de Fomento* 1, 4 (1905): 106, AGN.

31. Schneider, "Puericulture"; Lefaucheur, "La Puériculture d'Adolphe Pinard"; Offen, "Depopulation, Nationalism, and Feminism." Medical advice for the protection of pregnant, potentially pregnant, and puerperal women took on various shapes throughout the world. See, for example, Pieper Mooney, *The Politics of Motherhood*; Bock and Thane, *Maternity and Gender Policies*; Koven and Michel, *Mothers of a New World*; Klaus, *Every Child a Lion*; Arnup, *Education for Motherhood*; Pedersen, *Family, Dependence*; Apple, *Perfect Motherhood*; Hodges, *Reproductive Health in India*.

32. Avendaño and Fernandez Dávila, *La Despoblación*, n.p. Italics in the original.

33. Ibid. See also Archivo Histórico del Ministerio de Hacienda, Dirección de Salubridad Pública, Rómulo Eyzaguirre, "Demografía Sanitaria," *Boletín del Ministerio de Fomento* 2, 1 (1906): 1–22, AGN.

34. Deustua, "Higiene de la Lactancia," 6.

35. Lawezzari, "Algunas Consideraciones sobre la Protección de la Infancia en Lima," 52.

36. Guevara Chacabana, "Aspectos Históricos de la Enseñanza de la Pediatría."

37. Paz Soldán, *La Protección a la Infancia en el Perú*.

38. Román Arredondo, "Contribución al Mejoramiento de la Asistencia Médico-Social del Niño Chalaco."

39. Ley 2851, "Trabajo de los Niños y Mujeres por Cuenta Ajena" (November 23, 1918), ACP. See also Barandiarán, "Descanso y Protección de la Mujer Embarazada."

40. Guevara Chacabana, "Aspectos Históricos de la Enseñanza de la Pediatría."

41. Paz Soldán, *Actas y Trabajos de la Primera Conferencia Nacional sobre el Niño Peruano*.

42. *Boletín del Departamento de Protección Materno Infantil* 1, 1 (1922).

43. "La Profesión de Obstetriz y Su Papel en la Demogénesis Peruana," *La Reforma Médica* 33, 492–93 (February 1947): 77–87.

44. "Hacia la Reforma Universitaria: La Enseñanza de la Obstetricia," *La Acción Médica* (March 17, 1928): 3.

45. See various issues of *La Acción Médica*, for example, "La Maternidad y la Alimentación" (March 23, 1929): 6; "Educacion Física Femenina" (September 28, 1929): 4–5; Samuel Gajardo, "Las Deficiencias del Hogar como Factor de Delincencia de Menores," *La Acción Médica* (November 2, 1929): 1–2, 15; "Aspectos Sociales de la Educacion Sexual" (November 9, 1929): 3; and "El Papel Preponderante de la Madre en la Educación Sexual de sus Hijos" (November 16, 1929): 10–11. See also issues of *Acción Católica Peruana* (February 12, 1933): 27; and (November 26, 1933): 191; as well as "Orígenes, Desarrollo y Finalidades de la Cruz Roja: A los Pueblos de América," *Anales de la Cruz Roja Peruana* 31 (August 1934): 35–44.

46. On midwifery in Peru, see Rabí Chara, *De la Casa de Maternidad de Lima al Instituto Nacional Materno Perinatal*.

47. "Acción Social de las Visitadoras de Higiene Infantil," *Boletín del Instituto Nacional del Niño* 1, 1 (June 1933): 12–14. See also González, "Contribución a la Maternología Nacional."

48. Contreras, "Sobre los Orígenes de la Explosión Demográfica en el Perú," 10.

49. Ministerio de Hacienda, David Matto, *Memoria del Ministro de Fomento a la Legislatura Ordinaria de 1909*, AGN. See point 228, on "Atribuciones de las Obstetrices Titulares," 295.

50. "La Profesión de Obstetriz y Su Papel en la Demogénesis Peruana," *La Reforma Médica* 33, 492–93 (February 1947): 77–87.

51. Ministerio de Hacienda, Carta de Abel Olaechea, Dirección de Salubridad Pública, al Ministerio de Hacienda (January 23, 1917), AGN.

52. Furthermore, according to Dr. Hipólito Larrabure, of the 33,124 births registered in Lima between 1914 and 1922, 14,605 did not receive any medical attention at all. For this reason, he insisted on the need to train more midwives. See Larrabure's intervention in Paz Soldán, *Actas y Trabajos de la Primera Conferencia Nacional sobre el Niño Peruano*. See also López Cornejo, "Las Realidades de la Asistencia del Parto en el Perú."

53. See Bowser, *African Slave in Colonial Peru*; Aguirre, *Breve Historia de la Esclavitud en el Perú*; Cadena, *Indigenous Mestizos*; and Chambers, *De Súbditos a Ciudadanos*.

54. Alberto Flores Galindo traces these back at least to the Tupac Amaru II rebellion in the 1780s. See Flores Galindo, *Buscando un Inca*.

55. Mallon, *Peasant and Nation*; Thurner, *From Two Republics to One Divided.*

56. See Herzog, "Percibir el Otro."

57. Daniel Laborería, "El Arte de Curar entre los Antiguos Peruanos," *Anales de la Universidad Nacional Mayor de San Marcos* 29 (1902): 59–263; "Vida Física de la Mujer," *La Acción Médica* (September 22, 1928): 11; Lucio Castro Medina, "La Obstetricia en la Raza Indígena," *Actualidad Médica Peruana* 5, 2 (June 1939): 44–50; "Medicina y Antropología," *Actualidad Médica Peruana* 2, 2 (1936): 1–2; *Actualidad Médica Peruana* 1, 11 (1936): 617–19; "La Unificación del Idioma como Medida de Higiene Mental en el Perú," *Actualidad Médica Peruana* 4, 9 (January 1939): 310; "La Influencia del Bilingüismo en la Mentalidad del Pueblo Peruano,"*Actualidad Médica Peruana* 6, 5 (September 1940): 131–33; "Las Fantasias Medico-Sociales del Congreso Indigenista de Pátzcuaro," *La Reforma Médica* 26, 351 (March 15, 1941): 187–89; Kuczynski Godard, *La Vida en la Amazonía Peruana.*

58. Paz Soldán, "La Medicina Militar y los Problemas Nacionales," 13–14. See also Tudela, *El Problema de la Población el el Perú*; León García, "Las Razas en Lima"; "Un Significado Ejemplo de los Progresos de la Higiene Rural," *Anales de la Cruz Roja Peruana* 2 (September–October 1934): 19–21.

59. Zárate, *Dar a Luz en Chile, Siglo XIX*; Carrillo, "Nacimiento y Muerte de una Profesión"; Clark, *Gender, State, and Medicine.*

60. See, for example, José B. Jimenez Camacho, "El Ejercicio de la Profesión Médica en Provincias: Obstetricia Rural en la Sierra del Perú," *Actualidad Médica Peruana* 6, 3 (July 1940): 74–79.

61. Carlos A. Bambarén, "Labor y Finalidades de la Liga Nacional de Higiene y Profilaxia Social," *Anales de la Cruz Roja Peruana* 4 (December 1934–January 1935): 9–11; Arias Schreiber Pezet, "Los Médicos Peruanos en la Guerra del Pacífico."

62. Catálogo de los expedientes del Congreso y de la Cámara de Diputados, libro 12, legajo 9, cuaderno 1, "Asuntos de interés general pendientes en comisiones: Principal de legislación, exp. 16: Represión del alcoholismo" (1905), ACP.

63. *La Temperancia* 8, 17 (May 20, 1922): 41–42; ley 4950, "Declarando obligatoria en los colegios y escuelas en general la enseñanza de la higiene, enfermedades infecto contagiosas, alcoholismo y puericultura," (February 16, 1924), ACP.

64. Macera, "Sexo y Coloniaje"; Drinot, "Moralidad, Moda y Sexualidad."

65. Gil Cárdenas, "El Matrimonio Civil"; Guzmán Rodriguez, "Profilaxis de las Enfermedades Venéreas"; Merkel, "Reglamentación de la Prostitución en Lima"; Casas, "La Delincuencia Infantil."

66. Archivo Histórico del Ministerio de Hacienda, Juan Manuel García, "Memoria del Ministro de Fomento a la Legislatura Ordinaria de 1912," AGN. See also Colina, "Contribución al Estudio de la Profilaxia de las Enfermedades Venéreas."

67. González, "La Prostitución Reglamentada en Lima."

68. See Guy, *Sex and Danger in Buenos Aires*; Bliss, *Compromised Positions*; Levine, *Prostitution, Race, and Politics*; Donovan, *White Slave Crusades.*

69. J. L. Pando Baura, "Editorial," *La Acción Médica* (June 29, 1929): 8.

70. "Sifilicomio," *Boletín de la Academia Nacional de Medicina* (1922–23): 1–2; Espinosa Palacios, "La Sífilis en las Clases Trabajadoras."

71. Gerardo Alarco, "Programa General para la Lucha Antivenérea," *Revista de la Sanidad Militar del Perú* 1, 1–2 (January–June 1928): 56–61; Luis Arias Schreiber, "La Profilaxia de las Enfermedades Venéreas en el Ejército," *Revista de la Sanidad Militar del Peru* 1, 3 (July–September 1928): 172–95; Melgar Menéndez, "Profilaxia Social de las Enfermedades Venéreas"; R. Angulo, "La Profilaxia Antivenérea entre Nosostros," *Revista Médica Peruana* 5, 58–59 (October–November 1933): 1414–24; Corrales Diaz, "Estadística y Profilaxia de las Enfermedades Venéreas en la Armada Peruana"; Latorre, "El Preventivo Antivenéreo Civil en Lima"; Rosa Cáceres Silva, "Rol de la Enfermera en la Profilaxia de las Enfermedades Venéreas," *Boletín del Enfermero de la Sanidad de Gobierno y Policía* 1, 6 (September–October 1946): 15–19.

72. "Estatutos de la Liga Nacional Antivenérea," *Boletín de la Dirección General de Salubridad Publica* (1927): 213–15.

73. Enrique B. Rubin, "Discurso con Motivo de la Inauguración del Museo Nacional de Profilaxis Antivenérea," *La Reforma Médica* 18, 147 (September 15, 1932): 226–28.

74. Ley 8124, "Ministerio de Salud Pública, Trabajo y Previsión Social" (October 5, 1935), ACP.

75. Lip, Lazo, and Brito, *El Trabajo Médico en el Perú.*

76. "La Lucha Anti-venérea en Lima y Labor de los Puestos de Socorro," *Boletín de la Dirección General de Salubridad* 1, 3 (1935): 9.

77. Pilares Polo Escalante, "La Profilaxis de la Sífilis en el Ejército."

78. "Dia Antivenéreo," *La Reforma Médica* 24, 290 (September 1, 1938): 672, 706.

79. An important parallel is the discussion of the "cult of masculinity" that emerged with the Mexican Revolution. See Bliss, *Compromised Positions.*

80. See Mannarelli, *Pecados Públicos*; Hunefeldt, *Liberalism in the Bedroom.*

81. Gloria Gray, "Bolivar Odicio, El Cashibo Civilizador," *Perú Indígena* 4, 9 (April 1953): 146–55.

82. *Boletín de la Dirección General de Salubridad* 1943 and 1944, AGN; and Cueto, "Social Medicine and 'Leprosy.'"

83. "El Certificado Médico Pre-Nupcial," *Educación Sanitaria* 2, 14 (November 1942–June 1943): 5. Prenuptial certificates were first mandated by the civil matrimony law of 1931, though the 1936 civil code made them a less strict requirement.

84. Bustíos Romaní, "Historia de la Educación Médica, Segunda Parte."

85. Peru, Instituto Nacional de Estadística e Informática, "Historia de los Censos en el Perú."

86. Aramburú, *Migración Interna en el Perú.*

87. Necochea López, "Demographic Knowledge and Nation-Building."

88. Arévalo Ruiz, "La 'Barriada' Carmen de la Legua."

89. Altuna del Valle, "Una Concentración Sub-Urbana Peligrosa para la Sanidad de Lima." See also Suarez Camargo, "Una Visita a 'Ciudad de Dios'"; and Alayza Tejada, "Estudio Médico Social del Distrito de Pachacamac."

90. Monge Raguz, "El Avecindamiento Humano en el Cerro San Cosme," 11.

91. Morales Martinez, "Eugenesia, Matrimonio y Convivencia," 59–60. See also Arroyo Posadas, "Infancia y Pro-biofilaxis, Dos Mil Niños y su Destino Socio Vital en 'El Montón.'"

92. Vílches Bedoya, "Capacidad para el Matrimonio."

93. Stepan, *The Hour of Eugenics*.

## Chapter 2

1. Interviews with Elsa Lescano (Lima, July 7, 2010) and Alfredo Larrañaga Leguía (Lima, July 11, 2006); and Larrañaga and Kesserü, "Dos Años de Experiencia Clínica con el Enantato de Noretisterona como Anticonceptivo Inyectable de Depósito."

2. Mörner, *Race Mixture*.

3. Chambers, *De Súbditos a Ciudadanos*; Borchart de Moreno, "Words and Wounds."

4. See also Ehrick, "Affectionate Mothers and the Colossal Machine"; Nari, *Políticas de Maternidad y Maternalismo Político*; and Freire, *Mulheres, Mães e Médicos*.

5. Miller, *Latin American Women*, 74. On the 1919 protest organized by the Comité Femenino Pro Abaratamiento de las Subsistencias, see Perú, MIMDES, Cincuenta Años del Voto Femenino en el Perú, 31. See also Chaney, "Old and New Feminists"; Stevens, "Marianismo"; Barrig, *Cinturón de Castidad*; Palmer and Rojas Chaves, "Educating Señorita"; Guy, *White Slavery and Mothers*; O'Phelan and Zegarra, *Mujeres, Familia y Sociedad en la Historia de América Latina*; and Pieper Mooney, *The Politics of Motherhood*.

6. Augusto Alvarez Rodrich, "La Sagrada Familia," *La República* (February 14, 2013): 5.

7. Dalurzo, *Homenaje en Buenos Aires a Irene Silva de Santolalla*; "Irene Santolalla, 90, Peruvian Specialist on Children Is Dead," *New York Times* (August 4, 1992): B6.

8. Interview with Irene Santolalla Silva (Chosica, July 16, 2010).

9. Santolalla, *Mi Aporte a la Educación Familiar*, 9, 13. Hereafter *MAEF*.

10. Francisco P. Cabrejas to Irene S. de Santolalla (Buenos Aires, March 22, 1938, and April 27, 1938), in *MAEF*, 13–14.

11. Peru, *Anteproyecto de una Ley de Elecciones, Cámara de Diputados, Exposición de Motivos*, 43.

12. Wicht, "La Situación Demográfica del Perú."

13. Portal, "Hacia la Mujer Nueva," cited in Barrig, *Cinturón de Castidad*, 26; and Portal, *El Aprismo y la Mujer*. See also Reedy, *Magda Portal*. Interestingly, Luis Alberto Sánchez, fellow APRA leader and member of the congressional committee in question, voted against granting women the vote.

14. Perú, MIMDES, Cincuenta Años del Voto Femenino en el Perú, 32.

15. Santolalla, *Por la Felicidad de Nuestros Hijos*.

16. Aída Berza to Irene S. De Santolalla (Buenos Aires, June 24, 1940), and Ernesto Goldschmidt, "Mensaje Transmitido por CX48, Radio Femenina del Uruguay," (October 4, 1956), in *MAEF*, 24, 102.

17. Santolalla, *Hacia un Mundo Mejor*, 164, 138.

18. Women were permitted to obtain a university education starting in 1908. The first public high school for women opened in 1928. See Barrig, *Cinturón de Castidad*, 23. On women's social advancement through education, see Zegarra, "Roles Femeninos y Perspectivas Sociales en las Décadas Iniciales de la República."

19. Gonzalez de Fanning, "Concerning the Education of Women," 31.

20. Santolalla, *Hacia un Mundo Mejor*, 117.

21. Ibid., 128–29. The Pan American Child Congresses have met since 1916 and, from their beginnings, have enjoyed substantial female participation. See Guy, "The Politics of Pan-American Cooperation"; Birn, "Uruguay on the World Stage."

22. Santolalla, *¡El Gran Problema!*, 7.

23. Santolalla, *Hacia un Mundo Mejor*, 103, 145, 263.

24. Josermo Murillo Vacareza, president of the Sociedad Boliviana de Eugenesia, to Irene Silva de Santolalla (Oruro, February 28, 1945); Carlos Bernardo de Quiroz, president of the Sociedad Argentina de Eugenesia to Irene Silva de Santolalla (August 1, 1949); Paul Popenoe to Irene Silva de Santolalla (Los Angeles, July 27, 1946, and September 28, 1948), in *MAEF*, 385, 43, 208, 212.

25. García y García, *La Mujer y el Hogar*, 40.

26. Cosamalón, "Soy Yo la que Sostengo la Casa."

27. Manuel Salcedo, "Discurso de Transmisión de Cargo en la Sociedad Peruana de Pediatría," *Boletín del Departamento de Protección Materno Infantil* 4, 15–16 (1944): 11–32.

28. Santolalla, *Perú, País Pionero*, 13; Hampe Martínez, "La Universidad Católica de Lima y la Evolución de las Universidades Privadas en el Perú Contemporáneo"; "Las Primeras Parlamentarias Peruanas," in www.congreso.gob.pe/museo/mujeres -Parlamentarias.pdf (accessed March 8, 2011).

29. "Conclusiones del 1er Congreso Internacional de Madres, Buenos Aires, Julio 1948," in *MAEF*, 32

30. "Entrevista de Josefina Escoté Hernández a Irene Silva de Santolalla," *Margarita* (1948), in *MAEF*, 147.

31. Santolalla, *¡El Gran Problema!*, 30.

32. Carlos Bernardo de Quiroz, president of the Sociedad Argentina de Eugenesia, to Irene Silva de Santolalla (Buenos Aires, October 15, 1949), in *MAEF*, 44.

33. Santolalla, *¡El Gran Problema!*, 126–28.

34. Ibid., 7; Vera Zouroff to Irene S. de Santolalla (Santiago, Chile, April 19, 1950), in *MAEF*, 150.

35. Ley 12391, "Sustituyendo los Artículos 84, 86 y 88 de la Constitución del Estado, para Conceder la Ciudadanía a la Mujer" (September 7, 1955), ACP.

36. Santolalla, *Perú, País Pionero*, 9.

37. Interview with Irene Santolalla Silva (Chosica, July 16, 2010).

38. Santolalla, *Perú, País Pionero*, 41, 42, 14.

39. Santolalla, *¡El Gran Problema!*, 205.

40. Marina Bermejo and Tony Rodriguez, "Mujer de las Américas," *Ecos de Nueva York* (1956), in *MAEF*, 233, 242–43.

41. Ana María Perera Moya, president of the Inter-American Commission of Women of the Organization of American States, to Irene Silva de Santolalla (New York, August 14, 1956), in *MAEF*, 235; Perú, MIMDES, "Cincuenta Años del Voto Femenino en el Perú," 5.

42. Leyes 13923, 14000, 13517, and 14084, ACP. Santolalla's effort to censor movies also failed. See "Producción Legislativa del Ex-Representante Irene Silva Linares

de Santolalla," in www.congreso.gob.pe/archivo/damas/01-Silva-Irene-Senadora/
Produccion-Legislativa.pdf (accessed October 4, 2010).

43. Santolalla, *Perú, País Pionero*, 45; Motion 24 in "Producción Legislativa."

44. Law 12818 in "Producción Legislativa."

45. "Ley de Educación Familiar," in *MAEF*, 105.

46. Interview with Irene Santolalla Silva (Chosica, July 16, 2010).

47. Santolalla, *Perú, País Pionero*, 17.

48. Ricardo Pollo Darraque, Uruguay Cultural Attaché, "Educación Familiar," *La Crónica* (January 6, 1957), in *MAEF*, 119; and Dalurzo, *Homenaje*, 28.

49. "Resolución Suprema 27, creando el Instituto de Educacion Familiar y Matrimonial" (January 30, 1959), in Santolalla, *Perú, País Pionero*, 9, 18–20; María Teresa de Valverde, consulate general of Bolivia in New York, to Irene Silva de Santolalla (New York City, August 15, 1963), in *MAEF*, 273.

50. Woolsey Teller, "Peruvian Woman Wins Family Education Battle," *Indianapolis Star* (February 7, 1971), in *MAEF*, 297; Guillermina Paredes de Alcázar, president of the Peruvian Association of Family Education Professionals, to Irene Silva de Santolalla (April 23, 1982), in Santolalla, *Perú, País Pionero*, n.p.; see also Susana Villarán public profile at www.munlima.gob.pe/contenidos/biografia.aspx (accessed January 28, 2011).

51. Ley 2851, "Trabajo de los Niños y Mujeres por Cuenta Ajena" (November 23, 1918), ACP.

52. Villavicencio, *Del Silencio a la Palabra*. See also Drinot, *The Allure of Labor*.

53. Zegarra, "María Jesús Alvarado y el Rol de las Mujeres en la Construcción de la Patria."

54. Drinot, "Creole Anti-Communism."

55. Escuela Sindical Autonoma de Lima, "Mujeres: Trabajadoras . . . Ciudadanas" (1958): 78, 30.

56. Helio Castellón, "¿Está Masculinizándose la Mujer que Trabaja?" *Ñusta* 1, 5 (November 1957): 7–9, 8.

57. Instituto Interamericano de Ciencias Agrícolas, "Simposio de Educación para el Hogar," 2.

58. Avabai Wadia to Irene Santolalla Silva (Bombay, February 2, 1967) in *MAEF*, 566.

59. Avabai Wadia, *The Light Is Ours*, 255.

60. See "De la Mujer Peruana" section in *Plan Inca Elaborado por el Gobierno Revolucionario de la Fuerza Armada, 1968*.

61. Gobierno del Perú, Comisión Nacional de la Mujer Peruana, "Programa Operativo de Control Antivenéreo en Lima y Callao" (Lima, October 30, 1969), CENDOC.

62. Barrig, *Cinturón de Castidad*; Saporta Sternbach, Navarro-Aranguren, Chuchryk, Alvarez, "Feminisms in Latin America"; Vargas, "Los Feminismos Peruanos."

63. Orvig, "Tambien Antes Hubo Algo."

64. Portugal, "El Retorno de las Brujas"; Trapasso, "Romper la Invisibilidad."

65. Violeta Sara-Lafosse, "Dinámica de Población y Relaciones Sociales," in CISEPA-Pontificia Universidad Católica del Perú (Lima, November 1974), CENDOC.

66. ALIMUPER, "¿Quienes Controlan la Fertilidad de la Mujer?" (Lima, 1970), CENDOC.

67. ALIMUPER, "Legalización del Aborto en el Perú" (Lima, August 1977, 3); Maria Guisán, "Liberación de la Mujer y el Rol Materno," in ALIMUPER, *Madre Solo Hay Una* (Lima, May 1976, 19–20), CENDOC.

68. Violeta Sara-Lafosse, "La Familia y la Mujer en Contextos Sociales Diferentes" (Lima, November 1978), CENDOC.

69. "Ley General de Educación, Decreto Ley 19326," Sección Considerandos 1, ACP.

70. *Boletín Informativo de la Unión Popular de Mujeres Peruanas* (1972).

71. *Boletín de la Secretaría de Prensa de la Unión Popular de Mujeres Peruanas* 1, 2 (March 8, 1971): 6.

72. Rosa Villarán, "Me Lincharían Si Les Digo 'Planifica tu Familia,'" *La Tortuga* 20 (1987): 13–20, 16.

73. Rosa Alba Mendieta de Bernhoeft to Irene Silva de Santolalla (São Paulo, October 26, 1970), in *MAEF*, 485; Centre for Population Activities and Asociación para el Desarrollo Integral de la Mujer, "Primer Seminario Taller de Mujeres en Dirigencia" (Lima, January 14–February 1, 1980), CENDOC.

74. Interview with Dr. Alfredo Larrañaga Leguía, former director of the Marcelino Institute (Lima, July 11, 2006).

75. Interview with Dr. Carmen Delgado de Thays (Lima, June 27, 2010). See also "Carmen Delgado curriculum vitae" and "Estrategia de desarrollo de la oficina ejecutiva de APPF," CDT.

76. Interview with Elsa Lescano (Lima, July 7, 2010), italics indicate words she emphasized.

77. "Se Dice Planificación Familiar, Paternidad Responsable, Protección Familiar, Pero Jamás Control de la Natalidad," *Patricia* 1, 7 (March 24, 1971): 21–25. See also "Guía para la visita," CDT.

78. Interview with Rosa Motta (Lima, July 6, 2010). See also "La consulta de planificación familiar"; "Programa de supervisión" (1972); and "Funcionamiento de un centro de protección familiar tipo I," CDT.

79. "Asistencia total en las acciones educativas por año, según tipo de acción" (1973), CDT.

80. "Estrategia para el desarrollo de los centros de protección familiar" CDT.

81. Interviews with former APPF midwives Luisa Parra (Lima, July 6, 2010) and Manuela Araujo (Lima, July 1, 2010).

82. Interviews with Rosa Motta (Lima, July 6, 2010) and Elsa Lescano (Lima, July 7, 2010).

83. In this vein, see Offen, "Defining Feminism"; Cott, "What's in a Name?" Kampwirth and Rodríguez, *Radical Women in Latin America*; Morcillo, *True Catholic Womanhood*; and Power, *Right-Wing Women in Chile*; Mayes, "Why Dominican Feminism Moved to the Right."

84. Note the parallels with the more recent U.S. maternalist tradition, described in Ladd-Taylor, "Toward Defining Maternalism in US History."

85. Microfilm reel 3525, grant 65-358, Mayor Grl. FAP Eduardo Montero to José Donayre, December 16, 1968; and microfilm reel 3446, grant 65-358, Richard Dye and Antonio Muñoz Najar to William Carmichael, May 3, 1973, FF.

86. Drysdale, "Education Approaches to Population Problems."

87. Unpublished reports, box 19112, folder 11899, "Observations on sex education in Peru, November 29th, 1974," FF.

88. See the intervention of Ricardo Morales, SJ, Presidente del Consejo Superior de Educación, in Peru, "Informe Final del Primer Seminario Nacional sobre Politica de Poblacion" (1976).

89. Roldán, "El Peligro Venéreo y su Profilaxia en el Ejército"; Vega Gamarra, "Contribución al Estudio de la Mortalidad Infantil en Huaraz"; Herón Frisancho, "Mortalidad Infantil y Movimiento Demográfico en la Ciudad de Puno"; Ruiz, "Evolución Demográfica de Chiclayo"; Villavicencio, *La Vida Sexual del Indígena Peruano.*

## Chapter 3

The quotation from Magda Portal comes from Andradi and Portugal, *Ser Mujer en el Perú*, 230.

1. López Cornejo, "Las Realidades de la Asistencia del Parto en el Perú"; Quintanilla Paulet, "Algunos Problemas Médicos en Relación con el Subdesarrollo Económico del Perú"; Arroyo Posadas, "Infancia y Pro-biofilaxis"; Burgos Amaya, "La Procreación Consciente en Nuestro País"; Bedoya Hevia, "Social Problems of Abortion."

2. Rice-Wray, "The Provoked Abortion"; Mendoza, "Population Growth and Family Planning"; Armijo and Monreal, "The Problem of Induced Abortion"; Gaslonde Sainz, "Abortion Research in Latin America"; Viel, *The Demographic Explosion*; Figa-Talamanca, "Health and Economic Consequences"; Corvalan, "The Abortion Epidemic."

3. Crane, "The Transnational Politics of Abortion"; Singh and Wulf, *Clandestine Abortion in Latin America*; Yam, Dries-Daffner, and García, "Abortion Opinion Research"; Ferrando, *El Aborto Clandestino en el Perú*; and Brooke, "High Rate of South American Abortion Ills."

4. Scholars writing in this vein include Stern, *The Secret History of Gender*; Reagan, *When Abortion Was a Crime*; Bart, "Seizing the Means of Reproduction"; Solinger, *The Abortionist*; Cline, *Creating Choice*; Usborne, *Cultures of Abortion in Weimar Germany*; and Schoen, *Choice and Coercion.*

5. The soul entering the body was what defined an "animated fetus." This Catholic thesis has existed at least since the eleventh century. See Coriden, "Church Law and Abortion."

6. Código Penal del Estado Sud Peruano 1836, libro III, título 1, capítulo 1, arts. 516 and 517.

7. Código Penal del Perú 1862, libro 2, sección 7, título 3, arts. 243–45.

8. Código Penal del Perú 1862, libro 2, sección 7, título 2, art. 242.

9. Prison (*prisión*) terms were different from jail (*cárcel*) terms, even though time served as inmates might be similar. Prison terms carried, in addition to the time served, the suspension of civil rights during imprisonment and for up to seven years after release from prison, as well as a probation period of up to five years, depending on good behavior. Jail terms carried the suspension of civil rights during confinement and a probation period of up to two and a half years.

10. Cáceres, "Patogenia y Etiología del Aborto"; Gavidia, "El Aborto como Accidente Espontáneo o Patológico"; and Guzmán Rodriguez, "Profilaxis de las Enfermedades Venéreas."

11. Pedro Villanueva, "Estenosis del Orificio Uterino y Sífilis Conyugal," *La Reforma Médica* 2, 26–28 (September 30, 1916): 99–100.

12. Basadre, "Ligeras Consideraciones sobre el Uso Prematuro y el Abuso del Corsé," 4.

13. Brölmann, Dijkhuizen, and Mol, "The Clinical Importance of the Microcurettage."

14. Molina, "El Curetaje Uterino," 39.

15. Beraún, "Curetaje Uterino y sus Aplicaciones Terapeuticas."

16. Ugarte Taboada, "Historia de los Servicios de Emergencia de Lima y Callao."

17. Chiri, "Consideraciones sobre la Sífilis y el Embarazo entre Nosotros." See also Barandiarán, "Descanso y Protección de la Mujer Embarazada."

18. Portillo, "El Problema de la Natimortalidad en Lima"; Avendaño and Fernandez-Dávila, *La Despoblación*; Herón Frisancho, "Mortalidad Infantil y Movimiento Demográfico en la Ciudad de Puno."

19. Obladen, "History of Surfactant up to 1980."

20. On infanticides in Lima, see Changanaquí, "Algunos Casos de Infanticidio en Lima"; and Mercado, "Contribución al Estudio del Infanticidio en Lima."

21. Avendaño and Fernandez-Dávila, *La Despoblación*.

22. *Anales de la Facultad de Medicina de la Universidad de San Marcos* (1913): 106.

23. Víctor Maúrtua, "Proyecto de Ley sobre el Infanticidio, Artículos 129 y 130," (1916), ACP.

24. Código Penal del Perú 1924, libro 2, sección 1, título 2, arts. 159–64.

25. Código Penal del Perú 1924, libro 2, sección 1, art. 155.

26. Código Penal del Perú 1924, libro 2, sección 1, art. 163.

27. Fernández Dávila, *El Delito de Aborto*, 22.

28. Fosalba y Muro, "La Excusa Absolutoria del Aborto Científico."

29. Several other physicians shared this view. See Tello Morales, "Causas de Muerte Materna en la Maternidad de Lima"; Amorín V., "Causas de la Mortalidad Fetal y la Neonatal en el Callao"; Quintana Flores, "Contribución al Estudio del Problema Social y Médico Legal del Aborto."

30. Escudero Villar, "Contribución al Estudio del Aborto," 3.

31. Olascoaga Mar, "Estudio Médico Social del Problema Materno-Infantil en la Ciudad de Tacna."

32. Busalleu, "Lección Inaugural del Curso de Obstetricia," 231.

33. Gajardo, "Las Deficiencias del Hogar como Factor de Delincencia de Menores"; Herón Frisancho, "Mortalidad Infantil y Movimiento Demográfico en la Ciudad de Puno."

34. "Aspectos Sociales de la Educación Sexual," *La Acción Médica* (November 9, 1929): 3; "El Papel Preponderante de la Madre en la Educación Sexual de sus Hijos," *La Acción Médica* (November 16, 1929): 10–11.

35. Avendaño, "¿Hay Jerarquía en la Sociedad Conyugal?"; Castellón, "¿Está Masculinizándose la Mujer que Trabaja?"

36. Salcedo F., "Infancia Abandonada en Peligro y Peligrosa," 13.

37. Valle Medina, "Contribución al Estudio del Problema Social y Médico-Legal del Aborto en el Callao."

38. Cited by Vidal, *Historia de la Obstetricia y Ginecología en el Perú*, 49. Though undated, this statement was most likely made by Avendaño while he was a professor of legal medicine at the Faculty of Medicine of Lima between 1919 and 1930.

39. Vargas Prada, "Circular No. 7 a los Médicos Directores de Hospitales" (April 10, 1933), cited in *La Reforma Médica* 19, 165 (June 15, 1933): 197.

40. Paz Soldán, "Editorial," 198.

41. However, the Penal Archive of Lima does not have the records between the years of 1933 and 1938. Thus, it is possible that some of Paz Soldán's accusations have been lost.

42. "Decreto Presidencial del 24 de Mayo de 1946," cited in "Regulación de la Fecundidad" (1979), CENDOC.

43. López Cornejo, "Las Realidades de la Asistencia del Parto en el Perú"; Barreto P., "Problema Materno-Infantil en Iquitos"; Landaburú Soubise, "Contribución al Estudio de la Mortalidad Materna"; Untiveros Morales, "La Frecuencia de los Abortos en Lima"; Frías Ocampo, "Causas de Internamiento y de Muerte en la Maternidad de Lima"; Neyra Mosquera, "El Problema Médico Legal y Médico Social del Aborto en el Perú"; Quintana Flores, "Estudio Estadístico de la Ciudad de Pisco."

44. Landaburú, "Contribución al Estudio de la Mortalidad Materna," 42, 100.

45. Frías Ocampo, "Causas de Internamiento y de Muerte en la Maternidad de Lima," 33-34.

46. Landaburú, "Contribución al Estudio de la Mortalidad Materna," 173. Vaginal tears were the next most common intervention, making up 25 percent of all surgeries.

47. Frías Ocampo, "Causas de Internamiento y de Muerte en la Maternidad de Lima," 11. Vaginal tears were the next most common intervention, making up 19 percent of all surgeries.

48. Tello Morales, "Causas de Muerte Materna en la Maternidad de Lima."

49. On the introduction of antibiotics in Peru, see Instituto Nacional de Planificación, "Plan Nacional de Desarrollo Económico y Social del Perú, 1962-1971."

50. On the Prado presidency, see Portocarrero, *El Imperio Prado, 1890-1970*.

51. Established in 1942, the SCISP operated in several Latin American countries as a dependency of local health ministries. Most SCISP employees were local health workers, but a few, especially the top decision makers, were highly trained U.S. experts paid by the U.S. government. On the health care assistance Peru received from the United States, see Cueto, *The Value of Health*.

52. The 1940 census was the first conducted in the twentieth century. Cajamarca, Cuzco, Junin, and Ancash were more populous than Piura, Ayacucho, and La Libertad. However, the regional archives at the former group of four departamentos either failed to respond to my queries or informed me they did not have the criminal records I requested. Lima criminal records are split between the Archivo General de la Nación (1895-1921) and the Archivo Penal (1961-79). Unfortunately, no archivist has been able to account for the missing Lima records between 1922 and 1960.

53. Montoya, "Estudio Médico Legal sobre un Caso de Pseudo-Embarazo y Pseudo-Aborto," 3–4.

54. Indeed, Peru's 1936 Civil Code, article 1136 stipulated that "anyone who by his acts, carelessness or imprudence, causes a damage to another, is obligated to indemnify it." In this case, the misdiagnosis could be interpreted as careless and damaging to the marriage.

55. Cáceres, "Patogenia y Etiología del Aborto," Observación VI.

56. Ibid., Observación I. On attempts to get truthful accounts about miscarriages from women, and women's efforts to thwart such attempts, see also Reagan, "About to Meet Her Maker."

57. Castellares, "Abortos Espontáneos y Abortos Provocados."

58. Untiveros Morales, "Frecuencia de los Abortos en Lima," 13.

59. Cabrera, "Ensayo de Clasificación de la Etiología del Aborto," 44.

60. Escudero Villar, "Contribución al Estudio del Aborto," 3, 81.

61. Quinine can act as an emmenagogue only when taken in large quantities that make it very toxic. See McGready, "Effects of Quinine and Chloroquine Antimalarial Treatments."

62. Beraún, "Curetaje Uterino," 45.

63. Gavidia, "Aborto como Accidente," 70.

64. Valdizán and Maldonado, *La Medicina Popular Peruana, Volumen 1*, 343.

65. Antúnez de Mayolo, *Cuadernos de Medicina Popular Peruana*, 5.

66. Carter, "Trial Marriage in the Andes?"; Berlin, "Aspects of Fertility Regulation"; Millones and Pratt, *Amor Brujo*.

67. Calle, *Anotaciones y Concordancias al Código Penal*, 138.

68. See ads in *La Prensa* (August 31, 1916): 3; and *La Prensa* (February 3, 1920): 6.

69. Gavidia, "Aborto como Accidente," 70.

70. Molina, "El Curetaje Uterino," n.p.

71. Beraún, "Curetaje Uterino," 45.

72. Cáceres, "Patogenia y Etiología del Aborto," Observación III, IV, and V.

73. Untiveros Morales, "Frecuencia de los Abortos en Lima," 47. However, within just a few years, falls were no longer deemed so innocent and began to be listed alongside oxytocic drugs, uterine irrigation, and the introduction of solid bodies in the uterus as the most common methods for the inducement of illegal abortions. See Neyra, "El Problema Médico Legal y Médico Social del Aborto en el Perú," 45.

74. Mexican scholars have also documented the belief that physical exhaustion causes abortions, as well as the technique of lifting heavy weights to induce a miscarriage. See Valle Prieto, "Parto y Aborto en Algunas 'Ciudades Perdidas' de México."

75. Contra Angélica Fernandes por infanticidio, Declaración de Angélica Fernandes, June 26, 1920; and Informe del Fiscal, July 7, 1920, ARL.

76. Representative of state interests.

77. Rosa Huamán contra Rosa Valderrama, 1940, Informe del Fiscal, January 13, 1941, ARL.

78. Contra Alejandro Cedamanos, 1937, Reporte del Fiscal, September 14, 1938, ARL.

79. Piccato, *City of Suspects*; Rodríguez, *Civilizing Argentina*.

80. Juzgado Penal 7, Grupo 48, No. 16, Exp. 221-1975, Aborto consentido de Gladys Castillo; Juzgado Penal 13, Grupo 66, No. 16, Exp. 241-1976, Aborto a Ana María Torres; Juzgado Penal 12, Grupo 99, No. 7, Exp. 8764-1977, Aborto de Eva Salazar; Juzgado Penal 12, Grupo 84, Exp. 9000-1977, Aborto de Doraliza Vega, APL.

81. Juzgado Penal 13, Grupo 66, No. 16, Exp. 241-1976, Aborto a Ana María Torres, Testimonio de Carlos García, and Testimonio de Maria Isabel Lavalle, May 17, 1976, APL.

82. Juzgado Penal 7, Grupo 48, No. 16, Exp. 221-1975, Aborto consentido de Gladys Castillo, Fallo del Juez, June 9, 1981, APL.

83. Juzgado Penal 12, Grupo 99, No. 7, Exp. 8764-1977, Aborto de Eva Salazar, Declaración de Antonio Mendoza, April 6, 1977, APL.

84. Causas criminales, legajo 14, Contra Eudosia Mendoza por aborto, 1901, AGN; and Contra Felícita Cisneros, 1946, ARA.

85. Contra Leocadia Riveros por aborto en agravio de Teófila Gavilán, 1936, Reporte del Fiscal, August 14, 1942, ARA.

86. See, for example, Juzgado Penal 2, Grupo 87, Exp. 166-1973, Contra Dra. Natividad Acosta Pinto; and Juzgado Penal 2, Grupo 82, N. 127, Exp. 733-1975, Contra Silvia Manchego de Urday, APL.

87. Contra Jacinto Huaynacho por aborto y homicidio, 1977, ARPu.

88. Contra Celia Jara Sanchez y un Boliviano desconocido, 1940, Informe final del Fiscal, February 3, 1941, ARL.

89. Contra Manuel Bocanegra y Ofelina Espejo, 1926, Carta del Dr. Hildebrando Ortiz, August 11, 1926, and Declaración del Dr. Hildebrando Ortiz, May 9, 1927, ARL.

90. Causas criminales, legajo 14, Contra Eudosia Mendoza por aborto (1901), Declaración de Don Anselmo Mendoza al Juez de Paz Gabriel Lira, November 23, 1900, AGN.

91. Platt, "El Feto Agresivo." On the spiritual liminality of fetuses in the Andes, see also Morgan, "Imagining the Unborn."

92. Contra Ignacio Quecara, 1976, Declaración de Catalina Machaca, February 7, 1977, ARPu.

93. Contra Angélica Fernandes por infanticidio, 1920, Declaración de Angélica Fernandes, June 26, 1920, ARL.

94. Contra Juan Roca por aborto en agravio de Magdalena Nuñez, 1943, ARPu; Juzgado Penal 2, Grupo 82, No. 127, Exp. 733-1975, Silvia Manchego; and Juzgado Penal 12, Grupo 108, Exp. 10007-1979, Contra Mercedes Díaz, APL.

95. Contra Manuel Díaz en agravio de Felícita Rebaza por aborto, 1940, Declaración de Manuel Díaz, May 15, 1940, ARL. On the link between the satisfaction of pregnant women's cravings and good births and maternal health in Spanish Latin America, see Valdizán and Maldonado, *Medicina Popular Peruana, Vol. 1*, 343; Flores Cisneros, "Saber Popular y Prácticas de Embarazo"; and Mendoza González, "¿Dónde Quedó el Arbol de las Placentas?"

96. Causas criminales, legajo 28, 1903-1904, No. 55, Contra Ismael Ramón por maltrato, Declaración de Ismael Ramón, August 13, 1904, AGN.

97. Rosa Huamán contra Rosa Valderrama, 1940, Manifestación de Rosa Valderrama, January 3 and 8, 1940, and Declaración de testigo Rosa Vaquedano, January 4, 1940, ARL. On the practice of honoring birth attendants through gifts rather than payment, see Vargas and Naccarato, *Allá, las Antiguas Abuelas Eran Parteras*; and Sáenz, *Partos y Parteras en la Cuenca del Rio Marcará*.

98. Juzgado Penal 7, Grupo 48, No. 16, Exp. 221–1975, Confrontación entre Gladys Castillo y María Gutierrez, May 29, 1975, APL.

99. Rosa Huamán contra Rosa Valderrama (1940), Declaración de testigo Rosa Vaquedano, January 4, 1940, and Manifestación de Vicente Wong, January 11, 1940, ARL.

100. Juzgado Penal 2, Grupo 82, No. 127, Exp. 733–1975, Instructiva de Amparo Burgos, October 1, 1975, APL.

101. Juzgado Penal 12, Grupo 85, No. 4, Exp. 10069–1979, Muerte de Genara Umiña, APL; Contra Jacinto Huaynacho por aborto y homicidio, 1977, ARPu; Contra Blanca Romero, Genoveva Juarez y Alfonso Farro por aborto en agravio de Fredesvinda Lara Ramirez, 1959, ARPi.

102. Contra Marcos Carbajal por delitos contra la vida, 1926, Carta del Fiscal, May 12, 1930, ARA.

103. Contra Nicolas Pancca y otros por lesiones y subsiguiente aborto, 1920, Reporte del Fiscal Zuñiga Bejar, July 13, 1921; Contra Luciano Apaza for infanticidio y lesiones, 1930, Reporte del Fiscal M. Pinera del Carpio, December 4, 1931, ARPu.

104. Causas criminales, legajo 28, 1903–1904, No. 55, Contra Ismael Ramón por maltrato, Declaraciones de Filomena Ramón y de Ismael Ramón, August 13, 1904, AGN.

105. Contra Manuel Díaz en agravio de Felícita Rebaza por aborto, 1940, Preventiva de Felícita Rebaza, May 20, 1940; Testimonio de testigo Fidencio Moreno, May 20, 1940; and Declaración de Manuel Díaz, May 15, 1940, ARL.

106. Sección Nulidad, leg. 77, exp. 5, César Málaga vs. Sara Sevilla, 1913, AAL; Contra Remberto Acevedo por tentativa de aborto, 1938, ARL; Contra Luis Vignolo por lesiones a Manuel Hidalgo y tentativa de aborto en agravio de Tomasa Hidalgo, 1943, ARPi; and Sección Causas de Divorcios, leg. 86, exp. 97, Don Carlos Dogni con Doña Helen Kramer, 1946, AAL.

107. Warshaw, *Encyclopedia of Surfing*, 126, 158–59.

108. Contra Wilfredo Tapia por tentativa de aborto, 1952, ARPu; and Contra Hermilio Morales por lesiones graves y aborto, 1924, Carta de Maximiana Zorrilla, June 18, 1924, ARA.

109. Sección causas de divorcios, leg. 119, exp. 25, Hortensia Noriega vs. Cristóbal Mendizábal, Cartas de Hortensia Noriega, November 15 and 16, 1905, AAL.

110. Causas criminales, Doña Julia Izquierdo contra José Aguilar por maltratos, 1901, Parte médico, February 12, 1901; Declaración de Julia Izquierdo, February 16, 1901; Comparece José Aguilar, January 9, 1902; and Carta de Julia Izquierdo, January 9, 1902, ARL.

111. Ruggiero, *Modernity in the Flesh*; Urías Horcasitas, "Eugenesia y Aborto en México."

112. Gotkowitz, "Trading Insults."

113. Stern, *Secret History of Gender.*

## Chapter 4

1. See, for example, Robinson, "Algunas Observaciones acerca de Nuestro Problema Racial," 58.

2. Pastor Padierna, "El Control Sanitario del Matrimonio"; Cademártori, "La Asistencia Médico-Social del Niño en el Callao"; Fosalba, "Ideas Generales sobre la Herencia"; Lewis, "El Problema de la Esterilización," 364; Mac-Lean y Estenos, "La Eugenesia en América."

3. Compare with Germain, "Women at Mexico," 235–38; Pedro, "A Experiência com Contraceptivos no Brasil"; Felitti, "El Debate Médico sobre Anticoncepción en Buenos Aires"; Langland, "Birth Control Pills and Molotov Cocktails."

4. Ley 8124, "Ministerio de Salud Pública, Trabajo y Previsión Social" (October 5, 1935), ACP.

5. On the Pan-American Health Organization, see Cueto, *The Value of Health.*

6. "Origenes, Desarrollo y Finalidades de la Cruz Roja: A los Pueblos de América," *Anales de la Cruz Roja Peruana* 31 (August 1934): 35–44; Flores S., "El Hogar Infantil y su Rendimiento de Bien Médico Social"; Luna Vegas, *Factores Etiológicos de la Peligrosidad en los Menores*; Salcedo, "Infancia Abandonada en Peligro y Peligrosa"; Linares Lizárraga, "Contribución al Estudio Médico Social de la Madre Lactante."

7. Valle Medina, "Problema Social y Médico-Legal del Aborto en el Callao"; Untiveros Morales, "La Frecuencia de los Abortos en Lima"; Monge Raguz, "El Avecindamiento Humano en el Cerro San Cosme"; Altuna del Valle, "Una Concentración Sub-Urbana Peligrosa para la Sanidad de Lima"; Arroyo Posadas, "Infancia y Pro-Biofilaxis."

8. José Alcántara La Torre, "El Nuevo Planeta," *Variedades* 25, 1150 (March 19, 1930): 3.

9. Jiménez Camacho, "El Ejercicio de la Profesión Médica en Provincias," 74–79.

10. Neira, *Huillca*, 10–11.

11. Mazzi, *Poesía Proletaria del Perú*, 107.

12. Tello Morales, "Causas de Muerte Materna en la Maternidad de Lima." The total number of women who gave birth at the Maternidad de Lima in this period was 101,859. National maternal mortality rates are only available from 1980. In that year, Peru's maternal mortality rate was 318 per 100,000 births. See http://www.unfpa.org .pe (accessed November 2, 2007).

13. Paz Soldán, "El Magno Problema," 10.

14. Paz Soldán, "¿Será Mejor que No Nazcan?" 40.

15. Quintanilla, "Problemas Médicos," 90.

16. Burgos Amaya, "La Procreación Consciente en Nuestro País."

17. The rhythm method of birth control was based on Kyusaku Ogino's and Hermann Knaus's near-simultaneous findings about the infertility periods in women's menstrual cycles in the mid-1930s. This research was the basis for a method that relies on the identification of segments in the menstrual cycle during which a pregnancy

is unlikely to occur. See Ogino, *The Conception Period of Women*. Hermann Knaus's research was published as *Die periodische Fruchtbarkeit und Unfruchtbarkeit des Weibes*.

18. "El Inquietante Problema de la Prole a Voluntad," *La Reforma Médica* 20, 181 (February 1934): 111–12.

19. Burgos Amaya, "La Procreación Consciente en Nuestro País," 52; Ostolaza, "Estudio del Chancro"; and López, "Diagnóstico de los Flujos Utero-Vaginales en las Enfermedades Venéreas."

20. Bambarén, "Algunas Consideraciones sobre las Perversiones Sexuales y la Delincuencia," 21. See also "Have Spermatozoa Functions or Effects Other than Fertilization?" 42–43.

21. Avendaño and Fernández Davila, *La Despoblación*, 27. See also Paz Soldán, "La Decadencia de la Maternidad," *La Reforma Médica* 20, 194 (September 1934): 561–68, 589–90.

22. "La Venta de Preservativos en la Vía Pública," *Boletín de la Dirección General de Salubridad Publica* (1940): 75.

23. See ads for Tuxedo, Romeo, Convoys, Koin Pack, and Sultán condoms in the *Revista Farmaceutica Peruana* 23, 275 (March 1955): 6; ibid. 24, 277 (May 1955): 13; and ibid. 25, 289 (May 1956): 22.

24. Caravedo, *Burguesía e Industria en el Perú*; Caravedo, *Desarrollo Desigual y Lucha Política en el Perú*; Pareja, *Aprismo y Sindicalismo en el Perú*; and Portocarrero, *De Bustamante a Odría*.

25. Aramburú, Bedoya, and Recharte, *Colonización en la Amazonía*.

26. Interview with Dr. Alfredo Larrañaga Leguía (Lima, July 11, 2006).

27. *Boletín CEPD* 3, 11 (March 1969): 3–6. See also interview with social worker Emperatriz Matallana (Lima, July 6, 2010).

28. Interview with Dr. Luis Fernández (Trujillo, July 13, 2010).

29. Interview with Dr. Alfredo Larrañaga Leguía (Lima, July 11, 2006).

30. Email from Dr. Luz Jefferson to the author (Lima, February 21, 2009).

31. Interview with Dr. Victor Díaz (Lima, June 30, 2010).

32. Interview with social worker Rosa Motta (Lima, July 6, 2010).

33. Email to the author from Dr. René Cervantes, who completed his residency training under Dr. Abraham Ludmir (Lima, December 16, 2008). See also Pieper Mooney, *The Politics of Motherhood*.

34. Interview with midwife Luisa Parra (Lima, July 6, 2010).

35. Interviews with Dr. Nazario Carrasco (Lima, June 28, 2010); Dr. Doris Chang León (Lima, June 25, 2010); Dr. Hugo Oblitas (Lima, July 19, 2004); and Dr. Hugo Calle (Lima, July 6, 2010).

36. Interview with Dr. Delia Moreno (Lima, July 5, 2010).

37. Carlos Uriarte, "Planificación Familiar: Dos Tendencias," *Boletín CEPD* 2, 7 (March 1968): 11. See also interview with social worker Natalia Romero (Lima, July 5, 2010).

38. PPFA II Series, box 204, folder 17, Distributor list of Enovid, Establecimientos Leonard, S.A., Casilla 2554, Lima, PPFA. See also advertisements for Anovlar 21 in the *Revista Médica del Hospital Central del Empleado* 5, 4 (October 1965).

39. "Un Problema de Conciencia," *Intima* 3, 22 (February 1966): 7–10.

40. Larrañaga and Kesserü, "Dos Años de Experiencia Clínica con el Enantato de Noretisterona."

41. Interview with Dr. Alfredo Larrañaga Leguía (Lima, July 11, 2006). See also Winterhalter, "Un Nuevo Contraceptivo Oral"; Hurtado, Kesserü, and Larrañaga, "D-Norgestrel, un Progestágeno a Microdosis"; Kesserü, Larrañaga, and Parada, "Postcoital Contraception with D-Norgestrel"; Larrañaga, Winterhalter, and Natal, "Evaluation of d-Norgestrel 1.0mg as a Postcoital Contraceptive."

42. Interview with Oswaldo Vasquez Cerna, Junta de Asistencia Nacional (National Welfare Board) 1972–76 (Lima, July 5, 2010); interview with social worker Elsa Lescano (Lima, July 7, 2010).

43. "La Planificación Familiar," *Patricia* 1, 7 (March 1971): 21–25.

44. Interview with former Schering Peru sales chief Carlos García San Martín (June 30, 2010).

45. Interview with Dr. Augusto Chávez (Lima, July 7, 2010).

46. See Necochea López, "A History of the Medical Control of Fertility in Peru," 184.

47. Notestein, "Demography in the United States," 684.

48. Hill, Stycos, and Back, *The Family and Population Control*; Stycos, *The Control of Human Fertility in Jamaica*.

49. Stycos, *Human Fertility in Latin America*, 147–61.

50. Hall, "Control de la Natalidad en Lima, Perú."

51. Interview with Dr. Marie-Françoise Hall (February 20, 2009).

52. "La Encuesta Hall," *Caretas* 296, 14 (August 1964): 30–38. See also "¿Demasiados Niños?" *Caretas* 260, 13 (February 1963): 11–14; "La Iglesia y los Anticonceptivos," *Caretas* 261, 13 (February 1963): 15, 54; "Editorial," *Boletin CEPD* 2, 7 (March 1968): 1, 8–9; José Adolph, "Natalidad y Revolución," *Expreso* (August 10, 1970); "El Retorno de lo Absurdo," *Caretas* 20, 423 (September 30–October 14, 1970): 14–16; Luis Rey de Castro, "¿Anti-Política Demográfica?" *Revista 7 Días* (October 1970); "Inquietante Pregunta: ¿Píldora o Dispositivo Intrauterino?" *Fémina* 1, 4 (January 1975): 12–13; and Bonfiglio, "Veinticinco Años de Debates de Población en la Prensa Peruana."

53. Iannacone Martínez, "Vida Reproductiva en las Mujeres de 20 a 39 Años"; Silva Valladares, "Vida Reproductiva de las Mujeres de 20–39 Años"; Navas Mena, "Planificación Familiar en el Medio Policial"; Bustamante de Montalvan, "Algunos Aspectos de Planificación Familiar en Trujillo."

54. Rice-Wray, "The Provoked Abortion." See also *Proceedings of the 4th IPPF/WHR Conference*, particularly the papers by Gómez and García on Argentina, Rozada on Uruguay, and Merchan, on Venezuela.

55. See, for example, Warwick, *Bitter Pills*, especially chapter 7.

56. Interview with midwife Luisa Parra (Lima, July 6, 2010).

57. "Informe de Sociedad Civil sobre Avances y Retrocesos en Salud Reproductiva y Equidad de Género" (June 15, 2003), CENDOC.

58. Williams, *Obstetrics*, 408.

59. Berkeley and Bonney, *Difficulties and Emergencies of Obstetric Practice*; DeLee, *Principles and Practice of Obstetrics*; Eden and Holland, *A Manual of Midwifery*; Adair, *Obstetrics and Gynecology*.

60. Eastman, *Williams Obstetrics*, 1046.

61. Landauro Valentini, "La Esterilización Quirúrgica en Obstetricia."

62. Interview with Dr. Victor Díaz (Lima, June 30, 2010).

63. Moreno, "Esterilización Tubárica Bilateral por Pinzamientos Sucesivos."

64. Interview with Dr. Ramiro Yanque (Lima, July 2, 2010).

65. Interview with Dr. Delia Moreno (Lima, July 5, 2010).

66. Interview with Dr. Luis Fernández (Trujillo, July 13, 2010); and Dr. Doris Chang León (Lima, June 25, 2010).

67. Interview with Dr. Miguel Exebio (Lima, July 1, 2010).

68. Interview with Dr. Ramiro Yanque (Lima, July 2, 2010).

69. Chávez and Bachmann, "Esterilización Quirúrgica en Pacientes Cesareadas."

70. Halton, Dickinson, and Tietze, "Contraception with an Intrauterine Silk Coil"; Oppenheimer, "Prevention of Pregnancy by the Gräfenberg Ring Method." On the history of the IUD, see Thiery, "Pioneers of the Intrauterine Device"; and Os, "The Intrauterine Device and Its Dynamics."

71. Tietze and Lewit, *First International Conference on Intra-Uterine Devices*, 7.

72. Berelson, "National Family Planning Programs," 8.

73. Tietze and Lewit, *First International Conference on Intra-Uterine Devices*, 57–59. Zipper went on to obtain a Population Council fellowship, which allowed him to spend 1962 at the Worcester Foundation in Shrewsbury, Massachusetts, working under Gregory Pincus, the inventor of the contraceptive pill. There he discovered the role of metal ions such as copper in preventing the implantation of fertilized eggs in the uterus, which led to his invention of the copper-T IUD in 1968, for which he received numerous patents: U.S. Patent 3,563,235, "Intrauterine Contraceptive Method" (September 18, 1968); U.S. Patent 28,399, "Intrauterine Contraceptive Method (reissued April 29, 1975); U.S. Patent 4,040,417, "Intrauterine Device" (August 9, 1977).

74. Segal, Southam, and Shafer, *Second International Conference on IUDs*, 90–92.

75. Interview with Dr. Delia Moreno (Lima, July 5, 2010).

76. Interview with Dr. Hugo Calle (Lima, July 6, 2010).

77. Interview with Dr. Hugo Oblitas (Lima, July 19, 2004); and Dr. Luis Fernández (Trujillo, July 13, 2010).

78. Bachmann, "El Aborto Inducido como Problema Social," 6.

79. Gavidia Lino, "El Aborto como Problema de Seguridad Social"; Medel, "Avances en Anticoncepción Intrauterina"; "Inquietante Pregunta: ¿Píldora o Dispositivo Intrauterino?" *Fémina* 1, 4 (January 1975): 12–13.

80. Microfilm reel 3472, grant 65-358, "Proyecto de Ampliación del Programa Materno-Infantil del Hospital de Torax, Bravo Chico, Octubre 1966," FF.

81. Interview with midwife Luisa Parra (Lima, July 6, 2010).

82. Interviews with Dr. Delia Moreno (Lima, July 5, 2010); Dr. Doris Chang León (Lima, June 25, 2010); midwife Manuela Araujo (Lima, July 1, 2010); and Dr. Luis Fernandez (Trujillo, July 13, 2010).

83. Necochea López, "La Asociación Peruana de Protección Familiar."

84. Ministerio de Trabajo to APPF, July 18, 1970; and "Convenio entre el Concejo Distrital de San Miguel y la APPF" (June 2, 1972), MRZ.

85. Alfaro, "La Asociación Peruana de Protección Familiar y la Planificación Familiar."

86. PPFA II Series, box 83, folder 27, UPCH request for renewal of funds to Family Planning International Assistance, February 1976; folder 28, UPCH request for renewal of funds to Family Planning International Assistance, February 1978; and Dr. Daniel Weintraub, FPIA chief operating officer, to Gerard Bowers, chief of the Grants Management Branch of the Family Planning Services Division, Office of Population, USAID, March 2, 1978, PPFA.

87. Telephone interview with Dr. Walter Llaque Dávila (Lima, July 12, 2006).

88. "Resolution Ministerial 000293-73-SA/DS," *El Peruano*, December 21, 1973: 1.

89. See the handwritten note from Robbins in memorandum from Daniel Weintraub to John Robbins, January 14, 1975, in PPFA II, box 83, folder 27, PPFA.

90. Barnes, "United States Private Agencies' Contributions to Population Programs," 664.

91. Interviews with Dr. Carmen Delgado de Thays, former APPF director of education (Lima, June 27, 2010); and social worker Emperatriz Matallana (Lima, July 6, 2010).

92. Interview with Dr. Nazario Carrasco (Lima, June 28, 2010).

93. Interview with midwife Luisa Parra (Lima, July 6, 2010).

94. Interview with Dr. Ramiro Yanque (Lima, July 2, 2010). See also interviews with Dr. Victor Díaz (Lima, June 30, 2010); Dr. Doris Chang León (June 25, 2010); Dr. Delia Moreno (Lima, July 5, 2010); and Dr. Miguel Exebio (Lima, July 1, 2010).

95. Quotes from interviews with Dr. Nazario Carrasco (Lima, June 28, 2010) and social worker Martha de Laudi (Lima, April 14, 2006), respectively.

96. See interviews with Dr. Carmen Delgado de Thays, former APPF director of education (Lima, June 27, 2010); midwife Luisa Parra (Lima, July 6, 2010); social worker Rosa Motta (Lima, July 6, 2010); and Dr. Augusto Chávez (Lima, July 7, 2010).

97. Interview with Consuelo Castillo, family planning volunteer (Lima, June 22, 2006).

98. Interviews with Dr. Helí Cancino (Lima, July 19, 2004); social worker Rosa Motta (Lima, July 6, 2010); Dr. Alfredo Larrañaga Leguía (Lima, July 11, 2006); Dr. Hugo Oblitas (Lima, July 19, 2004); and Dr. Nazario Carrasco (Lima, June 28, 2010).

99. Interview with Dr. Doris Chang León (Lima, June 25, 2010).

100. Andradi and Portugal, *Ser Mujer en el Perú*, 45.

101. Ibid., 60, 187. Teresa Dávila is likely referring to the hormonal secretions that help ovarian follicles mature into human eggs. The pill was designed to interfere with that cycle.

102. Berelson, "National Family Planning Programs," 6; "The First Forty Years"; Wulf, "Overcoming Circumstances."

103. Montero Mogollón, "Motivaciones de las Pacientes con DIU Perdidas al Seguimiento," 43.

104. Echandía et al., "Pueblo Joven El Planeta," 6.

105. Interview with Carlos García San Martín (Lima, June 30, 2010).

106. See, for example, Vicuña, Kesserü, and Larrañaga, "Evaluación del Uso del Dispositivo Intrauterino"; Guardia, "Evaluación de Dispositivos Intrauterinos en Pamplona Alta"; Martínez Valdez, "Anticoncepción Intrauterina."

107. Telephone interview with Dr. Walter Llaque Dávila (Lima, July 12, 2006); interview with Dr. Delia Moreno (Lima, July 5, 2010).

108. Interview with Dr. Jorge Ascenzo (Lima, May 4, 2006).

109. Interview with Dr. Delia Moreno (Lima, July 5, 2010). See also interview with social worker Emperatriz Matallana (Lima, July 6, 2010).

110. Interviews with Dr. Nazario Carrasco (Lima, June 28, 2010); and midwife Luisa Parra (Lima, July 6, 2010).

111. Interview with social worker Martha de Laudi (Lima, April 14, 2006).

112. See Pieper Mooney, *The Politics of Motherhood*; and Felitti, *La Revolución de la Píldora*.

113. Viel, "Family Planning in Chile"; and Ott, "Population Policy Formation in Colombia."

## Chapter 5

1. Notestein, "Reminiscences."

2. Prebisch, *The Economic Development of Latin America*.

3. CEPAL, *Análisis y Proyecciones del Desarrollo Económico*; and especially CEPAL, *Desarrollo Humano, Cambio Social y Crecimiento en América Latina*.

4. Symonds and Carder, *The United Nations and the Population Question*.

5. Stavenhagen, "Social and Demographic Research."

6. Ferrando and Aramburú, "The Fertility Transition in Peru."

7. On the 1940 census, see Necochea López, "Demographic Knowledge and Nation-Building."

8. Perú, Instituto Nacional de Planificación, "Plan Nacional de Desarrollo Económico y Social del Perú, 1962–1971"; *Boletín de Noticias del Instituto Nacional de Planificación* 2 (December 1965); Perú, Instituto Nacional de Planificación y Oficina Nacional de Estadística y Censos, *Estudio sobre la Población Peruana*.

9. Wilmoth and Ball, "The Population Debate in American Popular Magazines, 1946–90." Reverend Thomas Malthus in the late eighteenth century was arguably the first to suggest population growth was a threat to the collective well-being of society. Hence, proponents of population reduction through birth control were often referred to as "neo-Malthusianists" by their opponents. See Malthus, *An Essay on the Principle of Population*. Exemplary of the contempt some felt toward "neo-Malthusianism" is Mass, *Population Target*.

10. Notestein, "Population: The Long View"; Vogt, *Road to Survival*; Nelson, "Low-Level Equilibrium Trap in Underdeveloped Economies"; Coale and Hoover, *Population Growth and Economic Development*; Sharpless, "Population Science, Private Foundations and Development Aid."

11. On the Vicos Project, see Bolton, *50 Años de Antropología*.

12. Box 10, folder 38, diary notes, meeting with Ofelia Mendoza, New York, October 24, 1963, 39, JMS.

13. Box 10, folder 42, diary notes, Peru, February 6–12, 1964, and April 4, 1964, JMS.

14. Folder correspondence, reports, studies, FC-S-Peru 58–66, J. Mayone Stycos to Dr. David Tejada de Rivero, July 23, 1964, PC.

15. Created in 1936, the Ford Foundation grew to one of the United States' largest private philanthropies in the early 1960s, donating over US$1.5 billion. In the early 1950s, it began to invest strongly in the social and behavioral sciences. Its Population Program made grants to the field for over US$21 million by 1964, including academic and research programs at Johns Hopkins, Harvard, the Worcester Foundation, and the Population Council, as well as national governments, particularly those of India, Pakistan, and Tunisia. See Caldwell and Caldwell, *Limiting Population Growth*.

16. Reel 3472, grant 65–358, Nick Eastman to Oscar Harkavy, September 10, 1964, FF.

17. Reel 3472, grant 65–358, "Preliminary Outline: Organization of a Program for Studies on Population Dynamics in Peru" (October 5, 1964), FF.

18. Box 10, folder 40, diary notes, Lima, Peru, November 16, 1964, 311, JMS.

19. Box 10, folder 40, diary notes, Lima, Peru, October 6, 1964, JMS.

20. "Decreto Supremo 244/64-DGS: Centro de Estudios de Población y Desarrollo," *El Peruano*, December 5, 1964: 1.

21. Reel 3472, grant 65–358, Alberto Arca Parró to Peter Fraenkel, January 14, 1965, FF.

22. Reel 1722, grant 65–358, John Hilliard to Harry Wilhelm, June 3, 1965, FF.

23. Reel 1722, grant 65–358, Ford Foundation to Alberto Arca Parró, September 23, 1965, FF.

24. Unpublished reports, box 18712, folder 4518, Peru log notes by Lyle Saunders, 1965, FF.

25. CEPD, *Primer Seminario de Población y Desarrollo*, xxxi–xxxii.

26. Reel 3472, grant 65–358, Ozzie Simmons to Alberto Arca Parró, December 14, 1965, FF; accession 1, box 66, folder 1156, Frank Notestein to Alberto Arca Parró, December 22, 1965, PC.

27. On Pincus's and the Worcester Foundation's role developing the contraceptive pill, see Watkins, *On the Pill*.

28. Reel 3472, grant 65–358, Ozzie Simmons to executive director, president, and members of the Consejo Directivo of the CEPD, March 21, 1966, FF.

29. Donaldson, "United States Government's International Population Policy."

30. Box 10, folder 42, diary notes, Peru, February 6–12, 1964; and April 4, 1964, 72, JMS.

31. Green, "The Evolution of US International Population Policy, 1965–92," 305.

32. Folder USAID, Dr. Jonathan Fine, Public Health Officer, USAID Bureau for Latin America, to Bernard Berelson, Population Council, Washington, March 11, 1966, PC.

33. See part 2, section II, p. 129 of U.S. Department of State, "National Security Study Memorandum 200."

34. On the PAHO's policy reversal, note the priorities set out by PAHO director Abraham Horwitz in 1959 in his "Relaciones entre Salud y Desarrollo Económico," and compare them with his own position by 1967 in "La Salud Hemisférica y la Reunión de Jefes de Estado Americanos," 65. On the WHO's reversal, see Resolution 1.43 in World Health Organization, *Handbook of Resolutions and Decisions, 1948–1972*; and "Administration of Maternal and Child Health Services," 5; and compare them with

World Health Assembly resolution 18.49 of May 1965, reaffirmed as WHA 19.43 in May 1966, and WHA 20.41 in May 1967, in WHO, *Handbook of Resolutions and Decisions, 1948–1972.*

35. Unpublished reports, box 18826, folder 6781, John Saunders, "CEPD Report" (September 1968), FF.

36. "Nota Editorial," *Boletín CEPD* 1, 1 (June 1966): 1.

37. Reel 3472, grant 65–358, "CEPD Informe #1, Octubre 1966"; unpublished reports, box 18826, folder 6781, John Saunders, "CEPD Report" (September 1968), FF.

38. Unpublished reports, box 18826, folder 6779, Robert Wickham to Peter Fraenkel, December 6, 1967, FF.

39. Reel 3472, grant 65–358, "Funcionamiento de un Consultorio Materno-Infantil y de Planeamiento Familiar" (June 30, 1966); and "Proyecto de Ampliación del Programa Materno-Infantil del Hospital de Torax, Bravo Chico" (October 1966), FF.

40. Folder US Government, Dept. of State, AID Peru, 67–68, Jonathan Fine to Gonzalo Echeverri, November 8, 1967, PC. See also reel C1573, grant 65–358, section Peru, Population, Lyle Saunders to Peru File, January 11, 1967, FF; folder Centro de Estudios de Población y Desarrollo, FC-O-Peru 67–68, Clifford Pease to José Donayre, May 2, 1967, PC; and reel 3472, grant 65–358, Draft of Letter of Understanding CEPD-AID, February 17, 1967, FF.

41. "Meeting on Population Policies in Relation to Development in Latin America: Recommendations," 1–4.

42. Prebisch, *Towards a New Trade Policy for Development*, 116.

43. Reel 3472, grant 65–358, Javier Arias Stella to Alberto Arca Parró, January 24, 1968; and field trip report of Dr. William Moore to Peter Fraenkel, April 18, 1968, FF.

44. Unpublished reports, box 18826, folder 6781, John Saunders "CEPD Report" (September 1968), FF; accession 2, box 43, folder US Government, Dept. of State, AID Peru, 67–68, William Dentzer Jr. to Dr. Oscar Harkavy, February 7, 1968, PC.

45. Reel 3472, grant 65–358, field trip report of Dr. William Moore to Peter Fraenkel, April 18, 1968, FF.

46. Reel 3472, grant 65–358, Clifford Pease to Javier Arias Stella, January 30, 1968, FF.

47. Reel 1722, grant 65–358, Peter Fraenkel to the files, March 9, 1968, 3–4, FF.

48. Reel 3472, grant 65–358, Dr. William Moore to Peter Fraenkel, April 18, 1968, 8, FF.

49. Reel 1722, grant 65–358, John Saunders to William Moore, May 27, 1968; unpublished reports, box 18826, folder 6781, John Saunders "CEPD Report" (September 1968), FF.

50. Accession 2, box 43, folder US Government, Dept. of State, AID Peru, 67–68, William T. Dentzer Jr. to Dr. Oscar Harkavy, February 7, 1968, PC.

51. President Bustamante announced the projected conduction of this census in 1948. See "Mensaje del Presidente Constitucional del Perú, Dr. José Luis Bustamante y Rivero, ante el Congreso Nacional" (July 28, 1948), ACP. On the Odría presidency, see Caravedo, *Desarrollo Desigual y Lucha Política en el Perú, 1948–1956*; Pareja, *Aprismo y Sindicalismo en el Perú*; and Portocarrero, *De Bustamante a Odría.*

52. Decreto Ley 11298, "Estableciendo que las Remuneraciones Denominadas 'Racionamiento,' 'Asistente,' 'Remuneración por Tiempo de Servicios' y 'Gratificación

por Familia Numerosa,' que se Abonan a los Miembros de los Institutos Armados, Están Comprendidas en la Exoneración del Impuesto a los Sueldos que Estatuye el Decreto Ley 11213" (March 10, 1950); Ley 12175, "Crédito Suplementario a la Partida 77 del Pliego de Salud Pública del Presupuesto de 1954, Destinada a Abonar las Bonificaciones del 25% sobre los Primeros 400 Soles de Sueldo, y por Familia Numerosa y Tiempo de Servicios" (December 27, 1954); Ley 12280, "Crédito Suplementario a la Partida 28 del Pliego de Educación Pública del Presupuesto de 1954, Destinado al Pago de la Bonificación a los Maestros por Familia Numerosa" (March 31, 1955), ACP. See also Ayala Villanueva, "Estudio Médico Social del Agrupamiento Hipólito Unánue o Risso."

53. On the CAEM, see Villanueva, *El CAEM y la Revolución de las Fuerzas Armadas*; Stepan, "New Professionalism of Internal Warfare"; Rodriguez Beruff, *Los Militares y el Poder*.

54. On APRA's history, see Haya de la Torre, *El Antimperialismo y el APRA*; Klaren, *Formación de las Haciendas Azucareras y Orígenes del APRA*.

55. Decreto Ley 14220, "Sistema Nacional de Planeamiento Económico y Social" (October 1962), ACP.

56. On Belaúnde's incomplete reforms, see Caballero, *Economía Agraria de la Sierra Peruana*.

57. The vast literature on the 1968–80 military governments includes Lowenthal, *The Peruvian Experiment*; Pease, *El Ocaso del Poder Oligárquico*; McClintock and Lowenthal, *The Peruvian Experiment Reconsidered*; and Mayer, *Cuentos Feos de la Reforma Agraria*.

58. Reel 3525, grant 65–358, Mayor Grl. FAP Eduardo Montero Rojas to José Donayre, December 16, 1968, FF.

59. *Boletín CEPD* 3, 11 (March 1969): 26.

60. Reel 3525, grant 65–358, John Saunders to Abraham Lowenthal, John Nagel, and Harry Wilhelm, August 4, 1969, FF.

61. Reel 3525, grant 65–358, John Saunders to Abraham Lowenthal, John Nagel, and Harry Wilhelm, October 13, 1969, FF.

62. Unpublished reports, box 18524, folder 1477, John Saunders to José Donayre Valle, May 13, 1969; reel 3525, grant 65–358, John Nagel to the files, July 9, 1969, FF.

63. Unpublished reports, box 18826, folder 6775, Ozzie Simmons to Abraham Lowenthal, July 27, 1970, FF.

64. Reel 1722, grant 65–358, John Nagel to Abraham Lowenthal, June 30, 1970, FF.

65. Reel 3525, grant 65–358, Otoniel Velasco to José Donayre, November 9, 1970, FF.

66. Reel 1722, grant 65–358, Antonio Muñoz Najar to John Nagel, August 3, 1971, FF.

67. Reel 1722, grant 65–358, Santiago Salinas to Richard Dye, August 18, 1971, FF.

68. Reel 3525, grant 65–358, Richard Dye to Santiago Salinas, October 11, 1971; reel 1722, grant 65–358, Antonio Muñoz Najar to John Nagel, March 8, 1972, FF.

69. See *Boletín CEPD* 6, 24 (August 1972).

70. Reel 1722, grant 65–358, Robert Blomberg to Richard Dye, November 2, 1972, FF.

71. Reel 1722, grant 65–358, John Nagel to Richard Dye, May 20, 1975, FF. See also "El Largo Brazo Yanqui LLegó al Perú a Través del CEPD," *Expreso*, April 25, 1975; reel

1722, grant 65–358, Antonio Muñoz Najar to William Carmichael, April 28, 1975; and reel 1722, grant 65–358, Richard Dye to William Carmichael, May 7, 1975, FF.

72. Reel 3525, grant 65–358, Antonio Muñoz Najar to files, June 21, 1973; and reel 1722, grant 65–358, Antonio Muñoz Najar to William Carmichael, July 24, 1973, FF.

73. Demographer Kingsley Davis denounced vigorously this idea in the 1940s, calling it one of the region's "great myths." See Davis, "Latin America's Multiplying Peoples."

74. Decreto Ley 19394, "Prorrogan por Un Año Término Fijado en Art. 4 de D.L. 18788 sobre Inscripción de Nacimiento" (May 9, 1972); Decreto Ley 19987, "Municipios del País Harán Inscripción sobre Nacimientos sin Mediar Declaración" (April 13, 1973); Decreto Ley 20223, "Abren Inscripción Extraordinaria del Nacimiento de Peruanos en los Registros del Estado Civil" (November 20, 1973), ACP.

75. Perú, Instituto Nacional de Planificación, *Plan Nacional de Desarollo, 1971–1975*, vol. 1, p. 9.

76. Bustíos Romaní, *Crisis de los Sistemas de Salud.*

77. Perú, INPROMI, Programa Nacional de Salud Materno-Infantil, 1973, parte III.

78. Decreto Supremo 055-71-SA; Resolución Suprema 00034-72-SA/DS, "Regionalización Docente y Asistencial" (March 1972), ACP.

79. Decreto Ley 17505, "Código Sanitario" (1969), ACP.

80. Decreto Ley 18949, "Instituto de Neonatología y Protección Materno-Infantil" (1971), ACP.

81. "Los Ministros de Salud de las Américas Aprueban las Metas para el Decenio 1971–1980."

82. Cueto, *The Value of Health.*

83. Perú, INPROMI, Programa Nacional de Salud Materno-Infantil, 1973, parte V.

84. Ibid., parte III.

85. Unpublished reports, box 19110, folder 11869, Robert Blomberg to James Trowbridge and Antonio Muñoz Najar, October 9, 1973, FF.

86. Perú, INPROMI, Programa Nacional de Salud Materno-Infantil, 1973, parte IV.

87. Perú, INPROMI, Normas y Procedimientos para la Atención de la Madre, 1972, 76; Perú, INPROMI, Programa Nacional de Salud Materno-Infantil, 1973, parte V.

88. "Oficina Sanitaria Panamericana."

89. Box 10, folder 39, diary notes February 4, 1965, OAS-PAHO, 328, JMS. See also Davis, Third Pan-American Sanitary Bureau Conference on Population Dynamics.

90. Davis, Third Pan-American Sanitary Bureau Conference on Population Dynamics, 2–3.

91. Interview with former PAHO adviser for Peru and Bolivia Duncan Pedersen (Montreal, December 3, 2008).

92. Perú, INPROMI, Normas y Procedimientos para la Atención de la Madre, 1972, 29.

93. Ibid., 75–76.

94. Perú, INPROMI, Programa Nacional de Salud Materno-Infantil, 1973, parte V.

95. Interviews with former PAHO adviser to INPROMI Duncan Pedersen (Montreal, December 3, 2008) and former INPROMI director René Cervantes (Lima, December 16, 2008).

96. "Proyecto de la APPF de extensión de servicios materno-infantiles y de bienestar familiar en la zona de salud Nor-occidental" (April 5, 1974), CDT.

97. Bustíos Romaní, *Crisis de los Sistemas de Salud*, 178.

98. USAID, Office of Health and Population, Peru, "History of Family Planning in Peru, 1997."

99. On population policymaking in Peru in the 1980s and beyond, see Cueto, "La Vocación por Volver a Empezar"; and Donayre, Guerra-García, and Sobrevilla, *Políticas y Programas de Población en el Perú*.

100. See, for example, Silva Colmenares, *No . . . Mas . . . Hijos!*; Malpica, *El Desarrollismo en el Perú*; and Mass, *Population Target*.

101. Sobrinho, *Estado e Populaçao*; Briggs, *Reproducing Empire*; Pieper Mooney, *The Politics of Motherhood*; Soto Laveaga, *Jungle Laboratories*; Felitti, *La Revolución de la Píldora*.

102. Hartmann, *Reproductive Rights and Wrongs*; Connelly, *Fatal Misconception*.

103. In all fairness, however, the notion of sexual and reproductive rights, and of birth control as one of those rights, was only in its infancy in 1970s Latin America. It has only become a prevalent aspect of human rights discussions since the 1994 International Conference on Population and Development of Cairo in 1994. On the growing prominence of the discourse of reproductive and sexual rights, see Ewig, *Second-Wave Neoliberalism*.

## Chapter 6

1. The original model is the New Testament's "Holy Family" made up of Jesus and his parents, Joseph and Mary. See CEP for Pope Pius XI's encyclical *Castii Connubii* (December 30, 1930); Pope Paul VI's *Humanae Vitae* (July 25, 1968) reaffirmed the value of this model.

2. Noonan refers to this as the "central theory on procreative purpose" of marriage, a concept developed early on in the history of Catholicism by Augustine, Bishop of Hippo, in the fourth century. Beginning in the sixteenth century, however, the numerical increase of educated urban Catholics, rivaling clerics in intellectual sophistication, led to greater confidence by Catholic theologians in the ability of lay people to make moral judgments. As a result, the former became less inclined to publicly insist on procreation as the exclusive lawful purpose of married intercourse. As Noonan notes, this may also have been related to the priesthood's unwillingness to alienate well-off Catholic patrons, who actively limited the size of their offspring, at a time when Protestantism was on the rise in Europe and was already dominant in North America. See Noonan, *Contraception*, 237, 409, 519. On the widespread use of coitus interruptus in Europe, see Schneider and Schneider, *Festival of the Poor*; and Fisher and Szreter, "They Prefer Withdrawal."

3. Gordon, *Woman's Body, Woman's Right*, xv, 4, 337.

4. Franco, "Defrocking the Vatican."

5. Davis, "Political Ambivalence in Latin America," 143.

6. Donaldson, "American Catholicism."

7. Piotrow, *World Population Crisis*, 90.

8. Rice-Wray, "The Provoked Abortion"; Acero and Dalle Rive, *Medicina Indígena*; Gervais and Gauvreau, "Women, Priests, and Physicians"; McCormmick, "The Scarlet Woman in the Flesh."

9. Jones and Nortman, "Roman Catholic Fertility."

10. Stycos, *Human Fertility in Latin America*, 4; Hall, "Population Growth"; Sobrinho, *Estado e Populaçao*, 79.

11. Fagley, *The Population Explosion*, 5–6.

12. The ACP was the national chapter of Catholic Action, a worldwide movement of lay Catholics established by Pope Pious XI in 1922. On Catholic Action, see Congar, *Lay People in the Church*.

13. Klaiber, "The Catholic Lay Movement in Peru"; Klaiber, *The Catholic Church in Peru*, 47.

14. See, for example, *Acción Católica Peruana* (January 24, 1932, and January 10, 1943).

15. Manuel Noriega, "Feminidad y Feminismo," *Sígueme* 9, 45 (September 1944): 6.

16. *Acción Católica Peruana* (November 26, 1933): 191.

17. Weigel, "The Church's Social Doctrine," 16.

18. Leo XIII, *Rerum Novarum* (May 15, 1891); Pius XI, *Quadragesimo Anno* (May 15, 1931), CEP.

19. Pius XI, *Castii Connubii*, point 59, CEP. These "natural reasons" and "defects" could include infertility, the postmenopausal period, and the infertile portion of a woman's menstrual cycle.

20. Ibid., points 10, 13, 16, 17, 24, 37, 80, 85, 89, and 90, CEP.

21. Ibid., point 121, CEP.

22. Juan Gualberto Guevara, "La Constitución Cristiana de la Familia: Resumen de una Carta Pastoral," *Gaceta Eclesiástica (Arzobispado de Arequipa)* 1, 2 (March–April 1947): 30–31, 31, CEP. See also "¿Demasiados Niños?" *Caretas* 260, 13 (February 1963): 11–14.

23. Pius XII's position in favor of the rhythm method for married couples became clear following an address to the Italian Catholic Union of Midwives on October 29, 1951. See Jones and Nortman, "Roman Catholic Fertility."

24. Villamón, "El Derecho de Nacer y la Conservación de la Especie," 7.

25. McGregor, "Posición de la Iglesia sobre la Regulación de los Nacimientos."

26. John XXIII, *Mater et Magistra* (May 15, 1961); John XXIII, *Pacem in Terris* (April 11, 1963); John XXIII, *Gaudium et Spes* (December 7, 1965), CEP. See also Wilde, *Vatican II*.

27. Marks, *Sexual Chemistry*; Kaiser, *The Encyclical That Never Was*.

28. Paul VI, *Humanae Vitae* (July 25, 1968), CEP.

29. Klaiber, "Prophets and Populists"; Klaiber, "The Catholic Lay Movement in Peru."

30. On liberation theology, see Gutierrez, *Teología de la Liberación*; Dussel, "A Note on Liberation Theology." On dependency theory, see Klaren and Bossert, *The Promise of Development*.

31. "Declaración de Sacerdotes Peruanos," *Oiga* 265, 6 (March 1968): 17, 33, 34.

32. Harold Griffiths, "Ya en el Perú se Respira el Clima Posconciliar," *Oiga* 266, 6 (March 1968): 12–13.

33. "Declaración del Episcopado Peruano sobre el Crecimiento Demográfico" (Lima, January 27, 1968), CEP.

34. Enrique Bartra, "Forum sobre Control de la Natalidad," *Revista de la Facultad de Farmacia y Bioquímica* 27, 98 (1965): 182–83. It was declarations such as this that buttressed McQuillan's argument regarding the similarities between Catholic and Marxist thought in relation to population growth. To both, population growth was an epiphenomenon caused by fundamental problems of inequality and insufficient planning that capitalism could not solve. See McQuillan, "Common Themes."

35. See pages 10 and 11 in Geusau, "International Reaction."

36. *Segunda Conferencia General del Episcopado Latinoamericano* (Medellín: Paulinas, September 1968): 17, CEP.

37. See the chapter on "Familia" in *Segunda Conferencia General del Episcopado Latinoamericano*, CEP.

38. *Segunda Conferencia General del Episcopado Latinoamericano*, 41–47, CEP.

39. "Their Choice: 'Ring of Misery,'" *Attleboro Sun*, January 14, 1967, 6, KP; interview with Joseph Kerrins (St. Petersburg, FL, March 3, 2005).

40. Dodge, *Becoming Global Citizens*.

41. Series 4, sub-series 4.2, box 186, folder 4, AID brochure, November 1963, NCWC.

42. Series 5, sub-series 5.2, box 194, folder 30, Len Peterson, "Papal Volunteers for Latin America," *IFNAID* 3, 1 (May–June 1961), NCWC.

43. Series 5, sub-series 5.2, box 194, folder 30, George Wolf, "The Peace Corps," *IFNAID* 3, 1 (May–June 1961), NCWC.

44. Series 5, sub-series 5.2, box 194, folder 30, NCWC News Service, "Relief Expert Notes Call for Cooperation between Private Groups and Government in Foreign Aid Law" (November 9, 1961), NCWC.

45. Series 5, sub-series 5.2, box 194, folder 30, NCWC News Service (Domestic), "Laymen Must Work to Promote Solutions to Latin Social Ills" (November 27, 1961), NCWC.

46. Series 4, sub-series 4.2, box 186, folder 3, Gerald Mische (AID) to Rev. John Considine, MM, Latin American Bureau, NCWC, March 11, 1962, NCWC.

47. Series 4, sub-series 4.2, box 186, folder 3, James Lamb, AID Director, to Rev. John Considine, MM, Latin American Bureau, NCWC, March 14, 1962, NCWC. See also interview with James Dette, former AID-Patterson volunteer (Montreal, May 30, 2006).

48. Series 4, sub-series 4.2, box 186, folder 4, James Lamb, AID Director, to AID membership, August 1963, NCWC.

49. Interview with Sal Piazza, former AID-Patterson volunteer (Montreal, June 17, 2006).

50. Letter from Fr. John Coss to the author (November 29, 2006).

51. Letter from Joseph Kerrins to Cardinal Juan Landázuri, Lima, December 28, 1967, KP.

52. Email from Br. Francisco Tanega to the author (April 17, 2006).

53. Rock, *The Time Has Come*; World Health Organization, "Clinical Aspects of Oral Gestogens."

54. Joseph Kerrins to Cardinal Juan Landázuri, Lima, December 28, 1967, KP.

55. Joseph Kerrins and Helen Kerrins, "'Responsible Parenthood Program in the Barriadas of Lima,' Report to the Association for International Development" (April–December 1967), KP.

56. Email from Br. Francisco Tanega to the author (April 17, 2006).

57. Yolande Murphy, "Humanitarian Obligation in Peru," *Attleboro Sun*, September 8, 1967, 3; and Yolande Murphy, "What He Witnessed Is Beyond Imagination," *Attleboro Sun*, March 9, 1968, 3.

58. William J. McIntire, M. M., "Responsible Parenthood in Lima," *America* 118 (October 1968): 380–82, KP.

59. Sanchez et al., *Tugurización en Lima Metropolitana*; Dietz, *Poverty and Problem-Solving*; Golte and Adams, *Los Caballos de Troya de los Invasores*.

60. Roy, "Aspectos Saltantes del Estudio de Fecundidad en El Agustino."

61. Joseph Kerrins letter to Gene and Joanne, June 9, 1967; and Joseph Kerrins letter, April 16, 1967, KP.

62. Joseph Kerrins letter, February 18, 1967, KP.

63. Joseph Kerrins to Gene and Joanne, June 9, 1967, KP.

64. Dean J. Campos Rey de Castro, Facultad de Medicina de la Universidad Nacional Mayor de San Marcos, to Joseph Kerrins, Lima, December 2, 1966. KP.

65. Letter from James Connolly, bishop of Fall River, to Joseph Kerrins, January 6, 1967, KP.

66. Jonathan Fine, M.D., human resources development officer, US Agency for International Development, to Joseph Kerrins, Lima, January 25, 1967, KP.

67. Joseph Kerrins, "'A Responsible Parenthood Program in the Barriadas of Lima,' Report to the Association for International Development (August 1968)," KP. See also interview with Joseph Kerrins (St. Petersburg, FL, March 3, 2005).

68. For a list of Lima parishes and the people responsible for them, see Secretariado del Episcopado Nacional del Perú, Anuario Eclesiastico del Perú, 1969, CEP.

69. Kerrins, "A Responsible Parenthood Program," KP.

70. Tone, *Devices and Desires*, 233.

71. Odell and Molitch, "The Pharmacology of Contraceptive Agents."

72. Maqueo-Topete et al., "A Pill-a-Month Contraceptive"; Rubio Lotvin and Berman, "Once-a-Month Oral Contraceptive"; Guiloff et al., "Once-a-Month Oral Contraceptive."

73. Kerrins and Kerrins, "Responsible Parenthood Program in the Barriadas of Lima," KP.

74. Federico and Laura Hurtado, presidents of the Archdiocesan Team of the Peruvian Christian Family Movement, to Cardinal Juan Landázuri, Lima, May 9, 1974, MFC.

75. Francisco Zarama and Consuelo Zarama, eds., *Este es el MFC: Décima Reunión de la Asamblea General del Movimiento Familiar Cristiano en América Latina* (Panama, 1979), MFC.

76. Interview with Mrs. Consuelo Castillo, former member of the MFC (Lima, June 22, 2006).

77. Joseph Kerrins to John and Pat, January 6, 1968, KP.

78. Joseph Kerrins to Father G., February 13, 1968, KP.

79. Joseph Kerrins to Cardinal Juan Landázuri, Lima, December 28, 1967, KP.

80. Kerrins and Kerrins, "Responsible Parenthood Program in the Barriadas of Lima"; see also Joseph Kerrins letter, June 9, 1968, KP.

81. "Gynecologist Hopeful Encyclical Won't Disrupt Family Planning," *Attleboro Sun,* August 3, 1968, 1, KP.

82. "Recomendaciones del Organismo Nacional de Desarrollo de Pueblos Jóvenes" (Lima, April 8, 1969), MFC.

83. Helí Cancino Izaguirre, Guillermo Tagliabue, Oscar Castillo, and Armando Tovar, "Promoción Conyugal, Familiar y de Investigación del MFC en Barrios Marginales (June 1968)," KP.

84. Reunión del equipo central arquidiocesano del MFC, Lima, January 14, 1970, MFC.

85. Pedro and Magdalena Pazos Gamio, directors, to Juan and Renata Idoña, Archdiocesan Presidents, MFC, Lima, February 18, 1970, MFC.

86. Pedro and Magdalena Pazos Gamio, directors, to Armando and Nelly Tovar, Archdiocesan Presidents, MFC, Lima, January 5, 1970, MFC.

87. Pazos et al., "Programas de Orientación Cristiana en Relación con la Regulación de la Natalidad en el Perú."

88. PPFAII, box 83, folder 22, memorandum from Harold Crow to John Robbins, Planned Parenthood Federation of America, October 12, 1973, PPFA.

89. PPFAII, box 83, folder 22, Harold Crow to Jake Harshbarger, Family Planning Services Division, Office of Population, USAID, August 13, 1973, PPFA.

90. Bartra, "Fundamentación Moral del Tratamiento Anovulatorio después del Parto," 426, 427.

91. Cardinal Juan Landázuri to Fr. Pedro Richards, Lima, February 3, 1977, MFC.

92. Reunión del Concejo del MFC, Lima, February 6, 1970, MFC.

93. Pedro Pazos, program director, to Drs. Heli Cancino and Guillermo Tagliabue, codirectors of the Medical Program, Lima, November 25, 1969, MFC.

94. Interview with Dr. Jorge Ascenzo, former PALF employee (Lima, July 19, 2004).

95. Interview with Dr. Hugo Oblitas, former PALF employee (Lima, July 19, 2004).

96. Interview with Ms. Martha de Laudi, former PALF employee (Lima, April 14, 2006).

97. "Familia y Población," *Iglesia en el Perú* 17 (April 1974): 1–8: 5, CEP.

98. Federico and Laura Hurtado, presidents of the Archdiocesan Team of the MFC, to Cardinal Juan Landázuri Ricketts, Lima, May 9, 1974, MFC.

99. Cardinal Juan Landázuri to Federico and Laura Hurtado, presidents of the Archdiocesan Team of the MFC, Lima, June 5, 1974, MFC.

100. PPFA II, box 83, folder 23, ATLF request for renewal of funds to FPIA, 1978. See also box 83, folder 25, ADIFAM request for renewal of funds to FPIA, 1978, PPFA.

101. PPFA II, box 83, folder 24, ATLF request for renewal of funds to FPIA, 1979, PPFA.

102. Interview with Dr. Guillermo Tagliabue, former PALF medical director (Lima, July 17, 2004).

103. Idígoras, "La Iglesia y la Regulación Racional y Cristiana de los Nacimientos."

104. Consejo Nacional de Población, "Experiencia Nacional en la Formulación y Ejecución de Políticas de Población, 1960–1976."

105. Gordon, *Woman's Body, Woman's Right*; Donaldson, "American Catholicism."

## Epilogue

1. Lineamientos de Política de Población en el Perú (hereafter "LPP"). The guideline was made public through Decreto Supremo 00625-75-SA (August 31, 1976).

2. UN, "World Population Plan of Action," Bucharest 1974, section A, points 1–13. See also Townley, "Government and Population"; Stycos, "Demographic Chic at the UN"; Finkle and Crane, "The Politics of Bucharest."

3. LPP, part I, section B, point 7.

4. LPP, part II.

5. Recently, it has reemerged as Peruvians debate the social legitimacy of emergency contraception, for example. An editorial in the left-leaning newspaper *La República* stressed that choosing a birth control method "ought to be the decision of a couple and their physician," without the "intromission" of religion. See "AOE Gana Batalla," *La República*, February 9, 2009, 18.

6. LPP, part III, section B, point 3.4.

7. Perú, Ministerio de Salud e Instituto Nacional de Planificación, *Primer Seminario Nacional sobre Política de Población*.

8. Perú, Resolución Ministerial 0018-77-SA/DS, February 17, 1977.

9. Perú, Consejo Nacional de Población, Decreto Supremo 049-80-PM, November 20, 1980.

10. Wicht, "La Situación Demográfica del Perú," 93; Wicht, *Dinámica Demográfica y Política de Población en el Perú*.

11. Cueto, "La Vocación por Volver a Empezar."

12. Espejo Núñez, "Estado Actual de la Población Peruana."

13. Luciana Biseo, email to the author (December 6, 2008).

14. Aramburú, "Is Population Policy Necessary?" Tsui, "Population Policies."

15. Gasman, Blandon, and Crane, "Abortion, Social Inequity, and Women's Health."

16. Guevara, "Mensaje a los Pueblos del Mundo a Través de la Tricontinental."

# Bibliography

## Primary Sources

*Archives*

Archivo Arzobispal de Lima, Lima
Archivo de la Conferencia Episcopal Peruana
Archivo del Congreso del Perú, Lima
Archivo del Movimiento Familiar Cristiano del Perú,
    c/o Mrs. Graciela de Leidinger, Lima
Archivo General de la Nación, Lima
Archivo Penal de Lima, Lima
Archivo Regional de Ayacucho, Ayacucho
Archivo Regional de La Libertad, Trujillo
Archivo Regional de Piura, Piura
Archivo Regional del Puno, Puno
Centro de Documentación de la Historia de la Mujer, Lima
Ford Foundation Papers at the Rockefeller Archive Center, Tarrytown, N.Y.
Joseph Stycos Papers, Cornell University, Ithaca, N.Y.
Papers of the National Catholic Welfare Council, Catholic University of America,
    Washington, D.C.
Personal archive of Dr. Carmen Delgado de Thays, former APPF director of education,
    Lima
Personal archive of Dr. Joseph Kerrins and Mrs. Helen Kerrins, St. Petersburg, Fla.,
    and East Falmouth, Mass.
Personal archive of Dr. Miguel Ramos Zambrano, former APPF director, Callao
Planned Parenthood Federation of America Archive, Sophia Smith Collection, Smith
    College, Northampton, Mass.
Population Council Papers at the Rockefeller Archive Center, Tarrytown, N.Y.

*Official Documents*

CEPAL. *Análisis y Proyecciones del Desarrollo Económico*. México: Naciones Unidas,
    1955.
———. *Desarrollo Humano, Cambio Social y Crecimiento en América Latina*. Santiago:
    CEPAL, 1975.
Fujimori, Alberto. "Discurso del Presidente en la 4ta Conferencia de la Mujer en
    Beijing, 15 de Setiembre de 1995." *Boletín del Consejo Nacional de Población* 4
    (Setiembre 1995): 13–14.

Pan American Health Organization (PAHO). "Gender, Health and Development in the Americas: Basic Indicators 2005."

———. "Health Situation in the Americas: Basic Indicators 2012."

Perú. "Amendment 155/95 to the National Population Policy (Decreto Ley 346)." Approved September 7, 1995.

———. *Anteproyecto de una Ley de Elecciones, Cámara de Diputados, Exposición de Motivos.* Lima: Hnos. Faura, 1931.

———. Código Civil de 1936.

———. Código Penal del Estado Sud Peruano de 1836.

———. Código Penal de 1862.

———. Código Penal de 1924.

———. Informe de la Defensoría del Pueblo 01–98: Anticoncepción Quirúrgica Voluntaria, January 26, 1998.

———. Informe Final del Primer Seminario Nacional sobre Política de Población, 1976.

———. Ley General de Educación, Decreto Ley 19326.

———. *Lineamientos de Política de Población en el Perú.* Lima: INP, 1976.

———. *Plan Inca Elaborado por el Gobierno Revolucionario de la Fuerza Armada, antes del 3 de Octubre de 1968.* Lima: Presidencia de la República, 1974.

———. "Producción Legislativa del Ex-Representante Irene Silva Linares de Santolalla." In www.congreso.gob.pe/archivo/damas/01-Silva-Irene-Senadora/Produccion-Legislativa.pdf

Perú, Centro de Estudios de Población y Desarrollo (CEPD). *Primer Seminario de Población y Desarrollo.* Lima: CEPD, 1966.

Perú, Consejo Nacional de Población. Decreto Supremo 049-80-PM approved November 20, 1980.

———. "Experiencia Nacional en la Formulación y Ejecución de Políticas de Población, 1960–1976." In *Antecedentes de la Política Peruana de Población.* Lima: 1978.

Perú, INPROMI. Normas y Procedimientos para la Atención de la Madre, 1972.

———. Programa Nacional de Salud e Instituto Materno-Infantil, 1973.

Perú, Instituto Nacional de Estadística e Informática. Historia de los Censos en el Perú.

Perú, Instituto Nacional de Planificación. Plan Nacional de Desarrollo, 1971–1975.

———. Plan Nacional de Desarrollo Económico y Social del Perú, 1962–1971.

Perú, Instituto Nacional de Planificación y Oficina Nacional de Estadística y Censos. *Estudio sobre la Población Peruana: Características y Evolución.* Lima: INP, 1973.

Perú, MIMDES. "Cincuenta Años del Voto Femenino en el Perú: Historia y Realidad Actual, 2005."

Perú, Ministerio de Salud e Instituto Nacional de Planificación. *Informe Final del Primer Seminario Nacional sobre Política de Población.* Lima: INP, 1976.

Perú, Resolución Ministerial 0018-77-SA/DS. Implementación de Lineamientos de Política de Población, February 17, 1977.

Taft-Morales, Maureen. "Peru in Brief: Political and Economic Conditions and Relations with the United States." US Congressional Research Service, October 18, 2012.

UN. "World Population Plan of Action." Bucharest, 1974.

UNFPA. "By Choice, Not by Chance: Family Planning, Human Rights, and Development: State of World Population 2012."

USAID, Office of Health and Population, Peru. "History of Family Planning in Peru, 1997."

U.S. Department of State. "National Security Study Memorandum 200: Implications of Worldwide Population Growth for US Security and Overseas Interests." In *Documents of the National Security Council, 7th Supplement,* 1974.

U.S. House of Representatives Committee on International Relations, Subcommittee on International Operations and Human Rights. "Hearing on the Peruvian Population Control Program." Washington, DC, February 25, 1998.

Villarán, Susana. Public profile at www.munlima.gob.pe/contenidos/biografia.aspx. Accessed January 28, 2011.

World Health Organization (WHO). "Administration of Maternal and Child Health Services." *Technical Report* 115 (1957).

———. "Clinical Aspects of Oral Gestogens." *Technical Report* 326 (1966).

———. *Handbook of Resolutions and Decisions of the World Health Assembly and the Executive Board, Volume 1: 1948–1972.* Geneva: WHO, 1973.


*Published Primary Sources*

Adair, Fred. *Obstetrics and Gynecology.* Philadelphia: Lea and Febiger, 1940.

Alberdi, Juan Bautista. *Bases y Puntos de Partida para la Organización Política de la República de Argentina.* Lima: n.p., 1879.

Alfaro, Carlos. "La Asociación Peruana de Protección Familiar y la Planificación Familiar." *Ginecología y Obstetricia* 16, 2 (1970): 145–52.

Andradi, Esther, and Ana María Portugal. *Ser Mujer en el Perú.* Lima: Mujer y Autonomía, 1978.

Antúnez de Mayolo, Santiago. *Cuadernos de Medicina Popular Peruana, 1977.*

Armijo, Rolando, and Tegualda Monreal. "The Problem of Induced Abortion in Chile." *Milbank Memorial Fund Quarterly* 43, 4 (1965): 263–80.

Avendaño, Jorge. "¿Hay Jerarquía en la Sociedad Conyugal?" *Nuestros Hijos* 3, 14 (December 1955): 7–8.

Avendaño, Leonidas, and Guillermo Fernandez Dávila. *La Despoblación en su Aspecto Social y Médico-Legal.* Lima: Sanmartí y Cia., 1922.

Bachmann, Carlos. "El Aborto Inducido como Problema Social: Su Prevención." *Tribuna Médica* 5, 222 (January 20, 1969): 1, 3, 6–7.

Barnes, Allan. "United States Private Agencies' Contributions to Population Programs." *International Journal of Health Services* 3, 4 (1973): 661–65.

Barrig, Maruja. *Cinturón de Castidad: La Mujer de Clase Media en el Perú.* Lima: Mosca Azul, 1979.

Bartra, Enrique. "Fundamentación Moral del Tratamiento Anovulatorio después del Parto." *Revista Teológica Limense* 7, 3 (1973): 425–31.

Bedoya Hevia, Mariano. "Social Problems of Abortion: Illegal Abortion." In *Proceedings of the 5th World Congress of Gynaecology and Obstetrics,* edited by C. Wood and W. A. W. Walters. London: Butterworths, 1967.

Berkeley, Comyns, and Victor Bonney. *The Difficulties and Emergencies of Obstetric Practice*. Philadelphia: P. Blakiston's Son, 1913.

Blacker, Charles. *Voluntary Sterilization*. London: Oxford University Press, 1934.

Borchart de Moreno, Christiana. "Words and Wounds: Gender Relations, Violence, and the State in Late Colonial and Early Republican Ecuador." *Colonial Latin American Review* 13, 1 (2004): 129–44.

Busalleu, Alejandro. "Lección Inaugural del Curso de Obstetricia." *Anales de la Facultad de Medicina de la Universidad de San Marcos* 21, 2 (1938): 225–36.

Calle, Juan José. *Anotaciones y Concordancias al Código Penal*. Lima: Congreso del Perú, 1924.

Capelo, Joaquín. *La Despoblación*. Lima: Sanmartí y Cia., 1912.

Carr-Saunders, Alexander. *World Population: Past Growth and Present Trends*. London: F. Cass, 1936.

Castellares Z., Marcelino. "Abortos Espontáneos y Abortos Provocados." *Actualidad Médica Peruana* 1, 6 (1935): 366–70.

Castellón, Helio. "¿Está Masculinizándose la Mujer que Trabaja?" *Ñusta* 1, 5 (November 1957): 7–9.

Chávez, Elmer, and Carlos Bachmann. "Esterilización Quirúrgica en Pacientes Cesareadas." *Revista del Hospital de Maternidad de Lima* 1, 1 (1975): 23–26.

Coale, Ansley, and Edgar Hoover. *Population Growth and Economic Development in Low Income Countries: A Case Study of India's Prospects*. Princeton: Princeton University Press, 1958.

Dalurzo, Beatriz F. *Homenaje en Buenos Aires a Irene Silva de Santolalla, Mujer de las Américas 1956*. Buenos Aires: Unión de Mujeres Americanas de la República Argentina, 1968.

Davis, Hugh, ed. *Third Pan-American Sanitary Bureau Conference on Population Dynamics, 13 February 1967*. Washington: PASB, 1967.

Davis, Kingsley. "Political Ambivalence in Latin America." *Journal of Legal and Political Sociology* 1 (1943): 127–50.

———. "Latin America's Multiplying Peoples." *Foreign Affairs* 25 (1946–47): 643–54.

Davis, Kingsley, and Ana Casis. "Urbanization in Latin America." *Milbank Memorial Fund Quarterly* 24 (1946): 186–207, 292–314.

DeLee, Joseph. *The Principles and Practice of Obstetrics*. Philadelphia: W. B. Saunders, 1913.

Dodge, Larry. *Becoming Global Citizens*. Cumberland, Wis.: Forum Publications, 2003.

Drysdale, Robert. "Education Approaches to Population Problems." In *Readings on Population Information and Education: Background Papers for a Ford Foundation Meeting on Population, Elsinore, Denmark—June 1972*. New York: Ford Foundation, 1973.

Eastman, Nicholson. *Williams Obstetrics*. New York: Appleton-Century-Crofts, 1950.

Eden, Thomas Watts, and Eardley Holland. *A Manual of Midwifery*. Toronto: Macmillan, 1925.

Escuela Sindical Autonóma de Lima. "Mujeres: Trabajadoras . . . Ciudadanas, 1958."

Fernández Dávila, Guillermo. *El Delito de Aborto*. Lima: Lux, 1926.

Finkle, Jason, and Barbara Crane. "The Politics of Bucharest: Population, Development and the New International Economic Order." *Population and Development Review* 1, 1 (1975): 87–114.

Gajardo, Samuel. "Las Deficiencias del Hogar como Factor de Delincencia de Menores." *La Acción Médica* (November 2, 1929): 1–2, 15.

Gálvez, José. *Una Lima Que Se Va*. Lima: Universitaria, 1913.

García y García, Elvira. *La Mujer y el Hogar*. Lima: Miranda, 1946.

Garland, Alejandro. *Reseña Industrial del Perú*. Lima: Imprenta La Industrial, 1905.

Gaslonde Sainz, Santiago. "Abortion Research in Latin America." *Studies in Family Planning* 7, 8 (1976): 211–17.

Germain, Adrienne. "Women at Mexico: Beyond Family Planning Acceptors." *Family Planning Perspectives* 7, 5 (1975): 235–38.

González de Fanning, Teresa. "Concerning the Education of Women." In *Confronting Change, Challenging Tradition: Women in Latin American History*, edited by Gertrude Yeager. Wilmington: Scholarly Resources, 1994.

González Prada, Manuel. *Pájinas Libres*. Lima: P. Dupont, 1894.

Graña, Francisco. *La Población del Perú a través de la Historia*. Lima: Torres Aguirre, 1916.

Guiloff, Enrique, Edel Berman, Alfredo Montiglio, Raul Osorio, and Charles Lloyd. "Clinical Study of a Once-a-Month Oral Contraceptive: Quinestrol-Quingestanol." *Fertility and Sterility* 21, 2 (1970): 110–18.

Hall, Marie-Françoise. "Control de la Natalidad en Lima, Perú." *Anales de la Facultad de Medicina* 49, 1 (1966): 1–27.

———. "Population Growth, US and Latin American Views: An Interpretation of the Response of the United States and Latin America to the Latin American Population Growth." *Population Studies* 27, 3 (1973): 415–29.

"Have Spermatozoa Functions or Effects Other Than Fertilization?" *Journal of the American Medical Association* 77, 1 (1921): 42–43.

Hill, Reuben, Joseph Stycos, and Kurt Back. *The Family and Population Control: A Puerto Rican Experiment in Social Change*. Chapel Hill: University of North Carolina Press, 1959.

Horwitz, Abraham. "Relaciones entre Salud y Desarrollo Económico." *Boletín de la Oficina Sanitaria Panamericana* 47 (Agosto 1959): 93–100.

———. "La Salud Hemisférica y la Reunión de Jefes de Estado Americanos." *Boletín de la Oficina Sanitaria Panamericana* 63, 1 (July 1967): 65.

Hurtado, Hilario, Esteban Kesserü, and Alfredo Larrañaga. "D-Norgestrel, un Progestágeno a Microdosis como Anticonceptivo Oral de Administración Continua." *Ginecología y Obstetricia* 16, 2 (1970): 119–26.

Idígoras, Jose Luis. "La Iglesia y la Regulación Racional y Cristiana de los Nacimientos." *El Mensajero del Corazón de Jesús* 20, 217–18 (August–September 1964): 219–24.

Instituto Interamericano de Ciencias Agrícolas de la OEA. "Simposio de Educación para el Hogar para Dirigentes de Programas de Enseñanza y Desarrollo, Lima, Peru, Febrero 15–28, 1967."

Jiménez Camacho, José. "El Ejercicio de la Profesión Médica en Provincias: Obstetricia Rural en la Sierra del Perú." *Actualidad Médica Peruana* 6, 3 (1940): 74–79.

Kesserü, Esteban, Alfredo Larrañaga, and Julio Parada. "Postcoital Contraception with
D-Norgestrel." *Contraception* 7, 5 (1973): 367–79.

Kessler, Alexander, and C. C. Stanley. "Human Reproduction and Family Planning:
Research Strategies in Developing Countries." *Nature* 251 (1974): 577–79.

Kiser, Clyde. "Population Trends and Public Health in Latin America." *Milbank
Memorial Fund Quarterly* 45 (1967): 43–59.

Knaus, Hermann. *Die periodische Fruchtbarkeit und Unfruchtbarkeit des Weibes*. Wien:
W. Maudrich, 1934.

Kuczynski Godard, Maxime. *La Vida en la Amazonía Peruana: Observaciones de un
Médico*. Lima: UNMSM, 1944.

Landauro Valentini, Alonso. "La Esterilización Quirúrgica en Obstetricia." *Boletín de la
Asociación de Médicos del Hospital de Mujeres y Maternidad del Callao*, 9, 7, 37 (1953):
857–63.

Landry, Adolphe. *La Révolution Démographique: Études et Essais sur les Problèmes de la
Population*. Paris: Institut Nationale d'Études Démographiques, 1934.

Larrañaga, Alfredo, and Esteban Kesserü. "Dos Años de Experiencia Clínica con
el Enantato de Noretisterona como Anticonceptivo Inyectable de Depósito."
*Ginecología y Obstetricia* 14, 2 (1968): 209–21.

Larrañaga, Alfredo, Max Winterhalter, and José Natal. "Evaluation of d-Norgestrel
1.0mg as a Post-coital Contraceptive." *International Journal of Fertility* 20 (1975):
156–60.

Lewis, José Guillermo. "El Problema de la Esterilización." *La Reforma Médica* 20, 189
(May 3, 1934): 364.

Lissón, Carlos. *Breves Apuntes sobre la Sociología del Perú en 1886*. Lima: Benito Gil,
1887.

"Los Ministros de Salud de las Américas aprueban las Metas para el Decenio 1971–
1980." *Boletín de la Oficina Sanitaria Panamericana* 74, 5 (Mayo 1973): 441–45.

Luna Vegas, Ricardo. *Factores Etiológicos de la Peligrosidad en los Menores*. Lima: La
Cotera, 1940.

Mac-Lean y Estenos, Roberto. "La Eugenesia en América." *Revista Mexicana de
Sociología* 13, 3 (1951): 359–87.

Maqueo-Topete, Manuel, Edel Berman, Javier Soberón, and Juan José Calderón. "A
Pill-a-Month Contraceptive." *Fertility and Sterility* 20, 6 (1969): 884–91.

Mazzi, Víctor, ed. *Poesía Proletaria del Perú, 1930–1976*. Lima: Biblioteca Universitaria,
1976.

McGregor, Felipe. "Posición de la Iglesia sobre la Regulación de los Nacimientos."
*Tribuna Médica* 2, 92 (June 6, 1966): 1, 13, 15.

Medel, Mario. "Avances en Anticoncepción Intrauterina." *Ginecología y Obstetricia* 21,
1–3 (1975): 244–59.

"Meeting on Population Policies in Relation to Development in Latin America:
Recommendations." *Studies in Family Planning* 1, 25 (1967): 1–4.

*Memorias del Segundo Congreso Médico Pan-Americano de México 16–19 de Noviembre de
1896*. Mexico: Hoeck & Hamilton, 1898.

Mendoza, Ofelia. "Population Growth and Family Planning in Latin America." *Journal
of Sex Research* 1, 2 (1965): 161–70.

Moreno, Javier. "Esterilización Tubárica Bilateral por Pinzamientos Sucesivos y Electrocauterización." *Tribuna Médica* 4, 157 (September 18, 1967): 1–7.

Neira Samanez, Hugo. *Huillca: Habla un Campesino Peruano*. Lima: Peisa, 1974.

Nelson, Richard. "A Theory of the Low-Level Equilibrium Trap in Underdeveloped Economies." *American Economic Review* 46, 5 (1956): 894–908.

Notestein, Frank. "Population: The Long View." In *Food for the World*, edited by Theodore Schultz. Chicago: University of Chicago Press, 1945.

———. "Reminiscences: The Role of Foundations, the Population Association of America, Princeton University and the United Nations in Fostering American Interest in Population Problems." *Milbank Memorial Fund Quarterly* 49, 4 (1971, part 2): 67–85.

Odell, W. D., and M. E. Molitch. "The Pharmacology of Contraceptive Agents." *Annual Review of Pharmacology* 14 (1974): 413–34.

"Oficina Sanitaria Panamericana." *Boletín de la Oficina Sanitaria Panamericana* 46, 2 (February 1959): 192–93.

Ogino, Kyusaku. *The Conception Period of Women*. Harrisburg: Medical Arts Publishing Company, 1934.

Oppenheimer, W. "Prevention of Pregnancy by the Gräfenberg Ring Method." *American Journal of Obstetrics and Gynecology* 78 (1959): 446–54.

Palma, Clemente. *El Porvenir de las Razas en el Perú*. Lima: Torres Aguirre, 1897.

Paz Soldán, Carlos Enrique. *La Protección a la Infancia en el Perú*. Lima: Centro Editorial, 1914.

———. "Editorial." *La Reforma Médica* 19, 165 (June 15, 1933): 198.

———. "El Magno Problema." *La Crónica* (May 5, 1949): 10.

———. "¿Será Mejor que No Nazcan?" *La Reforma Médica* 39, 577 (March–April 1953): 39–40.

———. *Heredia y sus Discípulos*. Lima: Instituto de Medicina Social, 1956.

———, ed. *Actas y Trabajos de la Primera Conferencia Nacional sobre el Niño Peruano*. Lima: Unión, 1922.

Pazos, Pedro, Helí Cancino, Guillermo Tagliabue, Carlos Flores-Guerra, and Enrique Bartra. "Programas de Orientación Cristiana en Relación con la Regulación de la Natalidad en el Perú." *Ginecología y Obstetricia* 16, 2 (1970): 153–68.

Prebisch, Raul. *The Economic Development of Latin America and Its Principal Problems*. New York: United Nations, 1950.

———. *Towards a New Trade Policy for Development*. New York: United Nations, 1964.

*Proceedings of the 4th IPPF/WHR Conference, San Juan, Puerto Rico, April 1964*. New York: IPPF, 1965.

Rice-Wray, Edris. "The Provoked Abortion—A Major Public Health Problem." *American Journal of Public Health* 54, 2 (1964): 313–21.

Robles Ramírez, Salvador. *Páginas de la Vida Real: Guía Matrimonial, Control de la Natalidad, Para Que?* Lima: Ediciones Luz, 1967.

Rock, John. *The Time Has Come: A Catholic Doctor's Proposals to End the Battle over Birth Control*. London: Longmans, 1963.

Rostow, Walt. *The Stages of Economic Growth, a Non-Communist Manifesto*. Cambridge: Cambridge University Press, 1960.

Rubio Lotvin, Boris, and Edel Berman. "Once-a-Month Oral Contraceptive: Quinestrol and Quingestanol." *Obstetrics and Gynecology* 35, 6 (1970): 933–36.

Salcedo, Manuel. "Infancia Abandonada en Peligro y Peligrosa." *Boletín del Departamento de Protección Materno Infantil* 4, 15–16 (1944): 11–32.

Santolalla, Irene Silva. *Por la Felicidad de Nuestros Hijos*. Buenos Aires, 1940.

———. *Hacia un Mundo Mejor*. Lima: Universal, 1943.

———. *Intentando la Solución de ¡El Gran Problema!* Lima: Salas, 1957.

———. *Mi Aporte a la Educación Familiar*. Lima: Universo, 1974.

———. *Perú, País Pionero en Educación Familiar Sistemática*. N.p.: Instituto Superior de Educacion Familiar, 1979.

Segal, S. J., A. L. Southam, and K. D. Shafer, eds. *Proceedings of the Second International Conference on Intra-Uterine Contraception*. Amsterdam: Excerpta Medica, 1965.

Stycos, Joseph. *The Control of Human Fertility in Jamaica*. Ithaca, N.Y.: Cornell University Press, 1964.

———. *Human Fertility in Latin America: Sociological Perspectives*. Ithaca, N.Y.: Cornell University Press, 1968.

———. "Demographic Chic at the UN." *Family Planning Perspectives* 6, 3 (1974): 160–64.

Thompson, Warren. *Danger Spots in World Population*. New York: A. A. Knopf, 1929.

Tietze, Christopher, and Sarah Lewit, eds. *Proceedings of the First International Conference on Intra-Uterine Devices*. Amsterdam: Excerpta Medica, 1962.

Townley, Ralph. "Government and Population: The World Population Conference, 1974." *International Journal of Health Services* 3, 4 (1974): 689–92.

*Transactions of the First Pan-American Medical Congress, Washington DC, 5–8 September 1893*. Washington D.C.: Government Printing Office, 1895.

Tudela, Francisco. *El Problema de la Población en el Perú*. Lima: San Pedro, 1908.

Valdizán, Hermilio, and Angel Maldonado. *La Medicina Popular Peruana, Volumen 1*. Lima: Torres Aguirre, 1922.

Vicuña, Juan Manuel, Esteban Kesseru, and Alfredo Larrañaga. "Evaluación del Uso del Dispositivo Intrauterino de Lippes como Método de Planificación Familiar." *Ginecología y Obstetricia* 16, 2 (1970): 101–18.

Villamón, Froilán. "El Derecho de Nacer y la Conservación de la Especie." *Revista Peruana de Obstetricia* 3, 1 (1955): 7–26.

Villavicencio, Victor. *La Vida Sexual del Indígena Peruano*. Lima: Barrantes Castro, 1942.

Vogt, William. *Road to Survival*. New York: William Sloane, 1948.

Wadia, Avabai. *The Light Is Ours: Memoirs and Movements*. N.p.: International Planned Parenthood Federation, 2001.

Williams, J. Whitridge. *Obstetrics*. New York: D. Appleton, 1904.

## Medical Theses

Alayza Tejada, Eleodoro. "Estudio Médico Social del Distrito de Pachacamac." Tesis de Grado, Facultad de Medicina de San Fernando, 1955.

Altuna del Valle, Enrique. "Una Concentración Sub-Urbana Peligrosa para la Sanidad de Lima." Tesis de Grado, Facultad de Medicina de San Fernando, 1955.

Amorín V., Antonio. "Causas de la Mortalidad Fetal y la Neonatal en el Callao." Tesis de Grado, Facultad de Medicina de San Fernando, 1953.

Arévalo Ruiz, Manuel. "La 'Barriada' Carmen de la Legua: Contribución al Estudio Médico Social de los Suburbios de Lima." Tesis de Grado, Facultad de Medicina de San Fernando, 1957.

Arroyo Posadas, Glicerio. "Infancia y Pro-biofilaxis (Dos Mil Niños y su Destino Socio Vital en El Montón)." Tesis de Grado, Facultad de Medicina de San Fernando, 1957.

Bambarén, Celso. "Algunas Consideraciones sobre las Perversiones Sexuales y la Delincuencia." Tesis de Grado, Facultad de Medicina de San Fernando, 1946.

Barandiarán, J. M. "Descanso y Protección de la Mujer Embarazada." Tesis de Grado, Facultad de Medicina de San Fernando, 1922.

Barreto P., David U. "Problema Materno-Infantil en Iquitos." Tesis de Grado, Facultad de Medicina de San Fernando, 1945.

Basadre, Eduardo. "Ligeras Consideraciones sobre el Uso Prematuro y el Abuso del Corsé." Tesis de Grado, Facultad de Medicina de San Fernando, 1907.

Beraún, A. A. "Curetaje Uterino y sus Aplicaciones Terapeuticas." Tesis de Grado, Facultad de Medicina de San Fernando, 1906.

Burgos Amaya, José. "La Procreación Consciente en Nuestro País y el Ritmo de la Esterilidad y de la Fecundidad en la Mujer." Tesis de Grado, Facultad de Medicina de San Fernando, 1957.

Bustamante de Montalvan, Tula. "Algunos Aspectos de Planificación Familiar en Trujillo." Tesis de Bachiller en Enfermería, U. Nacional de Trujillo, 1968.

Cabrera Castro, Francisco. "Ensayo de Clasificación de la Etiología del Aborto." Tesis de Grado, Facultad de Medicina de San Fernando, 1931.

Cáceres, Ismael. "Patogenia y Etiología del Aborto." Tesis de Grado, Facultad de Medicina de San Fernando, 1891.

Cademártori, Luis. "La Asistencia Médico-Social del Niño en el Callao." Tesis de Grado, Facultad de Medicina de San Fernando, 1928.

Casas, Alfonso de las. "La Delincuencia Infantil." Tesis de Grado, Facultad de Medicina de San Fernando, 1913.

Changanaquí E., Francisco. "Algunos Casos de Infanticidio en Lima." Tesis de Grado, Facultad de Medicina de San Fernando, 1916.

Chiri, Leoncio P. "Consideraciones sobre la Sífilis y el Embarazo entre Nosotros." Tesis de Grado, Facultad de Medicina de San Fernando, 1917.

Colina, Victor. "Contribución al Estudio de la Profilaxia de las Enfermedades Venéreas y de su Tratamiento Abortivo." Tesis de Grado, Facultad de Medicina de San Fernando, 1917.

Corrales Diaz, J. "Estadística y Profilaxia de las Enfermedades Venéreas en la Armada Peruana." Tesis de Grado, Facultad de Medicina de San Fernando, 1934.

Deustua, Luis Fidel. "Higiene de la Lactancia." Tesis de Grado, Facultad de Medicina de San Fernando, 1884.

Echandía, Juana, Giovanna Elescano, Dominga Dueñas, Elena Castillo, María Medina, Luis Sánchez, Clara Tasaico, Pablo Castro, Regina Arakaki, Rosa Agüero, and Esther Reyes. "Estudio de la Comunidad y Programación de Actividades de Salud del Pueblo Joven El Planeta." Tesis de Grado, Facultad de Enfermería de San Fernando, 1972.

Escudero Villar, Juan M. "Contribución al Estudio del Aborto." Tesis de Grado, Facultad de Medicina de San Fernando, 1930.

Espinosa Palacios, José Nicanor. "La Sifilis en las Clases Trabajadoras." Tesis de Grado, Facultad de Medicina de San Fernando, 1936.

Flores S., Elio. "El Hogar Infantil y su Rendimiento de Bien Médico Social." Tesis de Grado, Facultad de Medicina de San Fernando, 1936.

Fosalba, Rafael. "Ideas Generales sobre la Herencia." Tesis de Grado, Facultad de Medicina de San Fernando, 1928.

Fosalba y Muro, Daniel A. "La Excusa Absolutoria del Aborto Científico." Tesis de Grado, Facultad de Medicina de San Fernando, 1929.

Frías Ocampo, César. "Causas de Internamiento y de Muerte en la Maternidad de Lima." Tesis de Grado, Facultad de Medicina de San Fernando, 1951.

Gavidia, Agustín. "El Aborto como Accidente Espontáneo o Patológico en el Curso del Embarazo." Tesis de Grado, Facultad de Medicina de San Fernando, 1904.

Gavidia Lino, Victor Manuel. "El Aborto como Problema de Seguridad Social." Tesis de Grado, Facultad de Medicina de San Fernando, 1968.

Gil Cárdenas, José. "El Matrimonio Civil." Tesis de Grado, Facultad de Medicina de San Fernando, 1884.

González, Benigno. "Contribución a la Maternología Nacional." Tesis de Grado, Facultad de Medicina de San Fernando, 1929.

González, Juan N. "La Prostitución Reglamentada en Lima." Tesis de Grado, Facultad de Medicina de San Fernando, 1918.

Guardia Salas, Guillermo. "Evaluación Quirúrgica de Dispositivos Intrauterinos Aplicados en un Plan Piloto de Planificación Familiar en Pamplona Alta." Tesis Doctoral, Facultad de Medicina de San Fernando, 1971.

Guzmán Rodriguez, Manuel. "Profilaxis de las Enfermedades Venéreas." Tesis de Grado, Facultad de Medicina de San Fernando, 1905.

Herón Frisancho, Juan. "Mortalidad Infantil y Movimiento Demográfico en la Ciudad de Puno." Tesis de Grado, Facultad de Medicina de San Fernando, 1938.

Iannacone Martínez, Felipe. "Vida Reproductiva en las Mujeres de 20 a 39 Años." Tesis de Grado, Facultad de Medicina de San Fernando, 1964.

Landaburú Soubise, Juan E. "Contribución al Estudio de la Mortalidad Materna." Tesis de Grado, Facultad de Medicina de San Fernando, 1946.

Latorre, Rafael. "El Preventivo Antivenéreo Civil en Lima." Tesis de Grado, Facultad de Medicina de San Fernando, 1944.

Lawezzari, Alejandro. "Algunas Consideraciones sobre la Protección de la Infancia en Lima." Tesis de Grado, Facultad de Medicina de San Fernando, 1908.

León García, Enrique. "Las Razas en Lima." Tesis Doctoral, Facultad de Medicina de San Fernando, 1909.

Linares Lizárraga, Antonieta. "Contribución al Estudio Médico Social de la Madre Lactante." Tesis de Grado, Facultad de Medicina de San Fernando, 1947.

López, Mariano M. "Diagnóstico de los Flujos Utero-Vaginales en las Enfermedades Venéreas." Tesis de Grado, Facultad de Medicina de San Fernando, 1891.

López Cornejo, Félix. "Las Realidades de la Asistencia del Parto en el Perú." Tesis de Grado, Facultad de Medicina de San Fernando, 1940.

Martínez Valdez, J. Emilio. "Anticoncepción Intrauterina: Evaluación de los Dispositivos Intrauterinos en el Centro de Protección Familiar de Breña." Tesis de Grado, Facultad de Medicina de San Fernando, 1974.

Melgar Menéndez, Pedro. "Profilaxia Social de las Enfermedades Venéreas." Tesis de Grado, Facultad de Medicina de San Fernando, 1929.

Mercado B., Alejandro. "Contribución al Estudio del Infanticidio en Lima." Tesis de Grado, Facultad de Medicina de San Fernando, 1921.

Merkel, Felipe. "Reglamentación de la Prostitución en Lima." Tesis de Doctorado, Facultad de Medicina de San Fernando, 1908.

Molina, Wenceslao. "El Curetaje Uterino." Tesis de Doctorado, Facultad de Medicina de San Fernando, 1896.

Monge Raguz, Augusto. "El Avecindamiento Humano en el Cerro San Cosme." Tesis de Grado, Facultad de Medicina de San Fernando, 1954.

Montero Mogollón, María de los Angeles. "Motivaciones de las Pacientes con Dispositivo Intrauterino Perdidas al Seguimiento." Tesis de Grado, Facultad de Trabajo Social de la Universidad de San Marcos, 1972.

Montoya M., José Julio. "Estudio Médico Legal sobre un Caso de Pseudo-Embarazo y Pseudo-Aborto." Tesis de Grado, Facultad de Medicina de San Fernando, 1941.

Morales Martínez, Humberto. "Eugenesia, Matrimonio y Convivencia: Aspecto Médico Legal." Tesis de Grado, Facultad de Medicina de San Fernando, 1957.

Navas Mena, José P. "Planificación Familiar en el Medio Policial." Tesis de Grado, Facultad de Medicina de San Fernando, 1966.

Neyra Mosquera, Alejandro. "El Problema Médico Legal y Médico Social del Aborto en el Perú." Tesis de Grado, Facultad de Medicina de San Fernando, 1951.

Olascoaga Mar, Carlos. "Estudio Médico Social del Problema Materno-Infantil en la Ciudad de Tacna." Tesis de Grado, Facultad de Medicina de San Fernando, 1961.

Ostolaza, Mariano. "Estudio del Chancro." Tesis de Grado, Facultad de Medicina de San Fernando, 1889.

Pastor Padierna, Carlos. "El Control Sanitario del Matrimonio." Tesis de Grado, Facultad de Medicina de San Fernando, 1924.

Paz Soldán, Carlos Enrique. "La Medicina Militar y los Problemas Nacionales." Tesis de Grado, Facultad de Medicina de San Fernando, 1910.

Pilares Polo Escalante, Victor M. "La Profilaxis de la Sífilis en el Ejército." Tesis de Grado, Facultad de Medicina de San Fernando, 1947.

Portillo B., Humberto. "El Problema de la Natimortalidad en Lima." Tesis de Grado, Facultad de Medicina de San Fernando, 1925.

Quintana Flores, Carlos Alberto. "Contribución al Estudio del Problema Social y Médico Legal del Aborto: Estudio Estadístico de la Ciudad de Pisco." Tesis de Grado, Facultad de Medicina de San Fernando, 1955.

Quintanilla Paulet, Antonio. "Algunos Problemas Médicos en Relación con el Subdesarrollo Económico del Perú." Tesis de Grado, Facultad de Medicina de San Fernando, 1956.

Robinson, Fernando. "Algunas Observaciones acerca de Nuestro Problema Racial."
Tesis de Grado, Facultad de Medicina de San Fernando, 1936.
Roldán, Nestor P. "El Peligro Venéreo y su Profilaxia en el Ejército." Tesis de Grado,
Facultad de Medicina de San Fernando, 1914.
Román Arredondo, Manuel Salomón. "Contribución al Mejoramiento de la Asistencia
Médico-Social del Niño Chalaco." Tesis de Grado, Facultad de Medicina de San
Fernando, 1940.
Ruiz, José Alejandro. "Evolución Demográfica de Chiclayo." Tesis de Grado, Facultad
de Medicina de San Fernando, 1938.
Silva Valladares, Carlos Alberto. "Vida Reproductiva de las Mujeres de 20–39 Años."
Tesis de Grado, Facultad de Medicina de San Fernando, 1966.
Suarez Camargo, José. "Una Visita a 'Ciudad de Dios.'" Tesis de Grado, Facultad de
Medicina de San Fernando, 1955.
Tello Morales, Ernesto. "Causas de Muerte Materna en la Maternidad de Lima,
1947–1952." Tesis de Grado, Facultad de Medicina de San Fernando, 1953.
Untiveros Morales, Jesús. "La Frecuencia de los Abortos en Lima." Tesis de Grado,
Facultad de Medicina de San Fernando, 1946.
Valle Medina, Pedro. "Contribución al Estudio del Problema Social y Médico-Legal del
Aborto en el Callao." Tesis de Grado, Facultad de Medicina de San Fernando, 1946.
Vega Gamarra, Pedro. "Contribución al Estudio de la Mortalidad Infantil en Huaraz."
Tesis de Grado, Facultad de Medicina de San Fernando, 1929.
Vílches Bedoya, Harry. "Capacidad para el Matrimonio." Tesis de Grado, Facultad de
Medicina de San Fernando, 1956.
Winterhalter Uriarte, Max. "Un Nuevo Contraceptivo Oral." Tesis de Grado, Facultad
de Medicina de San Fernando, 1969.

### Periodicals and Internet Sites Cited

Acción Católica Peruana
Actualidad Médica Peruana
Anales de la Academia Nacional de Medicina de Lima
Anales de la Cruz Roja Peruana
Anales de la Facultad de Medicina de la Universidad de San Marcos
Anales de la Universidad Nacional Mayor de San Marcos
Anuario de la Academia Nacional de Medicina
Boletín CEPD
Boletín de la Academia Nacional de Medicina
Boletín de la Dirección General de Salubridad
Boletín de la Secretaría de Prensa de la Unión Popular de Mujeres Peruanas
Boletín de Noticias del Instituto Nacional de Planificación
Boletín del Departamento de Protección Materno Infantil
Boletín del Enfermero de la Sanidad de Gobierno y Policía
Boletín del Instituto Nacional del Niño
Boletín del Ministerio de Fomento
Boletín Informativo de la Union Popular de Mujeres Peruanas

*Caretas*
*Educación Sanitaria*
*El Comercio*
*El Peruano*
*El Universal*
*Expreso*
*Fémina*
*Intima*
*La Acción Médica*
*La Crónica Médica*
*La Prensa*
*La Reforma Médica*
*La República*
*La Temperancia*
*La Tortuga*
*La Unión Médica*
*New York Times*
*Oiga*
*Patricia: Para la Mujer Moderna*
*Perú Indígena*
*Revista 7 Días*
*Revista de la Facultad de Farmacia y Bioquímica*
*Revista de la Sanidad Militar del Perú*
*Revista Farmaceutica Peruana*
*Revista Médica del Hospital Central del Empleado*
*Revista Médica Peruana*
*Sígueme*
www.unfpa.org.pe
worldbank.org


## Interviews and Personal Communications (via Electronic Mail or Letter)

Midwife Manuela Araujo (Lima, July 1, 2010)

Dr. Jorge Ascenzo, obstetrician-gynecologist, formerly of the Proyecto de Apoyo Laico Familiar (Lima, July 19, 2004, and May 4, 2006)

Ms. Luciana Biseo, former member of the Commission for the Population Policy Guideline of 1976, email to the author (December 6, 2008)

Dr. Hugo Calle, obstetrician-gynecologist, retired (Lima, July 6, 2010)

Dr. Helí Cancino, former director of the Proyecto de Apoyo Laico Familiar (Lima, July 19, 2004)

Dr. Nazario Carrasco, obstetrician-gynecologist (Lima, June 28, 2010)

Mrs. Consuelo Castillo, former member of the Movimiento Familiar Cristiano (Lima, June 22, 2006)

Dr. René Cervantes Begazo, former director of the INPROMI (Lima, December 16, 2008)

Dr. Doris Chang León, obstetrician-gynecologist, retired (Lima, June 25, 2010)

Dr. Augusto Chávez, obstetrician-gynecologist, retired (Lima, July 7, 2010)

Fr. John Coss, Catholic priest, order of the Sons of Mary, letter to the author (November 29, 2006)

Dr. Carmen Delgado de Thays, former APPF director of education (Lima, June 27, 2010)

Mr. James Dette, former volunteer, Association for International Development (Montreal, May 30, 2006)

Dr. Victor Díaz, obstetrician-gynecologist, retired (Lima, June 30, 2010)

Dr. Miguel Exebio, obstetrician-gynecologist, retired (Lima, July 1, 2010)

Dr. Luis Fernández, obstetrician-gynecologist, retired (Trujillo, July 13, 2010)

Mr. Carlos García San Martín, former Schering Peru sales chief (June 30, 2010)

Dr. Marie-Françoise Hall, formerly of the International Health Program, Johns Hopkins University School of Medicine (February 20, 2009)

Dr. Luz Jefferson, former medical director of APPF clinic in Breña, email to the author (Lima, February 21, 2009)

Dr. Joseph Kerrins, obsterician-gynecologist, retired, and former volunteer, Association for International Development (St. Petersburg, Fla., March 3, 2005)

Dr. Alfredo Larrañaga Leguía, former director of the Instituto Marcelino (Lima, July 11, 2006)

Ms. Martha de Laudi, social worker, formerly of the Proyecto de Apoyo Laico Familiar (Lima, April 14, 2006)

Ms. Elsa Lescano, family educator, retired (Lima, July 7, 2010)

Dr. Walter Llaque Dávila, former dean, Universidad Nacional de Trujillo (Lima, July 12, 2006)

Ms. Emperatriz Matallana, social worker, retired (Lima, July 6, 2010)

Dr. Delia Moreno, obstetrician-gynecologist, retired (Lima, July 5, 2010)

Ms. Rosa Motta, family educator, retired (Lima, July 6, 2010)

Dr. Hugo Oblitas, obstetrician-gynecologist, formerly of the Proyecto de Apoyo Laico Familiar (Lima, July 19, 2004)

Dr. Duncan Pedersen, former PAHO Adviser for Peru and Bolivia (Montreal, December 3, 2008)

Midwife Luisa Parra (Lima, July 6, 2010)

Mr. Sal Piazza, former volunteer, Association for International Development (Montreal, June 17, 2006)

Ms. Natalia Romero, social worker, retired (Lima, July 5, 2010)

Ms. Irene Santolalla Silva, family educator, retired (Chosica, July 16, 2010)

Dr. Guillermo Tagliabue, obstetrician-gynecologist, formerly of the Proyecto de Apoyo Laico Familiar (Lima, July 17, 2004)

Br. Francisco Tanega, Catholic priest, order of the Sons of Mary, email to the author (April 17, 2006)

Mr. Oswaldo Vasquez Cerna, formerly of the Junta de Asistencia Nacional (Lima, July 5, 2010)

Dr. Ramiro Yanque, obstetrician-gynecologist, retired (Lima, July 2, 2010)

## Secondary Sources

Abel, Christopher. *Health, Hygiene and Sanitation in Latin America c. 1870 to 1950*. London: University of London Press, 1996.

Acero, Gloria, and María Dalle Rive. *Medicina Indígena: Cacha-Chimborazo*. Quito: Abya-Yala, 1992.

Agostoni, Claudia. "Las Mensajeras de la Salud: Enfermeras Visitadoras en la Ciudad de México durante la Década de los 20." *Estudios de Historia Moderna y Contemporánea de México* 33 (2007): 89–120.

Aguila, Alicia del. *Los Velos y las Pieles: Cuerpo, Genero y Reordenamiento Social en el Peru Republicano*. Lima: IEP, 2003.

Aguirre, Carlos. *Breve Historia de la Esclavitud en el Perú: Una Herida Que No Deja de Sangrar*. Lima: Fondo Editorial del Congreso del Perú, 2005.

Almeida, Marta de. "Circuito Aberto: Idéias e Intercâmbios Médico-Científicos na América Latina nos Primórdios do Século XX." *História, Ciências, Saúde* 13, 3 (2006): 733–57.

Anderson, Jeanine. *Tendiendo Puentes: Calidad de Atención desde la Perspectiva de las Mujeres Rurales y de los Proveedores de los Servicios de Salud*. Lima: Manuela Ramos, 2001.

Apple, Rima. *Perfect Motherhood: Science and Childrearing in America*. New Brunswick, N.J.: Rutgers University Press, 2006.

Aramburú, Carlos. *Migración Interna en el Perú*. Lima: INANDEP, 1981.

———. "Is Population Policy Necessary? Latin America and the Andean Countries." *Population and Development Review* 20 (1994 Supplement): 159–78.

Aramburú, Carlos, Eduardo Bedoya, and Jorge Recharte. *Colonización en la Amazonía*. Lima: Centro de Investigación y Población Amazónica, 1982.

Arana, Marie. "The Kids Left behind by the Boom." *New York Times* (March 21, 2013): A27.

Arias Schreiber Pezet, Jorge. "Los Médicos Peruanos en la Guerra del Pacífico." *Acta Médica Peruana* 2 (1979): 1–8.

Arias Stella, Javier. "Anatomía Patológica en el Perú: Un Enfoque Histórico." *Revista Médica Herediana* 9, 2 (1998): 81–83.

Ariès, Philippe. *Centuries of Childhood: A Social History of Family Life*. New York: Vintage Books, 1962.

Arnup, Katherine. *Education for Motherhood: Advice for Mothers in Twentieth-Century Canada*. Toronto: University of Toronto Press, 1994.

Bart, Pauline. "Seizing the Means of Reproduction: An Illegal Feminist Abortion Collective—How and Why It Worked." In *Women, Health and Reproduction*, edited by Helen Roberts. London: Routledge & Kegan Paul, 1981.

Bazul, Victor. "El Profesor Doctor Constantino T. Carvallo y la Creación de la Cátedra de Ginecología en la Facultad de Medicina." *Anales de la Facultad de Medicina* 57, 2–4 (1996): 40–42.

Berelson, Bernard. "National Family Planning Programs: A Guide." *Studies in Family Planning* 1, 5 (1964, Supplement): 1–12.

Berlin, Elois Ann. "Aspects of Fertility Regulation among the Aguaruna Jivaro of Peru." In *Women's Medicine: A Cross-Cultural Study of Indigenous Fertility Regulation*, edited by Lucile Newman. New Brunswick, N.J.: Rutgers University Press, 1985.

Birn, Anne-Emanuelle. "'No More Surprising Than a Broken Pitcher'? Maternal and Child Health in the Early Years of the Pan American Sanitary Bureau." *Canadian Bulletin of Medical History* 19 (2002): 17–46.

———. "Uruguay on the World Stage: How Child Health Became an International Priority." *American Journal of Public Health* 95, 9 (2005): 1506–17.

———. *Marriage of Convenience: Rockefeller International Health and Revolutionary Mexico.* Rochester, N.Y.: University of Rochester Press, 2006.

Blake, Stanley. "The Medicalization of Nordestinos: Public Health and Regional Identity in Northeastern Brazil, 1889–1930." *The Americas* 60, 2 (2003): 217–48.

Bledsoe, Caroline. *Contingent Lives: Fertility, Time and Aging in West Africa.* Chicago: University of Chicago Press, 2002.

Bliss, Katherine. *Compromised Positions: Prostitution, Public Health, and Gender Politics in Revolutionary Mexico City.* University Park: Penn State University Press, 2001.

Bock, Gisela, and Pat Thane, eds. *Maternity and Gender Policies: Women and the Rise of the European Welfare States, 1880–1950s.* London: Routledge, 1991.

Bolton, Ralph, and Enrique Mayer, eds. *Andean Kinship and Marriage.* Washington, D.C.: American Anthropological Association, 1977.

Bolton, Ralph, Tom Greaves, and Florencia Zapata. *50 Años de Antropología: Vicos y Otras Experiencias Aplicadas en el Perú.* Lima: IEP, 2010.

Bonfiglio, Giovanni. "Veinticinco Años de Debates de Población en la Prensa Peruana, 1974–1999." Mimeographed document, 1999.

———. *La Presencia Europea en el Perú.* Lima: Congreso del Perú, 2001.

Bonilla, Heraclio. *Un Siglo a la Deriva: Ensayos sobre el Perú, Bolivia y la Guerra.* Lima: IEP, 1981.

Borges, Dain. "'Puffy, Ugly, Slothful and Inert': Degeneration in Brazilian Social Thought, 1880–1940." *Journal of Latin American Studies* 25, 2 (1993): 235–56.

Bowser, Frederick. *The African Slave in Colonial Peru, 1524–1650.* Stanford: Stanford University Press, 1974.

Briggs, Laura. *Reproducing Empire: Race, Sex, Science and US Imperialism in Puerto Rico.* Berkeley: University of California Press, 2002.

Brölmann, H. A. M., F. P. H. L. J. Dijkhuizen, and B. W. J. Mol. "The Clinical Importance of the Microcurettage." *Reviews in Gynaecological Practice* 4 (2004): 58–64.

Brooke, James. "High Rate of South American Abortion Ills Seen." *New York Times* (November 23, 1993): C5.

Brouwere, Vincent de. "The Comparative Study of Maternal Mortality over Time: The Role of the Professionalization of Childbirth." *Social History of Medicine* 20, 3 (2008): 541–62.

Brown, Phil, and Edwin Mikkelsen. *No Safe Place: Toxic Waste, Leukemia, and Community Action.* Berkeley: University of California Press, 1990.

Bulmer-Thomas, Victor. *The Economic History of Latin America since Independence.* Cambridge: Cambridge University Press, 2003.

Burga, Manuel, and Alberto Flores Galindo. *Apogeo y Crisis de la República Aristocrática.* Lima: Rikchay, 1979.

Bustíos Romaní, Carlos. "Notas sobre la Historia de la Educación Médica en el Perú, Primera Parte, 1568–1933." *Acta Médica Peruana* 20, 2 (2003): 94–108.

———. "Notas sobre la Historia de la Educación Médica, 1933–1980, Segunda Parte." *Acta Médica Peruana* 20, 3 (2003): 133–49.

———. *Crisis de los Sistemas de Salud y de Seguridad Social en el Perú: 1968–1990.* Lima: Universidad Nacional Mayor de San Marcos, 2007.

Caballero, José María. *Economía Agraria de la Sierra Peruana antes de la Reforma Agraria de 1969.* Lima: IEP, 1969.

Cadena, Marisol de la. *Indigenous Mestizos: The Politics of Race and Culture in Cuzco, Peru, 1919–1991.* Durham, N.C.: Duke University Press, 2000.

Caldwell, John. "Toward a Restatement of Demographic Transition Theory." *Population and Development Review* 2, 3–4 (1976): 321–66.

Caldwell, John, and Pat Caldwell. *Limiting Population Growth and the Ford Foundation Contribution.* London: Frances Pinter, 1986.

Canguilhem, Georges. *Le Normal et le Pathologique.* Paris: Presses Universitaires Françaises, 1966.

Cañizares-Esguerra, Jorge. *Nature, Empire, and Nation: Explorations of the History of Science in the Iberian World.* Stanford: Stanford University Press, 2006.

Caravedo, Baltazar. *Burguesía e Industria en el Perú, 1933–1945.* Lima: IEP, 1976.

———. *Desarrollo Desigual y Lucha Política en el Perú, 1948–1956: La Burguesía Arequipeña y el Estado Peruano.* Lima: IEP, 1978.

Carrillo, Ana María. "Nacimiento y Muerte de una Profesión: Las Parteras Tituladas en México." *Dynamis* 19 (1999): 167–90.

Carter, W. E. "Trial Marriage in the Andes?" In *Andean Kinship and Marriage*, edited by Ralph Bolton and Enrique Mayer. Washington, D.C.: American Anthropological Association, 1977.

Casalino Sen, Carlota. "De Cómo los 'Chinos' Se Transformaron y nos Transformaron en Peruanos." *Investigaciones Sociales* 9, 15 (2005): 109–32.

Castañeda, Xochitl, Cecilia García, and Ana Langer. "Ethnography of Fertility and Menstruation in Rural Mexico." *Social Science and Medicine* 42, 1 (1996): 133–40.

Caulfield, Suann. *In Defense of Honor: Sexual Morality, Modernity, and Nation in Early-Twentieth-Century Brazil.* Durham, N.C.: Duke University Press, 2000.

Chambers, Sarah. *De Súbditos a Ciudadanos: Honor, Genero y Politica en Arequipa, 1780–1854.* Lima: Red para el Desarrollo de las Ciencias Sociales, 2003.

Chambi, Néstor, Walter Chambi, Víctor Quiso, Sabino Cutipa, Valeriano Gordillo, and Jorge Apaza. *Así Nomás Nos Curamos: La Medicina en los Andes.* Puno: Asociación Chuyma, 1997.

Chaney, Elsa. "Old and New Feminists in Latin America: The Case of Peru and Chile." *Journal of Marriage and the Family* 35, 2 (1973): 331–43.

———. *Supermadre: Women in Politics in Latin America.* Austin: University of Texas Press, 1979.

Chassen-López, Francie. "A Patron of Progress: Juana Catarina Romero, the Nineteenth-Century Cacica of Tehuantepec." *Hispanic American Historical Review* 88, 3 (2008): 393–426.

Clark, A. Kim. *Gender, State, and Medicine in Highland Ecuador: Modernizing Women, Modernizing the State, 1895–1950.* Pittsburgh: University of Pittsburg Press, 2012.

Cline, David. *Creating Choice: A Community Responds to the Need for Abortion and Birth Control, 1961–1973.* New York: Palgrave Macmillan, 2006.

Coale, Ansley, and Susan Cotts Watkins, eds. *The Decline of Fertility in Europe.* Princeton: Princeton University Press, 1986.

Congar, Yves M. J. *Lay People in the Church: A Study for a Theology of the Laity.* Westminster, Md.: Newman, 1962.

Connelly, Matthew. *Fatal Misconception: The Struggle to Control World Population.* Cambridge, Mass.: Harvard University Press, 2008.

Contreras, Carlos. "Sobre los Orígenes de la Explosión Demográfica en el Perú: 1876–1940." Documento de Trabajo 61, Serie Economía 21. Lima: IEP, 1994.

———. *El Aprendizaje del Capitalismo: Estudios de Historia Económica y Social del Perú Republicano.* Lima: IEP, 2004.

Coriden, James. "Church Law and Abortion." *The Jurist* 33 (1973): 184–98.

Corvalan, Hugo. "The Abortion Epidemic." In *Birth Control: An International Assessment*, edited by Malcolm Potts and Pouru Bhiwandiwala. Lancaster: MTP, 1979.

Cosamalón, Jesús. "'Soy Yo la que Sostengo la Casa': El Trabajo Femenino en Lima (Siglo XIX)." In *La Mujer en la Historia del Perú, Siglos XV al XX*, edited by Carmen Meza and Teodoro Hampe. Lima: Congreso del Perú, 2007.

Cott, Nancy. "'What's in a Name?' The Limits of Social Feminism." *Journal of American History* 76, 3 (1989): 809–29.

Crane, Barbara. "The Transnational Politics of Abortion." *Population and Development Review* 20 (1994 Supplement): 241–62.

Cuba, Juan Manuel. "Influencia de la Medicina Francesa en la Medicina Peruana." *Revista Peruana de Neurología* 8, 1 (2002): 31–40.

Cueto, Marcos. *El Regreso de las Epidemias.* Lima: IEP, 1997.

———. "Social Medicine and 'Leprosy' in the Peruvian Amazon." *The Americas* 61, 1 (2004): 55–80.

———. "La Vocación por Volver a Empezar: Las Políticas de Población en el Perú." *Revista Peruana de Medicina Experimental y Salud Pública* 23, 2 (2006): 123–31.

———. *The Value of Health: A History of the Pan American Health Organization.* Rochester, N.Y.: University of Rochester Press, 2007.

Cueto, Marcos, ed. *Missionaries of Science: The Rockefeller Foundation and Latin America.* Bloomington: Indiana University Press, 1994.

David, Henry. "Abortion in Europe, 1920–91: A Public Health Perspective." *Studies in Family Planning* 23, 1 (1992): 1–22.

Davis-Floyd, Robbie, and Carolyn Sargent, eds. *Childbirth and Authoritative Knowledge: Cross-Cultural Perspectives.* Berkeley: University of California Press, 1997.

Demeny, Paul. "Social Science and Population Policy." *Population and Development Review* 14, 3 (1988): 451–79.

Dietz, Henry. *Poverty and Problem-Solving under Military Rule: The Urban Poor in Lima, Peru*. Austin: University of Texas Press, 1980.

Donaldson, Peter. "American Catholicism and the International Family Planning Movement." *Population Studies* 42 (1988): 367–73.

————. "On the Origins of the United States Government's International Population Policy." *Population Studies* 44, 3 (1990): 385–99.

Donayre, José, Roger Guerra-García, and Luis Sobrevilla. *Políticas y Programas de Población en el Perú: Del Debate a la Acción*. Lima: UPCH, 2012.

Donovan, Brian. *White Slave Crusades: Race, Gender, and Anti-Vice Activism, 1887–1917*. Urbana: University of Illinois Press, 2006.

Dore, Elizabeth, and Maxine Molyneux, eds. *Hidden Histories of Gender and the State in Latin America*. Durham, N.C.: Duke University Press, 2000.

Drinot, Paulo. "Moralidad, Moda y Sexualidad: El Contexto Moral de la Creación del Barrio Rojo de Lima." In *Mujeres, Familia y Sociedad en la Historia de América Latina, Siglos XVIII-XXI*, edited by Scarlett O'Phelan and Margarita Zegarra. Lima: CENDOC-Mujer, 2006.

————. *The Allure of Labor: Workers, Race, and the Making of the Peruvian State*. Durham, N.C.: Duke University Press, 2011.

————. "Creole Anti-Communism: Labor, the Peruvian Communist Party, and APRA, 1930-1934." *Hispanic American Historical Review* 92, 4 (2012): 703–36.

Dussel, Enrique. "A Note on Liberation Theology." In *Ideas and Ideologies in Twentieth-Century Latin America*, edited by Leslie Bethell. Cambridge: Cambridge University Press, 1996.

Ehrick, Christine. "Affectionate Mothers and the Colossal Machine: Feminism, Social Assistance and the State in Uruguay, 1910-1932." *The Americas* 58, 1 (2001): 121–39.

Eraso, Yolanda. "Biotypology, Endocrinology and Sterilization: The Practice of Eugenics in the Treatment of Argentinian Women during the 1930s." *Bulletin of the History of Medicine* 81, 4 (2008): 793–822.

Espejo Núñez, Teobaldo. "Estado Actual de la Población Peruana." *Revista de la Academia Peruana de Salud* 13, 1 (2006): 40–64.

Ewig, Christina. *Second-Wave Neoliberalism: Gender, Race, and Health Sector Reform in Peru*. University Park: Penn State University Press, 2010.

Fagley, Richard. *The Population Explosion and Christian Responsibility*. New York: Oxford University Press, 1960.

Felitti, Karina. "El Debate Médico sobre Anticoncepción en Buenos Aires en los Años Sesenta del Siglo XX." *Dynamis* 27 (2007): 333–57.

————. *La Revolución de la Píldora: Sexualidad y Política en los Sesenta*. Buenos Aires: Edhasa, 2012.

Ferrando, Delicia. *El Aborto Clandestino en el Perú: Hechos y Cifras*. Lima: Flora Tristán and Pathfinder International, 2002.

Ferrando, Delicia, and Carlos Aramburú. "The Fertility Transition in Peru." In *The Fertility Transition in Latin America*, edited by José Miguel Guzmán, Susheela Singh, Germán Rodríguez, and Edith Pantelides. Oxford: Clarendon, 1996.

Few, Martha. *Women Who Live Evil Lives: Gender, Religion and the Politics of Power in Colonial Guatemala*. Austin: University of Texas Press, 2002.

Figa-Talamanca, Irene. "Health and Economic Consequences of Illegal Abortions: Preliminary Findings from an International Study." In *Pregnancy Termination,* edited by Gerald Zatuchni, John Sciarra, and J. Joseph Speidel. Hagerstown, Md.: Harper and Row, 1979.

Finkle, Jason, and C. Alison McIntosh. "The New Politics of Population." *Population and Development Review* 20 (1994 Supplement): 3–34.

"The First Forty Years." *IPPF/WHR Forum* 10, 1 (1994): 36–41.

Fisher, Kate. "Uncertain Aims and Tacit Negotiation: Birth Control Practices in Britain 1925–1950." *Population and Development Review* 26 (2000): 295–317.

———. *Birth Control, Sex, and Marriage in Britain.* Oxford: Oxford University Press, 2006.

Fisher, Kate, and Simon Szreter. "'They Prefer Withdrawal': The Choice of Birth Control in Britain, 1918–1950." *Journal of Interdisciplinary History* 34, 2 (2003): 263–91.

Flores Cisneros, Carmen. "Saber Popular y Prácticas de Embarazo, Parto y Puerperio en Yahuío, Sierra Norte de Oaxaca." *Perinatología y Reproducción Humana* 17 (2003): 36–52.

Flores Galindo, Alberto. *Buscando un Inca: Identidad y Utopía en los Andes.* Lima: SUR, 1986.

Franco, Jean. "Defrocking the Vatican: Feminism's Secular Project." In *Cultures of Politics, Politics of Cultures: Revisioning Latin American Social Movements,* edited by Sonia Alvarez, Evelina Dagnino, and Arturo Escobar. Boulder, Colo.: Westview, 1998.

Freire, Maria. *Mulheres, Mães e Médicos: Discurso Maternalista no Brasil.* Rio de Janeiro: FGV, 2009.

Gasman, N., M. M. Blandon, and B. B. Crane. "Abortion, Social Inequity, and Women's Health: Obstetrician-Gynecologists as Agents of Change." *International Journal of Gynecology and Obstetrics* 94 (2006): 310–16.

Gervais, Diane, and Danielle Gauvreau. "Women, Priests, and Physicians: Family Limitation in Quebec, 1940–1970." *Journal of Interdisciplinary History* 34, 2 (2003): 293–314.

Geusau, Leo Alting von. "International Reaction to the Encyclical *Humana Vitae.*" *Studies in Family Planning* 1, 50 (1970): 8–12.

Ginsburg, Faye, and Rayna Rapp, eds. *Conceiving the New World Order: The Global Politics of Reproduction.* Berkeley: University of California Press, 1995.

Golte, Jürgen, and Norma Adams. *Los Caballos de Troya de los Invasores: Estrategias Campesinas en la Conquista de la Gran Lima.* Lima: IEP, 1990.

Good, Byron. *Medicine, Rationality and Experience: An Anthropological Perspective.* Cambridge: Cambridge University Press, 1994.

Gordon, Linda. *Woman's Body, Woman's Right: A Social History of Birth Control in America.* New York: Grossman, 1976.

Gotkowitz, Laura. "Trading Insults: Honor, Violence, and the Gendered Culture of Commerce in Cochabamba, Bolivia, 1870s–1950s." *Hispanic American Historical Review* 83, 1 (2003): 83–118.

Graham, Richard, ed. *The Idea of Race in Latin America, 1870–1940.* Austin: University of Texas Press, 1990.

Graham, Sandra Lauderdale. *House and Street: The Domestic World of Servants and Masters in Nineteenth-Century Rio de Janeiro*. Cambridge: Cambridge University Press, 1988.

Green, Marshall. "The Evolution of US International Population Policy, 1965–92: A Chronological Account." *Population and Development Review* 19, 2 (1993): 303–21.

Guevara, Ernesto. "Mensaje a los Pueblos del Mundo a Través de la Tricontinental." In *Obras 1957–1967, Tomo II*. La Habana: Casa de las Américas, 1970.

Guevara Chacabana, Gamaniel. "Aspectos Históricos de la Enseñanza de la Pediatría y la Atención de la Salud Infantil en el Perú." *Paediatrica* 8, 1 (2006): 20–26.

Gutierrez, Gustavo. *Teología de la Liberación: Perspectivas*. Lima: CEP, 1971.

Guy, Donna. "Women, Peonage, and Industrialization: Argentina, 1810–1914." *Latin American Research Review* 16, 3 (1981): 65–89.

———. *Sex and Danger in Buenos Aires: Prostitution, Family, and Nation in Argentina*. Lincoln: University of Nebraska Press, 1990.

———. "The Politics of Pan-American Cooperation: Maternalist Feminism and the Child Rights Movement, 1913–1960." *Gender & History* 10, 3 (1998): 449–69.

———. *White Slavery and Mothers Alive and Dead: The Troubled Meeting of Sex, Gender, Public Health, and Progress in Latin America*. Lincoln: University of Nebraska Press, 2000.

Guzmán, José Miguel, Susheela Singh, Germán Rodríguez, and Edith Pantelides, eds. *The Fertility Transition in Latin America*. Oxford: Clarendon, 1996.

Hale, Charles. "Political Ideas and Ideologies in Latin America, 1870–1930." In *Ideas and Ideologies in Twentieth-Century Latin America*, edited by Leslie Bethell. Cambridge: Cambridge University Press, 1996.

Halperín Donghi, Tulio. *Historia Contemporánea de América Latina*. Madrid: Alianza, 1970.

Halton, M., R. L. Dickinson, and C. Tietze. "Contraception with an Intrauterine Silk Coil." *Human Fertility* 13 (1948): 10–13.

Hampe Martínez, Teodoro. "La Universidad Católica de Lima y la Evolución de las Universidades Privadas en el Peru Contemporáneo." *Revista de Historia de América* 110 (1990): 133–54.

Hartmann, Betsy. *Reproductive Rights and Wrongs: The Global Politics of Population Control and Contraceptive Choice*. New York: Harper & Row, 1987.

Haya de la Torre, Victor Raúl. *El Antimperialismo y el APRA*. Santiago: Ercilla, 1936.

Herzog, Tamar. "Percibir el Otro: El Código Penal de 1924 y la División de los Peruanos en Personas 'Civilizadas,' 'Semi-Civilizadas' y 'Salvajes.'" In *Observation and Communication: The Construction of Realities in the Hispanic World*, edited by Johannes-Michael Scholz and Tamar Herzog. Frankfurt: Vittorio Klostermann, 1997.

Hochman, Gilberto. *A Era do Saneamento: As Bases da Política de Saúde Pública no Brasil*. São Paulo: HUCITEC-ANPOCS, 1998.

Hochmann, Gilberto, and Diego Armus, eds. *Cuidar, Controlar, Curar: Ensaios Históricos sobre Saude e Doença na América Latina*. Rio de Janeiro: Fiocruz, 2004.

Hodges, Sarah. *Contraception, Colonialism, and Commerce: Birth Control in South India, 1920–1940*. Aldershot: Ashgate, 2008.

Hodges, Sarah, ed. *Reproductive Health in India: History, Politics, Controversies*. New Delhi: Orient Longman, 2006.

Hunefeldt, Christine. *Liberalism in the Bedroom: Quarreling Spouses in Nineteenth-Century Lima*. University Park: Pennsylvania State University Press, 2000.

Hunt, Nancy Rose. *A Colonial Lexicon of Birth Ritual, Medicalization, and Mobility in the Congo*. Durham, N.C.: Duke University Press, 1999.

Hutchison, Elizabeth Quay. "Add Gender and Stir: Cooking Up Gendered Histories of Modern Latin America." *Latin American Research Review* 38, 1 (2003): 266–87.

Inhorn, Marcia. *Local Babies, Global Science: Gender, Religion, and In Vitro Fertilization in Egypt*. New York: Routledge, 2003.

Iza, Agustín, and Oswaldo Salaverry. "El Hospital Real de San Andrés." *Anales de la Facultad de Medicina* 61, 3 (2000): 247–52.

Jeffery, Roger, and Patricia Jeffery. "Traditional Births Attendants in Rural North India: The Social Organization of Childbearing." In *Knowledge, Power, and Practice: The Anthropology of Medicine and Everyday Life*, edited by Shirley Lindenbaum and Margaret Lock. Berkeley: University of California Press, 1993.

Johnson-Hanks, Jennifer. "On the Modernity of Traditional Contraception: Time and the Social Context of Fertility." *Population and Development Review* 28, 2 (2002): 229–49.

Jones, Gavin, and Dorothy Nortman. "Roman Catholic Fertility and Family Planning: A Comparative Review of the Research Literature." *Studies in Family Planning* 1, 34 (1968): 1–27.

Kaiser, Robert Blair. *The Encyclical That Never Was: The Story of the Commission on Population, Family, and Birth, 1964–1966*. London: Sheed and Ward, 1987.

Kampwirth, Karen, and Victoria Rodríguez, eds. *Radical Women in Latin America, Left and Right*. University Park: Pennsylvania State University Press, 2001.

Klaiber, Jeffrey. "The Catholic Lay Movement in Peru: 1867–1959." *The Americas* 40, 2 (1983): 149–70.

———. "Prophets and Populists: Liberation Theology, 1968–1988." *The Americas* 46, 1 (1989): 1–15.

———. *The Catholic Church in Peru, 1821–1985: A Social History*. Washington D.C.: Catholic University Press, 1992.

Klaren, Peter. *Formación de las Haciendas Azucareras y Orígenes del APRA*. Lima: IEP, 1976.

Klaren, Peter, and Thomas Bossert, eds. *The Promise of Development: Theories of Change in Latin America*. Boulder, Colo.: Westview, 1986.

Klaus, Alisa. *Every Child a Lion: The Origins of Maternal and Infant Health Policy in the United States and France, 1890–1920*. Ithaca, N.Y.: Cornell University Press, 1993.

Klausen, Susanne. *Race, Maternity, and the Politics of Birth Control in South Africa, 1910–39*. New York: Palgrave Macmillan, 2004.

Kleinman, Arthur. *The Illness Narratives: Suffering, Healing, and the Human Condition*. New York: Basic Books, 1988.

Koven, Seth, and Sonya Michel, eds. *Mothers of a New World: Maternalist Politics and the Origins of Welfare States*. New York: Routledge, 1993.

Ladd-Taylor, Molly. "Eugenics, Sterilisation and Modern Marriage in the USA: The Strange Career of Paul Popenoe." *Gender & History* 13, 2 (2001): 298–327.

———. "Toward Defining Materialism in U.S. History." *Journal of Women's History* 5, 2 (1993): 110–13.

Langland, Victoria. "Birth Control Pills and Molotov Cocktails: Reading Sex and Revolution in 1968 Brazil." In *In from the Cold: Latin America's New Encounter with the Cold War*, edited by Gilbert Joseph and Daniela Spenser. Durham, N.C.: Duke University Press, 2008.

"Las Primeras Parlamentarias Peruanas." In www.congreso.gob.pe/museo/mujeres -Parlamentarias.pdf. Accessed March 8, 2011.

Latham, Michael. *Modernization as Ideology: American Social Science and Nation Building in the Kennedy Era*. Chapel Hill: University of North Carolina Press, 2000.

Lavrin, Asunción, ed. *Latin American Women: Historical Perspectives*. Westport, Conn.: Greenwood, 1978.

Leavitt, Judith. *Brought to Bed: Childbearing in America, 1750–1950*. New York: Oxford University Press, 1986.

Lefaucheur, Nadine. "La Puériculture d'Adolphe Pinard." In *Darwinisme et Societé*, edited by Patrick Tort. Paris: Presses Universitaires Françaises, 1992.

Levine, Philippa. *Prostitution, Race, and Politics: Policing Venereal Disease in the British Empire*. New York: Routledge, 2003.

Lewis, Jane. *The Politics of Motherhood: Child and Maternal Welfare in England, 1900–1939*. London: Croom Helm, 1980.

Lip, César, Oswaldo Lazo, and Pedro Brito. *El Trabajo Médico en el Perú*. Lima: Organización Panamericana de la Salud, 1990.

Lipset, Seymour Martin. "Some Social Requisites of Democracy: Economic Development and Political Legitimacy." *American Political Science Review* 53, 1 (1959): 69–105.

Lock, Margaret. *Encounters with Aging: Mythologies of Menopause in Japan and North America*. Berkeley: University of California Press, 1993.

Lock, Margaret, and Patricia Kaufert, eds. *Pragmatic Women and Body Politics*. Cambridge: Cambridge University Press, 1998.

Lowenthal, Abraham, ed. *The Peruvian Experiment: Continuity and Change under Military Rule*. Princeton: Princeton University Press, 1975.

Macera, Pablo. "Sexo y Coloniaje." In *Trabajos de Historia, vol. 3*. Lima: INC, 1977.

Macias, Anna. "Women and the Mexican Revolution." *The Americas* 37, 1 (1980): 53–82.

Mallon, Florencia. *Peasant and Nation: The Making of Postcolonial Mexico and Peru*. Berkeley: University of California Press, 1995.

Malpica Silva Santisteban, Carlos. *El Desarrollismo en el Perú: Década de Esperanzas y Fracasos, 1961–1971*. Lima: Horizonte, 1975.

Malthus, Thomas. *An Essay on the Principle of Population*. London: J. Johnson, 1798.

Mannarelli, María Emma. *Pecados Públicos: La Ilegitimidad en Lima, Siglo XVII*. Lima: Flora Tristán, 1993.

———. *Limpias y Modernas: Género, Higiene y Cultura en la Lima del Novecientos*. Lima: Flora Tristán, 1999.

Mariátegui, Javier. "Hermilio Valdizán y la Facultad de Medicina San Fernando." *Anales de la Facultad de Medicina* 58, 3 (1997): 1–4.

Marks, Lara. *Sexual Chemistry: History of the Contraceptive Pill*. New Haven: Yale University Press, 2001.

Martin, Emily. *The Woman in the Body: A Cultural Analysis of Reproduction*. Boston: Beacon, 1987.

Mass, Bonnie. *Population Target: The Political Economy of Population Control in Latin America*. Toronto: The Latin American Working Group and the Women's Press, 1976.

Mayer, Enrique. *Cuentos Feos de la Reforma Agraria*. Lima: IEP, 2009.

Mayes, April. "Why Dominican Feminism Moved to the Right: Class, Colour and Women's Activism in the Dominican Republic, 1880s–1940s." *Gender & History* 20, 2 (2008): 349–71.

Maynard Tucker, Gisele. "Barriers to Modern Contraceptive Use in Rural Peru." *Studies in Family Planning* 17, 6 (1986): 308–16.

———. "Haiti: Unions, Fertility and the Quest for Survival." *Social Science and Medicine* 43, 9 (1996): 1379–87.

McClintock, Cynthia, and Abraham Lowenthal, eds. *The Peruvian Experiment Reconsidered*. Princeton: Princeton University Press, 1983.

McCormick, Leann. "'The Scarlet Woman in the Flesh': The Establishment of a Family Planning Service in Northern Ireland, 1950–1974." *Social History of Medicine* 21, 2 (2008): 345–60.

McEvoy, Carmen. *La Utopía Republicana: Ideales y Realidades en la Formación de la Cultura Política Peruana, 1871–1919*. Lima: PUCP, 1997.

McGready, R. "The Effects of Quinine and Chloroquine Antimalarial Treatments in the First Trimester of Pregnancy." *Transactions of the Royal Society of Tropical Medicine and Hygiene* 96, 2 (2002): 180–84.

McQuillan, Kevin. "Common Themes in Catholic and Marxist Thought on Population and Development." *Population and Development Review* 5, 4 (1979): 689–98.

Meade, Teresa. *"Civilizing" Rio: Reform and Resistance in a Brazilian City, 1889–1930*. University Park: Pennsylvania State University Press, 1997.

Mendoza González, Zuanilda. "'¿Dónde Quedó el Arbol de las Placentas?' Transformaciones en el Saber acerca del Embarazo/Parto/Puerperio de Dos Generaciones de Triquis Migrantes a la Ciudad de México." *Salud Colectiva* 1, 2 (2005): 225–36.

Miller, Francesca. *Latin American Women and the Search for Social Justice*. Hanover, N.H.: University Press of New England, 1991.

Millones, Luis, and Mary Pratt. *Amor Brujo: Imagen y Cultura del Amor en los Andes*. Lima: IEP, 1989.

Morcillo, Aurora. *True Catholic Womanhood: Gender Ideology in Franco's Spain*. De Kalb: Northern Illinois University Press, 2000.

Morgan, Lynn. "Imagining the Unborn in the Ecuadorian Andes." *Feminist Studies* 23, 2 (1997): 323–50.

Mörner, Magnus. *Race Mixture in the History of Latin America*. Boston: Little, Brown, 1967.

Muñoz Cabrejo, Fanni. *Diversiones Públicas en Lima 1890–1920: La Experiencia de la Modernidad*. Lima: Red para el Desarrollo de las Ciencias Sociales, 2001.

Nari, Marcela. *Políticas de Maternidad y Maternalismo Político: Buenos Aires, 1890–1940*. Buenos Aires: Biblos, 2004.

Necochea López, Raúl. "Priests and Pills: Catholic Family Planning in Peru, 1967–1976." *Latin American Research Review* 43, 2 (2008): 34–56.

———. "A History of the Medical Control of Fertility in Peru, 1895–1976." Ph.D. diss., McGill University, 2009.

———. "La Asociación Peruana de Protección Familiar y los Inicios de la Anticoncepción en el Perú (1967–1975)." *Histórica* 33, 1 (2009): 87–130.

———. "Demographic Knowledge and Nation-Building: The Peruvian Census of 1940." *Berichte zur Wissenschaftsgeschichte* 33 (2010): 280–96.

Needell, Jeffrey. "The Revolta Contra Vacina of 1904: The Revolt against 'Modernization' in Belle-Epoque Rio de Janeiro." *Hispanic American Historical Review* 67, 2 (1987): 233–69.

Noonan, John, Jr. *Contraception: A History of Its Treatment by the Catholic Theologians and Canonists.* New York: New American Library, 1965.

Notestein, Frank. "Demography in the United States: A Partial Account of the Development of the Field." *Population and Development Review* 8, 4 (1982): 651–87.

Nye, Robert. *Crime, Madness, and Politics in Modern France: The Medical Concept of National Decline.* Princeton: Princeton University Press, 1984.

Obladen, Michael. "History of Surfactant up to 1980." *Biology of the Neonate* 87 (2005): 308–16.

Offen, Karen. "Depopulation, Nationalism, and Feminism in Fin-de-Siecle France." *American Historical Review* 89, 3 (1984): 648–76.

———. "Defining Feminism: A Comparative Historical Approach." *Signs* 14, 1 (1988): 119–57.

O'Phelan, Scarlett, and Margarita Zegarra, eds. *Mujeres, Familia y Sociedad en la Historia de América Latina, Siglos XVIII–XXI.* Lima: CENDOC-Mujer, 2006.

Ortiz Rescaniere, Alejandro. *La Pareja y el Mito: Estudios sobre las Concepciones de la Persona y de la Pareja en los Andes.* Lima: PUCP, 1993.

Orvig, Helen. "Tambien Antes Hubo Algo." In *25 Años de Feminismo en el Perú: Historia, Confluencias y Perspectivas,* edited by Gaby Cevasco. Lima: Flora Tristán, 2005.

Os, W. A. A. van. "The Intrauterine Device and Its Dynamics." *Advances in Contraception* 15 (1999): 119–32.

Ott, Emiline Royco. "Population Policy Formation in Colombia: The Role of ASCOFAME." *Studies in Family Planning* 8, 1 (1977): 2–10.

Palma, Hector. *"Gobernar es Seleccionar": Apuntes Sobre la Eugenesia.* Buenos Aires: Jorge Baudino, 2002.

Palmer, Steven. *From Popular Medicine to Medical Populism: Doctors, Healers, and Public Power in Costa Rica, 1800–1940.* Durham, N.C.: Duke University Press, 2003.

———. *Launching Global Health: The Caribbean Odyssey of the Rockefeller Foundation.* Ann Arbor: University of Michigan Press, 2010.

Palmer, Steven, and Gladys Rojas Chaves. "Educating Señorita: Teacher Training, Social Mobility, and the Birth of Costa Rican Feminism, 1885–1925." *Hispanic American Historical Review* 78, 1 (1998): 45–82.

Pamo Reyna, Oscar. "Estado Actual de las Publicaciones Periódicas Científicas Médicas del Perú." *Revista Médica Herediana* 16 (2004): 65–73.

Pareja, Piedad. *Aprismo y Sindicalismo en el Perú.* Lima: Rikchay, 1980.

Pease, Henry. *El Ocaso del Poder Oligárquico: Lucha Política en la Escena Oficial, 1968–1975*. Lima: DESCO, 1977.

Pedersen, Susan. *Family, Dependence, and the Origins of the Welfare State: Britain and France, 1914–1945*. Cambridge: Cambridge University Press, 1995.

Pedro, Joana Maria. "A Experiência com Contraceptivos no Brasil: Uma Questão de Geração." *Revista Brasileira de História (São Paulo)* 23, 45 (2003): 239–60.

Piccato, Pablo. *City of Suspects: Crime in Mexico City, 1900–1931*. Durham, N.C.: Duke University Press, 2001.

Pick, Daniel. *Faces of Degeneration: A European Disorder, 1848–1918*. Cambridge: Cambridge University Press, 1993.

Pieper Mooney, Jadwiga. *The Politics of Motherhood: Maternity and Women's Rights in Twentieth-Century Chile*. Pittsburgh: University of Pittsburgh Press, 2009.

Piotrow, Phyllis. *World Population Crisis: The United States Response*. New York: Praeger, 1973.

Platt, Tristan. "El Feto Agresivo: Parto, Formación de la Persona y Mito-Historia en los Andes." *Estudios Atacameños* 22 (2002): 127–55.

Polanyi, Michael. *Personal Knowledge: Towards a Post-Critical Philosophy*. Chicago: University of Chicago Press, 1958.

Portal, Magda. *El Aprismo y la Mujer*. Lima: Atahualpa, 1933.

Portocarrero, Felipe. *El Imperio Prado, 1890–1970*. Lima: CIUP, 1995.

Portocarrero, Gonzalo. *De Bustamante a Odría: El Fracaso del Frente Democrático Nacional, 1945–1950*. Lima: Mosca Azul, 1983.

Portugal, Ana María. "El Retorno de las Brujas." In *Movimiento Feminista en América Latina y el Caribe: Balance y Perpectivas*. Santiago: Isis Internacional, 1986.

Power, Margaret. *Right-Wing Women in Chile: Feminine Power and the Struggle against Allende, 1964–1973*. University Park: Pennsylvania State University Press, 2002.

Quevedo, Emilio, Catalina Borda, Juan Carlos Eslava, Claudia García, María del Pilar Guzmán, Paola Mejía, and Carlos Noguera. *Café y Gusanos, Mosquitos y Petroleo: El Tránsito desde la Higiene hacia la Medicina Tropical y la Salud Pública en Colombia, 1873–1953*. Bogotá: Universidad Nacional de Colombia, 2004.

Quijano, Aníbal. *La Emergencia del Grupo Cholo y sus Implicancias en la Sociedad Peruana*. Lima: IEP, 1967.

Rabí Chara, Miguel. *De la Casa de Maternidad de Lima al Instituto Nacional Materno Perinatal, 1826–2006*. Lima: Hospital Nacional San Bartolomé, 2006.

Ram, Kalpana, and Margaret Jolly, eds. *Maternities and Modernities: Colonial and Postcolonial Experiences in Asia and the Pacific*. Cambridge: Cambridge University Press, 1998.

Reagan, Leslie. "'About to Meet Her Maker': Women, Doctors, Dying Declarations, and the State's Investigation of Abortion, Chicago, 1867–1940." *Journal of American History* 77, 4 (1991): 1240–64.

———. *When Abortion Was a Crime: Women, Medicine and the Law in the United States, 1867–1973*. Berkeley: University of California Press, 1997.

Reber, Vera Blinn. "Blood, Coughs and Fever: Tuberculosis and the Working Class of Buenos Aires, Argentina, 1885–1915." *Social History of Medicine* 12, 1 (1999): 73–100.

Reedy, Daniel. *Magda Portal, la Pasionaria Peruana: Biografía Intelectual*. Lima: Flora Tristán, 2000.

Reher, David, and Pedro Iriso-Napal. "Marital Fertility and Its Determinants in Rural and Urban Spain, 1887–1930." *Population Studies* 43 (1989): 405–27.

Renne, Elisha. "The Pregnancy That Doesn't Stay: The Practice and Perception of Abortion by Ekiti Yoruba Women." *Social Science and Medicine* 42, 4, (1996): 483–94.

Reyes, Esperanza. "'No Somos Bultos Para Ser Tratados Así': El Programa de Planificación Familiar, 1996–1998." *Allpanchis* 31, 56 (2000): 107–28.

Riviale, Pascal. *Una Historia de la Presencia Francesa en el Perú, del Siglo de las Luces a los Años Locos*. Lima: IEP, 2008.

Rodríguez, Gustavo, and Sandro Venturo. *Ampay Mujer! Lo Mínimo que Debemos Saber sobre las Peruanas de Hoy*. Lima: Aguilar, 2009.

Rodríguez, Julia. *Civilizing Argentina: Science, Medicine, and the Modern State*. Chapel Hill: University of North Carolina Press, 2006.

Rodriguez Beruff, Jorge. *Los Militares y el Poder: Un Ensayo sobre la Doctrina Militar en el Peru, 1948–1968*. Lima: Mosca Azul, 1983.

Rodriguez Pastor, Humberto *Hijos del Celeste Imperio en el Perú, 1850–1900*. Lima: Instituto de Apoyo Agrario, 1989.

Rohden, Fabiola. *A Arte de Enganar a Natureza: Contracepção. Aborto e Infanticídio no Início do Século XX*. Rio de Janeiro: Fiocruz, 2003.

Rosemblatt, Karin. *Gendered Compromises: Political Cultures and the State in Chile, 1920–1950*. Chapel Hill: University of North Carolina Press, 2000.

Roy, Krishna. "Aspectos Saltantes del Estudio de Fecundidad en El Agustino." *Estudios de Población y Desarrollo* 3, 4 (1969): 1–8.

Ruggiero, Kristin. *Modernity in the Flesh: Medicine, Law, and Society in Turn-of-the-Century Argentina*. Stanford: Stanford University Press, 2004.

Sáenz, Tula. *Partos y Parteras en la Cuenca del Rio Marcará*. Huaraz: Asociación Urpichallay, 2000.

Sainz de la Maza Kaufmann, Marta. "Contraception in Three Chibcha Communities and the Concept of Natural Fertility (Guaymi, Hueter, Bribri, and Cabecar Indians)." *Current Anthropology* 38, 4 (1997): 681–87.

Salaverry, Oswaldo. "Los Orígenes del Pensamiento Médico de Hipólito Unanue." *Anales de la Facultad de Medicina* 66, 4 (2005): 357–70.

———. "El Inicio de la Educación Médica Moderna en el Perú: La Creación de la Facultad de Medicina de San Fernando." *Acta Médica Peruana* 23, 2 (2006): 122–31.

Sanchez, Abelardo, Raúl Guerrero, Julio Calderón, and Luis Olivera. *Tugurización en Lima Metropolitana*. Lima: DESCO, 1979.

Saporta Sternbach, Nancy, Marysa Navarro-Aranguren, Patricia Chuchryk, and Sonia Alvarez. "Feminisms in Latin America: From Bogotá to San Bernardo." *Signs* 17, 2 (1992): 393–434.

Sater, William. "The Politics of Public Health: Smallpox in Chile." *Journal of Latin American Studies* 35 (2003): 513–43.

Schneider, Jane, and Peter Schneider. *Festival of the Poor: Fertility Decline and the Ideology of Class in Sicily, 1860–1980*. Tucson: University of Arizona Press, 1996.

Schneider, William. "Puericulture, and the Style of French Eugenics." *History and Philosophy of the Life Sciences* 8 (1986): 265–77.

Schoen, Johanna. *Choice and Coercion: Birth Control, Sterilization, and Abortion in Public Health and Welfare*. Chapel Hill: University of North Carolina Press, 2005.

Schwartz, Ronald. "The Midwife in Contemporary Latin America." *Medical Anthropology* 5, 1 (1981): 51–71.

Sharpless, John. "Population Science, Private Foundations, and Development Aid." In *International Development and the Social Sciences*, edited by Frederick Cooper and Randall Packard. Berkeley: University of California Press, 1997.

Sherwin, Susan, ed. *The Politics of Women's Health: Exploring Agency and Autonomy*. Philadelphia: Temple University Press, 1998.

Shorter, Edward. *A History of Women's Bodies*. New York: Basic Books, 1982.

Silva Colmenares, Julio. *No . . . Mas . . . Hijos! Genocidio Preventivo en los Países Subdesarollados*. Bogotá: Paulinas, 1973.

Singh, Susheela, and Deirdre Wulf. *An Overview of Clandestine Abortion in Latin America*. New York: Alan Guttmacher Institute, 1996.

Skidmore, Thomas. *Black into White: Race and Nationality in Brazilian Thought*. Durham, N.C.: Duke University Press, 1998.

Sobrinho, Délcio da Fonseca. *Estado e Populaçao: Uma História do Planejamiento Familiar no Brasil*. Rio de Janeiro: Rosa dos Tempos, 1993.

Solinger, Rickie. *The Abortionist: A Woman against the Law*. Berkeley: University of California Press, 1996.

Soto Laveaga, Gabriela. *Jungle Laboratories: Mexican Peasants, National Projects, and the Making of the Pill*. Durham, N.C.: Duke University Press, 2009.

Sowell, David. "Contending Medical Ideologies and State Formation: The Nineteenth-Century Origins of Medical Pluralism in Contemporary Colombia." *Bulletin of the History of Medicine* 77 (2003): 900–926.

Stavenhagen, Rodolfo. "Social and Demographic Research in Latin American Universities." *Milbank Memorial Fund Quarterly* 42, 2 (1964, part 2): 148–74.

Stepan, Alfred. "The New Professionalism of Internal Warfare and Military Role Expansion." In *Armies and Politics in Latin America*, edited by Abraham Lowenthal. New York: Holmes and Meier, 1976.

Stepan, Nancy. *Beginnings of Brazilian Science: Oswaldo Cruz, Medical Research, and Policy, 1890–1920*. New York: Science History Publications, 1981.

———. *The Hour of Eugenics: Race, Gender, and Nation in Latin America*. Ithaca, N.Y.: Cornell University Press, 1991.

———. *Eradication: Ridding the World of Diseases Forever?* Ithaca, N.Y.: Cornell University Press, 2012.

Stern, Alexandra. "Buildings, Boundaries, and Blood: Medicalization and Nation-Building on the US-Mexico Border, 1910–1930." *Hispanic American Historical Review* 79, 1 (1999): 41–81.

Stern, Steven. *The Secret History of Gender: Women, Men, and Power in Late Colonial Mexico*. Chapel Hill: University of North Carolina Press, 1995.

Stevens, Evelyn. "Marianismo: The Other Face of Machismo in Latin America." In *Female and Male in Latin America*, edited by Ann Pescatello. Pittsburgh: University of Pittsburgh Press, 1973.

Suárez Findlay, Eileen. *Imposing Decency: The Politics of Sexuality and Race in Puerto Rico, 1870–1920*. Durham, N.C.: Duke University Press, 1999.

Summers, Carol. "Intimate Colonialism: The Imperial Production of Reproduction in Uganda, 1907–1925." *Signs* 16, 4 (1991): 787–807.

Symonds, Richard, and Michael Carder. *The United Nations and the Population Question, 1945–1970*. London: Sussex University Press, 1973.

Szreter, Simon. "The Idea of Demographic Transition and the Study of Fertility Change: A Critical Intellectual History." *Population and Development Review* 19, 4 (1993): 659–701.

Teitelbaum, Michael. "Relevance of Demographic Transition Theory for Developing Countries." *Science* 188, 4187 (1975): 420–25.

Thiery, M. "Pioneers of the Intrauterine Device." *European Journal of Contraception and Reproductive Health Care* 2, 1 (1997): 15–23.

Thurner, Mark. *From Two Republics to One Divided: Contradictions of Postcolonial Nationmaking in Andean Peru*. Durham, N.C.: Duke University Press, 1997.

Tone, Andrea. *Devices and Desires: A History of Contraceptives in America*. New York: Hill and Wang, 2001.

Trapasso, Rosa Dominga. "Romper la Invisibilidad." In *25 Años de Feminismo en el Perú: Historia, Confluencias y Perspectivas*, edited by Gaby Cevasco. Lima: Flora Tristán, 2005.

Tsui, Amy Ong. "Population Policies, Family Planning Programs, and Fertility: The Record." *Population and Development Review* 27 (2001): 184–204.

Ugarte Taboada, Claudia. "Historia de los Servicios de Emergencia de Lima y Callao." *Revista Médica Herediana* 11, 3 (2000): 97–106.

Urías Horcasitas, Beatriz. "Eugenesia y Aborto en México (1920–1940)." *Debate Feminista* 14, 27 (2003): 305–23.

Usborne, Cornelie. *Cultures of Abortion in Weimar Germany*. New York: Berghahn, 2007.

Valle Prieto, María Eugenia del. "Parto y Aborto en Algunas 'Ciudades Perdidas' de México." *Anales de Antropología (México)* 17, 2 (1980): 197–222.

Vargas, Rosana, and Paola Naccarato. *Allá, las Antiguas Abuelas Eran Parteras*. Lima: Flora Tristán, 1995.

Vargas, Virginia. "Los Feminismos Peruanos: Breve Balance de Tres Décadas." In *25 Años de Feminismo en el Perú: Historia, Confluencias y Perspectivas*, edited by Gaby Cevasco. Lima: Flora Tristán, 2005.

Vidal Amat y León, Jorge. *Historia de la Obstetricia y Ginecología en el Perú*. Lima: MAD, 2004.

Viel, Benjamin. *The Demographic Explosion: The Latin American Experience*. New York: Irvington, 1976.

———. "Family Planning in Chile." *Journal of Sex Research* 3, 4 (1967): 284–91.

Villanueva, Victor. *El CAEM y la Revolución de las Fuerzas Armadas*. Lima: IEP, 1972.

Villavicencio, Maritza. *Del Silencio a la Palabra: Mujeres Peruanas en los Siglos XIX y XX*. Lima: Flora Tristán, 1992.

Warren, Adam. *Medicine and Politics in Colonial Peru: Population Growth and the Bourbon Reforms.* Pittsburgh: University of Pittsburgh Press, 2010.

Warshaw, Mat. *The Encyclopedia of Surfing.* New York: Harcourt, 2005.

Warwick, Donald. *Bitter Pills: Population Policies and Their Implementation in Eight Developing Countries.* Cambridge: Cambridge University Press, 1982.

Watkins, Elizabeth. *On the Pill: A Social History of Oral Contraceptives, 1950–1970.* Baltimore: Johns Hopkins University Press, 1998.

Weigel, George. "The Church's Social Doctrine in the Twenty-First Century." *Logos: A Journal of Catholic Thought and Culture* 6, 2 (2003): 15–36.

Weismantel, Mary. *Cholas and Pishtacos: Stories of Race and Sex in the Andes.* Chicago: University of Chicago Press, 2001.

Wicht, Juan Julio. *Dinámica Demográfica y Política de Población en el Perú: Reflexiones Personales.* Lima: Centro de Estudios y Publicaciones, 1996.

———. "La Situación Demográfica del Perú." In *Reunión Nacional sobre Población: Problemas Poblacionales Peruanos.* Lima: AMIDEP, 1980.

Wilde, Melissa. *Vatican II: A Sociological Analysis of Religious Change.* Princeton: Princeton University Press, 2007.

Wilmoth, John, and Patrick Ball. "The Population Debate in American Popular Magazines, 1946–90." *Population and Development Review* 18, 4 (1992): 631–68.

Woodham, John. "The Influence of Hipólito Unanue on Peruvian Medical Science, 1789–1820: A Reappraisal." *Hispanic American Historical Review* 50, 4 (1970): 693–714.

Wulf, Deirdre. "Overcoming Circumstances." *International Family Planning Perspectives* 9, 1 (1983): 2–8.

Yam, Eileen, Ingrid Dries-Daffner, and Sandra García. "Abortion Opinion Research in Latin America and the Caribbean: A Review of the Literature." *Studies in Family Planning* 37, 4 (2006): 225–40.

Yon Leau, Carmen. *Hablan las Mujeres Andinas: Preferencias Reproductivas y Anticoncepción.* Lima: Manuela Ramos, 2000.

Zárate, Eduardo. *Los Inicios de la Escuela de Medicina de Lima: Cayetano Heredia, El Organizador.* Lima: Asamblea Nacional de Rectores, 2005.

Zárate, María Soledad. *Dar a Luz en Chile, Siglo XIX: De la "Ciencia de Hembra" a la Ciencia Obstétrica.* Santiago: Universidad Alberto Hurtado, 2007.

———, ed. *Por la Salud del Cuerpo.* Santiago: Universidad Alberto Hurtado, 2008.

Zegarra, Margarita. "María Jesús Alvarado y el Rol de las Mujeres en la Construcción de la Patria." In *Mujeres, Familia y Sociedad en la Historia de América Latina, Siglos XVIII al XXI,* edited by Scarlett O'Phelan and Margarita Zegarra. Lima: CENDOC-Mujer, 2006.

———. "Roles Femeninos y Perspectivas Sociales en las Décadas Iniciales de la República." In *La Mujer en la Historia del Perú, Siglos XV al XX,* edited by Carmen Meza and Teodoro Hampe. Lima: Congreso del Perú, 2007.

Zulawski, Ann. *Unequal Cures: Public Health and Political Change in Bolivia, 1900–1950.* Durham, N.C.: Duke University Press, 2007.

# Index

Caesarean surgery, 89, 91
Cajamarca, 34, 40, 41, 145
Callao, 55, 66, 110, 141, 142, 146
Callao Rotary Club, 14
Calle, Hugo, 92
Calle, Juan José, 66
Cancino, Helí, 96
Canguilhem, Georges, 7
Cano, Arnaldo, 116
Capelo, Joaquín, 19
Capitalism, 131, 185 (n. 34)
Caracas Report, 110
Carbajal, Mery, 75, 76
Cardinal, Cecilia, 50
Cardui, 67
*Caretas* (magazine), 88
Carlson, Bruce, 50
Caron, Alfred, 20
Carrasco, Nazario, 96
Carrillo, Ana María, 25
Carvallo, Constantino J., 30
Carvallo, Constantino T., 17
Casa del Buen Pastor, 75
Castellares, Marcelino, 65
*Castii Connubii* (encyclical, Pius XI), 129, 184 (n. 19)
Castilla, Ramón, 15
Castillo, Gladys, 72–73
Castro, Fidel, 40
Catholic Action, 37, 184 (n. 12). *See also* Acción Católica Peruana
Catholic Church, 34, 36; abortion and, 53, 58, 129, 130, 167 (n. 5); contraception and, 1, 86, 127, 128, 131, 141–48, 188 (n. 5); eugenics and, 38, 129; family education and, 39, 43, 142–43; family planning and, 3, 5, 12–13, 125, 126, 127, 129–30, 131, 132, 133–34, 136, 141–48, 154, 183 (n. 2); lay Catholics and, 5, 128–29, 130, 131–32, 133–34, 184 (n. 12); liberation theology and, 131, 132; marriage and, 58, 126–28, 129, 131, 132, 133, 136, 140, 141, 142, 147, 183 (nn. 1–2), 184 (nn. 19, 23); the pill and, 12, 13, 128, 136–37, 146, 147; population growth

and, 126, 127, 130–32, 133, 136, 145, 185 (n. 34); rhythm method and, 130, 136, 184 (n. 23); sex education and, 59–60; social doctrine and, 129, 130, 131, 146; sterilization and, 1, 90; women's legal rights and, 45, 128; women's roles and, 35, 43. *See also* Families; Latin America; United States
Catholic Church Responsible Parenthood program, 93, 94, 128, 140, 142, 146
Catt, Carrie Chapman, 40
Cayetano Heredia University, 107, 109, 116
Cedamanos, Alejandro, 69
Census: 1940, 62–63; 1950, 112, 180 (n. 51); 1961, 103
Center for Advanced Military Studies (CAEM), 113, 114, 123
Centro de Capacitación y Promoción Familiar (CCPF), 142
Centro de Estudios de Población y Desarrollo (Center for the Study of Population and Development, CEPD), 122, 151; creation of, 43, 113; demise of, 115–17, 119, 150; Family Planning, Genital Cancer Screening, and Abortion Prevention Project and, 110–11; U.S. funding and, 106–9, 112, 114, 124, 139, 142
Centro de la Mujer Peruana Flora Tristán, 49
Centro Latino Americano de Demografía (CELADE), 103, 107, 109, 123
Cervantes, René, 119
Cervical cancer screenings, 92, 94, 110–12, 114, 139
Cervical caps, 91, 136
Chang, Doris, 86, 96
Chávez, Augusto, 87
Chávez, Elmer, 91
Chávez, Gregoria, 75
Child health, 2, 22–23, 118, 119, 121, 123, 124, 125, 150
Children's Hospital (Hospital del Niño), 22, 119
Child's Week, 14

Chile, 16, 25, 36, 40, 57, 118, 140; Catholic Church and, 132, 144; family planning and, 47, 85, 92, 100; population growth and, 103, 108, 109, 123; Irene Silva de Santolalla and, 34, 35, 38

Chilean Association for Family Protection (Asociación Chilena para la Protección Familiar), 47

Chilean Federation of Women's Institutions, 38

Chimbote, 93

Chinese immigrants, 19, 159 (n. 25)

Chiri, Leoncio, 55–56

Christian Family Movement, 109, 115, 117, 134, 136

Cisneros, Felícita, 70

Civil Association for Family Welfare of Brazil (Sociedade Civil de Bem-Estar Familiar no Brasil, BEMFAM), 47

Civilista Party, 16, 22

Civil Service for Medical Graduates (SECIGRA), 118

Clark, Kim, 25

Coale, Ansley, 104

Coitus interruptus, 4, 83, 89, 130

Colareta, R., 64

Cold War, 2, 8, 9, 11, 12, 135, 147, 152, 153

Colegio de la Independencia, 15

Colombia: Catholic Church and, 132, 133; family education and, 41; family planning and, 47, 100, 109, 111, 123; population growth and, 105, 108

Columban order, 139

Comas, 139

Comité Pro-Abaratamiento de las Subsistencias, 42

Commission on Social Action, 144

Commission on Women, 42

Communism, 40, 42, 46, 108, 134, 135

Condoms, 27, 79, 83, 89, 136

Confederación Campesina del Perú (Peasant Federation of Peru), 47

Confederación de Trabajadores del Perú (Free Union School of the Workers' Federation of Peru), 42

Conference on Population and the Family, 109

Conference on the Family, Childhood, and Youth in National Development, 109

Contraception: 1950s and, 85, 89; 1960s and, 5, 43, 44, 47, 91–92, 110, 127, 136–37; 1970s and, 44, 45, 48, 94, 117, 121, 125, 145–46, 152, 183 (n. 103); abortion as, 4, 12, 52, 62, 78, 79, 88; breastfeeding and, 121, 143; Catholic Church and, 1, 86, 127, 128, 131, 141–48, 188 (n. 5); coitus interruptus, 4, 83, 89, 130; condoms, 27, 79, 83, 89, 136; emergency, 148, 154, 188 (n. 5); fertility surveys and, 87, 88; health workers and, 95, 96–98; injectable hormonal contraceptive trials, 32, 86, 93; Latin America and, 79, 92, 93, 144, 183 (n. 103); lay Catholics and, 136–37, 139, 140–41, 145; mass distribution of, 5, 8, 9, 50; medicinal herbs and, 5, 89; periodic abstinence, 131, 140, 143–44, 146; Peruvian rate of use of, 1–2; physicians and, 21, 85–87, 92–93, 94, 95, 144; pill trials and, 86, 139–40, 142, 154; population growth and, 4, 8, 43, 44, 86, 91–92, 104, 105, 106, 130, 146, 178 (n. 9); rhythm method, 83, 89, 130, 134, 136, 156 (n. 5), 173–74 (n. 17), 184 (n. 23); single women and, 48, 49, 50–51. *See also* Birth control organizations; Catholic Church; Family planning; IUDs; Marriage; Pill, the; Sterilization

Contreras, Carlos, 16

*Control de la natalidad*, 86

Copper, 112

Copper T IUDs, 98, 176 (n. 73)

Cornell University, 104

"Correcting Adult Behaviors to Educate Children" (Santolalla), 34

Corsets, 54

Coss, John, 135, 136–37

Costa Rica, 41

Crime, 81, 84, 96

CPSIA information can be obtained
at www.ICGtesting.com
Printed in the USA
LVHW110525011218
598842LV00006B/573/P

9 781469 618081